BEST PRACTICE FOR YOUTH SPORT

BEST PRACTICE FOR YOUTH SPORT

Robin S. Vealey, PhD

Miami University

Melissa A. Chase, PhD

Miami University

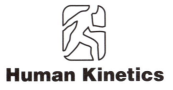

Human Kinetics

Library of Congress Cataloging-in-Publication Data

Vealey, Robin S., 1954-
 Best practice for youth sport / Robin S. Vealey and Melissa A. Chase.
   pages cm
 Includes bibliographical references and index.
 1. Sports for children. I. Chase, Melissa A., 1961- II. Title.
 GV709.2.V43 2016
 796.083--dc23

                          2015013239

ISBN: 978-0-7360-6696-9 (print)

The web addresses cited in this text were current as of June 2015, unless otherwise noted.

Acquisitions Editor: Myles Schrag
Developmental Editor: Kevin Matz
Managing Editor: B. Rego
Copyeditor: Joyce Sexton
Indexer: Laurel Plotzke
Permissions Manager: Dalene Reeder
Graphic Designer: Joe Buck
Cover Designer: Susan Rothermel Allen
Photograph (cover): Jaimie Duplass/Shutterstock
Photographs (interior): © Human Kinetics, unless otherwise noted
Photo Asset Manager: Laura Fitch
Photo Production Manager: Jason Allen
Art Manager: Kelly Hendren
Associate Art Manager: Alan L. Wilborn
Illustrations: © Human Kinetics, unless otherwise noted
Printer: Sheridan Books

Printed in the United States of America   10 9 8 7 6 5 4 3 2 1

The paper in this book is certified under a sustainable forestry program.

Human Kinetics
Website: www.HumanKinetics.com

United States: Human Kinetics
P.O. Box 5076
Champaign, IL 61825-5076
800-747-4457
e-mail: humank@hkusa.com

Canada: Human Kinetics
475 Devonshire Road Unit 100
Windsor, ON N8Y 2L5
800-465-7301 (in Canada only)
e-mail: info@hkcanada.com

Europe: Human Kinetics
107 Bradford Road
Stanningley
Leeds LS28 6AT, United Kingdom
+44 (0) 113 255 5665
e-mail: hk@hkeurope.com

Australia: Human Kinetics
57A Price Avenue
Lower Mitcham, South Australia 5062
08 8372 0999
e-mail: info@hkaustralia.com

New Zealand: Human Kinetics
P.O. Box 80
Mitcham Shopping Centre, South Australia 5062
0800 222 062
e-mail: info@hknewzealand.com

E3877

To our children, Jordan and Jackson Chase, our favorite youth sport athletes of all time. Thank you for the loving developmental experiences you have shared with us, which have made writing this book more personal and meaningful.

CONTENTS

ACKNOWLEDGMENTS

Thanks to Rainer Martens, who originally conceived the idea for this book and offered both his encouragement for us to write it and his needling to get it done. Rainer remained a helpful resource throughout the writing process. Thanks also to Myles Schrag, our acquisitions editor, for his steadfast support and patience over the years, waiting for us to commit to and finish this book. Myles' feedback and guidance throughout the writing process was superb, and we particularly appreciate that he supported our preferences and ideas for the book, even when his opinion differed from ours. Kevin Matz helped us through the final publication process as developmental editor, and we appreciate his timeliness, receptivity to our ideas, and continuous support.

Thank you to our many colleagues who helped us develop and enhance the content of the book. Lenny Wiersma served as reviewer of the initial book manuscript, and his feedback and suggestions as an expert on youth sport enabled us to significantly improve the content of the book. Thanks also to an anonymous second reviewer, who provided very helpful suggestions about the physical science content. Our Miami University colleague Thelma Horn was very helpful with her expertise in the area of physical growth, maturation, and readiness. Another Miami University colleague, Ron Cox, provided helpful guidance in the physical training chapter. Dan Gould, director of the Institute for the Study of Youth Sport at Michigan State University, provided useful suggestions for content, along with external reviewers.

We are grateful to graduate students Scott Pierce and Billy Lowe for helping us with background research, Justin DiSanti for his help in developing exam questions for the Instructor Guide, and Chris Hill for his assistance with the Resource Guide. Thanks also to the Miami University undergraduate students who "pilot tested" the book in class before it was published, and offered many useful suggestions to enhance its content. In particular, Ellie Prinster and Kevin Morris were highly engaged students who influenced the final content of the book. Former student Kevin Mallin sent us the letter written by his daughter Stasianne that leads off chapter 15. Thanks to Kevin and Stasianne for providing such a wonderful example of the parent–youth athlete relationship.

Thanks to our former youth sport coaches for providing us the opportunity to play and compete. Robin sends a special thanks to high school coach Sue Gregg for her wonderful leadership and support in the pre-Title IX era. Melissa recognizes Dee Knoblauch—friend, colleague, and former college basketball teammate—for helping her better understand how to be an effective coach and role model for athletes of all ages. We are also grateful to the hundreds of youth sport athletes we have coached, who taught us valuable lessons and helped us with the experiential knowledge to write this book.

Most of all, thanks to our families. Robin acknowledges the central role of her parents, Sherman and Mary Lou Vealey, in providing the unconditional love, support, and modeling that enabled her to enjoy and succeed in youth and college sport. Melissa thanks her mother, Jean Chase, her first and only youth sport coach for fighting for the opportunity for girls to play youth sports when no one else cared if girls played, and her father, Don Chase, for his constant support of her as an athlete, coach, and teacher and being her inspiration to work hard.

INTRODUCTION

It's all about the kid. This simple sentence conveys what we believe should be the focus of youth sport—the kids! It may sound obvious, yet this basic premise is often forgotten by adults based on their need to coach a championship team of 9- and 10-year-old soccer players or their desire to parent a child who wins a college athletic scholarship, Olympic medal, or professional sport contract.

There are many examples in communities across the nation and the world showing that youth sport works and truly is all about the kids. On almost any day, you can drive by facilities where kids are having fun, developing friendships with teammates, and learning valuable physical and mental skills that they can carry with them into adulthood. As parents of two youth sport participants, we have coached, cheered, spectated, carpooled, and provided postgame snacks. We have seen firsthand the fun, friendships, and skill development that our children and others have experienced via youth sport participation. Here are some of the many positive examples from the world of youth sport:

- Twin 8th-graders Claire and Chloe Gruenke finished the 800 meters together in last place at the Southern Illinois Class L state junior high meet after Chloe strained her right thigh muscle and Claire carried her the final 370 meters.

- When a referee barred a soccer player from competing in a game because she was wearing a *hijab* (a veil worn by Muslim females that covers the head and chest), all her teammates showed up at the next game wearing hijabs to show their support—and all were allowed to play.

- High school football coach Joe Ehrmann, a former professional athlete, implemented his InSideOut Coaching (2011) program to teach young male athletes how to move beyond stereotypical "manliness" to develop empathy skills, emotional connections with teammates, and respect for women.

So youth sport can and does work. However, there are also negative aspects of youth sport, usually the result of adults who twist our basic mantra "It's all about the kid" into something like "It's all about me and my need for my child to be great!" These negative aspects have been debated in many books about youth sports that discuss the "cheers and tears," the "dark side of youth sports," and "how to stop adults from ruining your child's fun and success in youth sports"—and ask "Whose game is it, anyway?" A quick perusal of the Internet can identify sensational examples of adults who have created negative consequences for youth involved in sport. These are some of them:

- A Michigan youth hockey coach allegedly directed teammates to conduct bare-knuckle fights as part of a practice session.

- Lincoln, Nebraska, police issued a ticket to a woman for leaving her daughter alongside Interstate 80 because of her unsatisfactory performance in a soccer game.

- A California high school football coach was caught on videotape moving a sideline yard marker so his team could gain a first down and win a league title.

- A Pennsylvania youth baseball coach was sent to prison for paying one of his players $25 to bean an autistic teammate to keep him out of the game in order to improve his team's chance to win.

Of course, these negative examples are extreme cases of an irrational minority of misled adults. They are misled by a youth sport culture that has become more specialized and professionalized. It is this emerging culture that makes it difficult for adults to know how to make decisions that are in the best interests of children. It is this culture that often results in forgetting that it should be all about the kids and their developmental needs.

Consider the following practices that have emerged based on the specialized and professionalized culture of youth sport. What is your opinion of these practices?

- Callaway Golf sponsors the Junior World Golf Championship for children 6 years and under. Is this a good idea? Should you start your child in golf early enough to compete in a world championship at age 6?

- Most major college basketball programs have identified the top-rated 10-year-old players in the country, because highly selective sport camps and Amateur Athletic Union (AAU) coaches showcase youngsters before they even reach middle school. Does that mean that your daughter must play on a nationally competitive AAU team and vie for a spot in a select camp, in addition to playing on a recreational team?

- Specialization in one sport for the purpose of gaining college scholarships and a life in professional sport is fast replacing participation in multiple sports in high school. Should a young athlete specialize exclusively and train in only one sport? And if so, at what age should he specialize? Should coaches have the authority to require that athletes participate only in their sport?

- Some young athletes live away from home to train in highly specialized sport schools and sacrifice a traditional childhood to pursue dreams of Olympic glory. If a young athlete shows early talent, is it the best thing for her to live apart from her family so she can reap the benefits of high-level training? Should the family sacrifice money and time together to allow one child to pursue her talent away from home?

These are questions emerging from the current landscape of youth sport. The purpose of this book is to provide you with the understanding needed to traverse this landscape. Our objective is to provide relevant sport science knowledge about youth sport, as well as practical tips and strategies for how to use this knowledge. That's why the book is titled *Best Practice for Youth Sport*—to emphasize our objective of offering you useful knowledge as you parent, coach, direct, or officiate kids within the youth sport culture. We hope that, armed with knowledge from this book, you will become an active social change agent in structuring and enhancing youth sport programs to meet the unique developmental needs of children.

The main theme of the book, illustrated in figure I.1, is that for youth sport programs to be all about the kid, they must be based on **developmentally appropriate practice.**

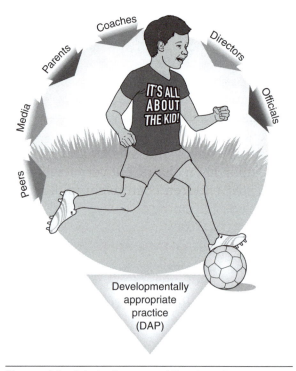

Figure I.1 Main theme of the book.

This is the DAP principle, and it is emphasized in every chapter of this book. For youth sport to serve the needs of our children and society, for it to be truly all about the kid, it must be based on a firm foundation of DAP (Copple, 2010).

Developmentally refers to the process of development, whereby humans grow into a more mature or advanced state. Child development research indicates that universal, predictable sequences of growth and change occur in children and youth as they age and mature. Significant physical, cognitive, and psychological changes occur between early childhood and early adulthood. These key developmental years are the years of youth sport participation, and adults involved in youth sport must understand the systematic changes that occur over time in the developing child. Would you believe that children with the same birthday may differ in physical maturation as much as five years? It's important to understand early and late maturation in youth athletes so you can teach, coach, and counsel children based on their unique maturational characteristics.

Appropriate refers to something that is fitting or just right. Adults organizing youth sport should focus on fitting the sport or activity to the child, as opposed to trying to fit the child into an adult-oriented activity that is not appropriate. Would you believe that tee ball is not an appropriate lead-up game to baseball or softball? Oh, it's great fun, with cheers and snacks and parents lined up in lawn chairs, but very few 5- and 6-year-old children cognitively understand defensive positioning or base running strategies, nor do they develop throwing and catching skills by participating in tee ball. In this book we continually encourage you to think outside of current practice and apply the DAP principle to make youth sport fitting, or just right for kids.

Practice refers to what we actually do. Putting it all together, developmentally appropriate practice is engaging in decisions, behaviors, and policies that meet the physical, psychological, and social needs of children and youth based on their ages and maturational levels. The point of this book is that best practice for youth sport is DAP.

As shown in figure I.1, multiple socializing agents surrounding youth sport athletes influence the practice of youth sport today. Parents are typically the most significant adults influencing the development of children, and children's interest in and responses to physical activity and sport are shaped as early as the toddler years by parents. Youth sport coaches influence children through the ways in which they design practices, teach skills, distribute awards, give feedback, and model appropriate behavior. Youth sport directors control the way youth sport is organized, and influence such practice decisions as whether boys and girls should play together and what sports and activities are offered for various age groups.

Youth sport officials must consider the best way to ensure fair and active play while allowing young athletes to play based on their maturational levels. Media are the public means of communication (television, Internet, newspapers, magazines) that influence people's perceptions of cultural events. Consider how public perception about youth sport was influenced when Tiger Woods appeared on the Mike Douglas television show as a 2-year-old golf phenomenon, or when LeBron James graced the cover of *Sport Illustrated* magazine as a high school junior. And finally, the friends, teammates, and siblings who make up the developing child's peer group are significant influences in the youth sport culture, particularly once children reach adolescence.

Notice that the youth pictured in figure I.1 is balancing precariously on the DAP foundation. We believe that the success of youth sport programs in helping kids develop their physical, psychological, and social skills is dependent on the ability of adult stakeholders to apply the DAP principle to developmentally "balance" the experience for kids. As you read through the book, you'll see that the chapters in each part of it serve as the bedrock upon which the DAP foundation rests. That is, by using the knowledge provided in the chapters to engage in DAP, you keep youth sport balanced and able to meet the unique needs of developing children and youth.

The book is divided into four parts. Part I provides the basics of youth sport, discussing who it includes, how it is structured, how it has evolved, and what its philosophies and purposes are and should be for society. Part II focuses on the key developmental concept of readiness in terms of knowing how and when children are ready to learn and compete. It places emphasis on shaping the youth sport culture through appropriate modification and skill teaching so that children's motivation to be physically active and competent is awakened and enhanced.

Part III asks the question "How much is too much in youth participation?" and is an attempt to assess how much physical and psychological intensity is appropriate for children at different developmental stages. For example, the negative consequences of the "overs" (overintensity, overspecialization, overstress, and overuse) are examined in relation to the negative youth sport consequences of injuries, burnout,

and overtraining. Part IV focuses on social considerations in youth sport, including the influence of coaches, parents, and stereotypical assumptions about gender and race.

To get started, we've created the Youth Sport IQ Test to raise your awareness about youth sport. Read and answer the following questions so you can get a feel for what the key issues are in the study of youth sport.

How did you do? You probably observed that some questions are straightforward, while others are more complex in that the correct answer seems to depend on various circumstances. If you observed this, then you're well on your way to understanding the youth sport culture. It is our hope that you can gain knowledge from the book to develop your own answers and solutions to the complex issues that we face in youth sport today.

So, read on. Our answers to the test are provided in the chapters of the book. We're hoping that your youth sport IQ is substantially increased through the knowledge you gain in reading this book. We urge you to harness this knowledge in thoughtful and innovative ways to create and maintain a youth sport culture that produces positive consequences for a better society. We hope you will use this knowledge not just for practice, but for best practice or DAP, so that youth sport truly will be all about the kid.

Youth Sport IQ Test

Answer true or false to the first five questions; choose one answer for the multiple-choice questions.

1. Competitive sport participation can stunt a child's growth.
2. Participation in youth sport builds character in kids.
3. Participation at a very young age is required to achieve high levels of sport proficiency.
4. Girls are less motivated and competent in sport than boys and thus should participate separately from boys.
5. Most injuries in youth sport occur as the result of collisions in contact sports (e.g., American football).
6. Which achievement area has been shown to create the most stress for children?
    a. competitive sport
    b. individual music solo
    c. academic test in school
7. The biggest problem in youth sports today is
    a. lack of facilities
    b. kids' lack of motivation
    c. overinvolvement of adults
8. The optimal age for children to learn fundamental motor skills is
    a. 2–8 years
    b. 8–10 years
    c. 10–12 years
9. For youth beginning organized sport, the best type of coach is someone who is
    a. very technically skilled
    b. very knowledgeable about the sport
    c. warm and supportive
    d. the same sex as the athletes (e.g., females coach females, males coach males)
10. Which of the following is NOT a strong motivator for children in youth sport?
    a. being with friends
    b. winning
    c. learning skills
    d. having fun

Youth Sport IQ Test answers: 1 (F), 2 (F), 3 (F), 4 (F), 5 (F), 6 (b), 7 (c), 8 (a), 9 (c), 10 (b).

LEARNING AIDS

Key Term

developmentally appropriate practice—Engaging in decisions, behaviors, and policies that meet the physical, psychological, and social needs of children and youth based on their ages and maturational levels.

Summary Points

1. "It's all about the kid" is the basic premise that adults should keep in mind about the needed focus in youth sport.

2. Best practice for youth sport means developmentally appropriate practice.

3. The success of youth sport programs in helping kids develop physical, psychological, and social skills is dependent on the ability of adult stakeholders (parents, coaches, directors, officials, media) to engage in developmentally appropriate practice.

Study Questions

1. Explain, providing a definition and using examples, what is meant by the term *developmentally appropriate practice*.

2. Explain why some adults, often well-meaning adults, fail to adhere to the premise that youth sport should be all about the kid. Identify some of the negative outcomes that could occur when adult stakeholders fail to remember this basic premise.

Reflective Learning Activities

1. Provide examples of developmentally appropriate practice in your youth sport experience, and also provide examples of developmentally inappropriate practice that you experienced. Describe the advantages or disadvantages (or both) that these types of practice provided for you. That is, how did these experiences affect your sport and personal development?

2. Pretend that you have unlimited financial and scientific resources to pursue the answer to any question about youth and sport. What would your burning research question be?

ANCILLARY SUPPORT

To ensure fully integrated support for instructors, the following ancillaries are available to course adopters of *Best Practice for Youth Sport* at www.HumanKinetics.com/BestPracticeForYouthSport:

- **Instructor guide.** Includes sample syllabuses, course outlines, a class project, and activity suggestions.

- **Test package.** Includes more than 200 true or false, multiple-choice, fill-in-the-blank, and short-answer questions.

- **Image bank.** The image bank includes most of the figures and tables from the text, sorted by chapters, that can be used to develop a customized presentation based on specific course requirements.

Youth Sport Basics

Welcome to part I of *Best Practice for Youth Sport,* where you'll get the "big picture" of youth sport. Here's a sampling of things you'll learn in the next three chapters on youth sport basics:

- How youth sport is organized, who participates and who doesn't, and why
- What youth sport looks like in different countries
- Why kids have moved from the "sandlot" to adult-organized sport
- Why the palm community beats the pyramid as a model for youth sport participation
- How to assess what type of program best fits specific types of kids
- How you can develop a sound philosophy and clear objectives for your youth sport program

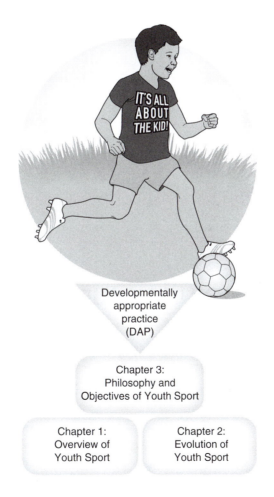

Developmentally
appropriate
practice
(DAP)

Chapter 3:
Philosophy and
Objectives of Youth Sport

Chapter 1:
Overview of
Youth Sport

Chapter 2:
Evolution of
Youth Sport

This part of the book is your boot camp, where you learn the youth sport basics that set you up to understand the rest of the material in the book. So no shortcuts! Take the time to complete your basic youth sport training by reading the next three chapters and be ready to use your knowledge for developmentally appropriate practice (DAP).

chapter 1

OVERVIEW OF YOUTH SPORT

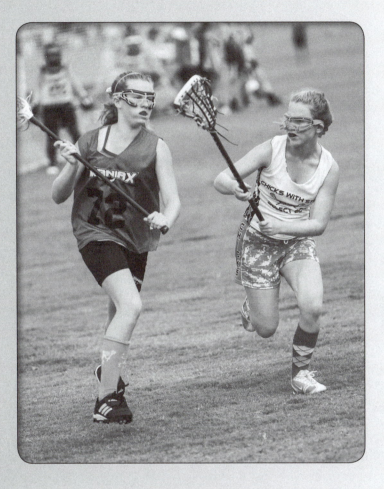

CHAPTER PREVIEW

In this chapter, you'll learn

» about different types of youth sports,

» what youth sport looks like in different countries,

» about barriers to youth sport participation, and

» about national and international organizations dedicated to the enhancement of youth sport.

What is this thing we call youth sport? Who does it include, and what types of activities qualify as youth sport? **Sport** can be defined as a game-like activity that is governed by specific rules, is competitive, and requires some form of physical exertion (Blanchard, 1995). Typically, sport involves a regularly scheduled progression of training and practices and competitive contests across a specified time frame, using such terms as *season* and *preseason*. A related term is **physical activity,** which is any bodily movement produced by skeletal muscles that results in energy expenditure (Caspersen, Powell, & Christenson, 1985). Sport is one type of physical activity; others include fitness activities like yoga or kayaking, leisure activities like gardening or hiking, transportation activities like biking and walking, and work activities like raking leaves or shoveling snow. Although the focus of this book is on sport, we refer to physical activity in relation to youth at times due to its importance for health and well-being. **Youth** refers to those individuals between early childhood and adulthood, typically 18 years and younger, who are undergoing significant physical and mental development.

Putting the terms *youth* and *sport* together complicates things more than these definitions might indicate. First, it's challenging for kids to engage in competitive social comparison with peers during a time of such drastic physical and emotional development. Second, adult coaches or instructors are designated as supervisors of most youth sport activities. Third, youth live in households with and are dependent on parents or guardians for decision making and resources related to sport participation. Fourth, sport is one of the most popular and widely publicized social institutions in the United States as well as around the world. Sport is one of the top 10 business industries in the United States, generating an estimated $400 billion worth of business in 2012 (Plunkett Research Ltd., 2013). Youth sport has been estimated to represent at least $5 billion annually as part of the overall U.S. sport industry (Wagner, Jones, & Riepenhoff, 2010).

It is easy for adult coaches, directors, and parents to lose sight of the importance of developmentally appropriate practice (DAP) based on the seductive pull of winning championships, gaining community prestige, profiting from pay-to-play club programs, securing athletic scholarships, and pursuing the fame and fortune of Olympic or professional sport status. So keep in mind that youth plus sport equals a unique subculture, a subculture that is very different from adult sport. As you read this book, continually consider the ways in which you can keep youth and sport compatible, and make youth plus sport a successful experience for the kids.

TYPES OF YOUTH SPORT

The term **youth sport** collectively applies to all of the programs that provide adult-supervised sport skill development sessions and competitive contests to children in the typical age range of 5 to 18 years. However, youth sport is structured in many different ways. For example, programs differ in their focus, objectives, and inclusion criteria. Some programs are open to all participants without regard to skill level and with a focus on enjoyment and participation. Other programs engage in skill-based selection of participants with an emphasis on identifying the best talent and on winning championships. Some programs focus on mastery-oriented skill improvement, a modest time commitment, and competitive events within a community, while other programs require a major commitment of training time and more extensive travel outside the community. Additional characteristics that vary across different types of youth sport programs include the length of competitive seasons, expected participation and training in the off-season, the qualifications of coaches and officials, and the amount of money required.

These variations in programs are confusing to parents, so we encourage youth sport directors and coaches to clearly market and explain the particular aspects of their programs. This way, parents and youth participants can make the best choices to meet their interests, motivation, current ability levels, and family resources. (In chapter 3, we provide some tips to help youth athletes and parents choose the program that best fits their needs and interests.)

As shown in the following list, youth sport can be generally divided into school-based and nonschool sports:

School Based

- Interscholastic competition
- Intramural games and sport competition
- Physical education (part of educational curriculum)
- Sport camps

Nonschool

- Local service club teams or leagues (Optimist youth hockey, Kiwanis baseball)
- National youth sport organization teams or leagues (American Youth Soccer Association and Soccer Association for Youth)
- National youth development organization programs (Boys and Girls Clubs, YMCA, Catholic Youth Organization)
- Community recreation department programs
- Olympic national governing bodies; national, state, and local programs (USA Wrestling)
- Club sports
- Sport academies (IMG Academy)
- Sport camps

From that initial division, youth sport may be further categorized into many different types of programs. This section explains these categories, with most of the examples coming from American sport. Later in the chapter, we provide some descriptions of youth sport practices in other countries in relation to these categories. We understand that our perspective is Western biased, even American biased, because that is the culture we know best. However, we acknowledge the importance of understanding the global aspects of youth sport and examining how knowledge is used for practice in different cultures.

School-Based Youth Sport

School-based youth sport includes interscholastic sport, intramural sport, physical education, and sport camps. *Interscholastic sport* involves athletes and teams competing against athletes and teams from other schools and typically requires tryouts in which a certain number of youth in a school are selected for participation. Due to the costs involved (travel, uniforms, coaches, officials), interscholastic youth sport usually offers only one or two teams per sport per school. American middle and high school interscholastic sport is coordinated by the National Federation of State High School Associations (NFHS), as well as each state's interscholastic sport governing association (e.g., Ohio High School Athletics Association). The NFHS and state associations establish standards such as eligibility, rules for competition, and coaching education requirements.

The term *intramural sport* is derived from the Latin *intra* and *muros,* meaning "within walls." Thus, intramural youth sports include games and sport competition for students within the school. Intramural sport is often offered to younger children before interscholastic sport is available, and also to adolescents in middle and high school as an alternative to interscholastic sport. Both interscholastic and intramural sports are extracurricular, or outside of the academic classes offered by the schools.

Physical education is part of the academic curriculum in most schools, and it is mandatory or optional based on the age of students and state or national guidelines. Physical education focuses on teaching physical skills and enhancing personal fitness; and although competitive activities may be part of physical education, skill development always supersedes competition. We include it as a category of youth sport because it is where many children first become involved in organized physical activity and because it is typically available to most children who attend school.

School-based sport camps are typically offered in the summer and directed by the school coaching staff and other coaches (often college athletes). Most school sport camps are focused on one sport and are offered at high schools or universities. School sport camps typically charge a fee and are open to all who wish to participate and improve their skills in the given sport.

Think about how wonderful it would be if all of these school-based categories of youth sport were fully funded, staffed with vibrant and competent adult leaders, based on DAP, innovative in meeting the interests and needs of youth, and integrative in working together to encourage all school-aged students to participate in some form of youth sport. Unfortunately, that is often not the case, based on such factors as the demise of funding for these programs as well as the social perceptions of youth that physical education and intramural participation are "uncool" compared to being on an interscholastic team. This is the traditional pyramid-structure problem in youth sport, with children dropping out in growing numbers past the age of 12 because they are not in the higher-ability group of athletes chosen for interscholastic teams.

Nonschool Sport

As shown on page 5, there are many types of nonschool youth sport programs, which have much higher participation numbers than school-based sport. We'll offer an overview of eight types of nonschool youth sport, which basically differ on who coordinates the programs and how they are structured.

1. **Local service club teams or leagues.** Local service club teams or leagues are organized and supported by community service clubs, such as Kiwanis or Optimist. These clubs sometimes sponsor one team for a certain age group, or they may coordinate an entire youth league (e.g., baseball, ice hockey) with multiple teams. These clubs have volunteer members and engage in local fund-raising to support community initiatives, like youth sport.

2. **National youth sport organization teams or leagues.** A very popular type of youth sport program in the United States is those teams and leagues affiliated with national youth sport organizations, such as the Soccer Association for Youth (SAY), American Youth Soccer Organization (AYSO—also known to parents as All Your Saturdays Are Over!), Little League baseball and softball, Pony Baseball and Softball, Pop Warner football, American Athletic Union (AAU) Basketball, and Biddy Basketball. There is a strong tradition of these youth sport organizations in the United States, and they are part of many community youth sport offerings.

3. **National youth development organization programs.** National youth development organizations were created to preserve and enhance the well-being of children. As one part of their broad mission, these organizations offer sport programs and other types of physical activity recreation for youth. Examples include the Boys and Girls Clubs of America, Young Men's Christian Association (YMCA), Young Women's Christian Association (YWCA), and the Catholic Youth Organization (CYO).

4. **Community recreation department programs.** Many towns and communities offer community recreation programs that include youth sport opportunities. For example, our local city parks and recreation department offers youth basketball, flag football, youth tennis lessons and competition,

and a summer swim team. It also offers the following programs affiliated with national sport organizations: SAY soccer; NFL and Pepsi Punt, Pass, and Kick competition; the First Tee golf program; and the Hershey Track & Field program. Community recreation centers also provide facilities such as basketball courts, tennis courts, and swimming pools, which are particularly vital to encourage physical activity in underserved youth.

5. **Olympic NGB national, state, and local programs.** National governing bodies (NGBs) of Olympic sports coordinate specific Olympic sports for a country, and also sponsor youth sport programs at national, regional, state, and local levels. A great example of this is the work dedicated to youth sports by USA Wrestling. USA Wrestling is responsible for the selection and training of teams to represent the United States in international competition, including world and Olympic competitions. An equal part of USA Wrestling's mission is to foster grassroots development for wrestling, which involves the sanctioning of age-group tournaments and the chartering of member clubs through established state associations. USA Wrestling also conducts regional and national championships for all age categories, national camps, clinics, and coaches' education programs.

6. **Club sports.** The type of private, non-school youth sport that began to proliferate in the 1990s and has changed the culture of American youth sport is **club sport.** American club sport is selective—kids try out for the team, and the best players are selected to be team members. The teams are also known as select teams (because athletes are selected for inclusion) or travel teams (because they play beyond the local communities where recreational and organization-sponsored youth sport teams play).

Club sport typically requires paying to play because most coaches are paid for their services—unlike the volunteer coach model seen in organization-sponsored and

community recreation programs. A coach, director, or manager registers a team name, purchases insurance through a sport organization provider, and then composes the team of any athletes he selects within age requirements. Usually, there are no geographic stipulations on team members, although some clubs have state boundary rules. Team sports (soccer, softball, baseball, basketball, and volleyball) have the largest numbers of participants in club sports, although individual-sport club sports, such as tennis, golf, gymnastics, and swimming, have historically been offered in the United States.

There are several pros and cons about American club sports for youth. In terms of pros, it makes sense to provide this opportunity to young athletes who seek higher levels of competition and more intensive skill development and training. Many of these young athletes seek to make high school teams and hope to participate in the collegiate version of their sports. Some club programs are administered full-time by coaches who receive salaries as high as $80,000 per year, which may advantage young athletes in learning from more knowledgeable and highly trained coaches. Clearly, athletes have the best chance of honing their sport skills in selective club sport programs that have professionally trained coaches.

Parents and athletes must weigh the costs associated with club sport participation, which often require thousands of dollars in fees as opposed to the modest fees (typically less than $50) assessed for traditional organization-sponsored or community recreation youth sport programs. In a survey of families in central Ohio, about one-third said they spent more than $1,500 a year on youth sports (Wagner et al., 2010). Some at the club level paid more than $10,000 per year. The other costs are in time, travel, and energy. It is not uncommon for parents to spend long hours driving club sport athletes to distant training sites and to spend every weekend at tournaments out of town. Another aspect

Growing Up With the Huddersfield Town Terrriers: A European Sport Club Example

Growing up in Manchester, England, Oli Templeton signed to play football (soccer) for his hometown Huddersfield Town Football Club (nicknamed the Terriers) when he was 12 years old. Continuing through high school, Templeton practiced with the club and played games on weekends against the youth teams of the clubs in the North England League. Templeton played for his high school soccer team as well, but he admitted that high school sports in England were definitely not taken as seriously as club sports. He played club competitions every Saturday and sometimes after school, while his high school team played about one game a month.

Templeton was not paid for playing for Huddersfield as a youth. Instead, he got free instruction from the club in return for his loyalty in continuing to play for them. Upon graduation from high school, the club offered him a two-year contract to play soccer instead of going to college. But this was not a pro contract and was minimal, including a small stipend to cover expenses and food. So even though Templeton was still playing for Huddersfield, he was never part of its top professional team. But he explains, "That two-year contract is what you want, but maybe out of ten guys, only one or two might sign a pro contract at the end of it. But people take

a shot at it because the reward can be massive if you make it." (For example, David Beckham signed with Manchester United on his 14th birthday and debuted with Man U's professional team when he was 17. Of course, Beckham went on to be an international soccer icon.) The players who don't make it to the professional team at the end of the two years sometimes head to college or begin jobs or careers in other areas.

Templeton decided to pursue a college education in the United States at Shippensburg University, because in the American system he could play soccer and attend college simultaneously. He describes the difference in systems: "In England you kind of have to make a decision of whether you want follow the athletic route or the school route. They are separate—one doesn't work with the other. In America, it's the best of both worlds—you can live the life of a student but the life of an athlete as well." College athletic scholarships are extremely rare in Europe, so while youth athletes try to get the attention of college recruiters in the United States, they seek to gain notice from professional sport clubs in Europe. Of course, in the United States, there is the inherent tension between academics and athletics in universities, which is not an issue in Europe. So indeed, perhaps there are merits to each system (Loh, 2011).

to consider is that in club sports, there are no organizational rules that require all athletes to participate in all competitions. So athletes may not get equal playing time, and they may not get to play at all on club teams. Overall, club sports are less regulated than other types of youth sports, so parents should be vigilant in assessing prospective club sport programs for their children.

Outside the United States, club sports (typically called sport clubs everywhere else) have historically been the main outlet for youth sport participation. They continue to dominate youth sports in Europe, Japan, North Africa, the Middle East, and Latin America and are also popular in Australia and New Zealand. These **sport clubs** around the world may be multisport or offer only one sport, and collectively they compete in regional, national, and even international sport federations (which govern competition via rules and standards).

Unlike the club system in the United States, the international sport club system is based on participation. These sport clubs are often formed by volunteers, are membership based (as compared to the private franchise club sports of the United States), and serve entire communities, with youth typically progressing through the ranks by playing for teams in different age-group categories until the age of 18. Even then, they may continue club participation as adults. Often, clubs have top selective teams, but overall the international version of club sports is based mainly on age-group participation, skill development, and community involvement. Sport clubs in countries other than the United States are significant for the development and maintenance of community identity in both urban and rural settings. For example, in Australia, rugby league and Australian rules football teams have fanatical community support and create strong identities for many country towns and city suburbs.

7. **Sport academies. Sport academies** are private or state-supported boarding schools that offer sport training along with academic schooling. But they are not traditional boarding schools that promise outstanding athletics to go with stringent academic standards (which is why we have categorized sport academies as a type of nonschool youth sport). The emphasis in sport academies is on *sport training*—that is why young people attend these academies. Most academies offer academic schooling on-site, which is practical in that it allows more sport training time, with the on-campus school much easier to include in the daily training schedules.

In the United States, the premier private sport academy is IMG Academy (see description in the Clipboard section). Another American example is the National Sports Academy (NSA) in Lake Placid, New York. The NSA offers high-performance training in 11 winter sports (alpine skiing, biathlon, boys' and girls' ice hockey, figure skating, freestyle skiing, luge, Nordic combined, Nordic skiing, ski jumping, and snowboarding). The United States Olympic Training Centers also offer resident athlete programs for young athletes chosen from their respective sport NGBs. These athletes board and train at one of the centers, and unlike the situation with IMG and NSA, they take academic classes at a nearby school while they are in resident sport training. Similar national sport academies include the Australian Institute of Sport (with many satellite campuses) and over 200 state-run sport academies in China.

8. **Sport camps.** Nonschool sport camps have become big business in the United States, as parents and youth look for off-season or summer opportunities to enhance sport skills. Traditional summer sport camps for children are local and broad based, offering many different types of sport and recreational activities. These types of camps are still offered by community recreation departments, university recreational services, private companies, and

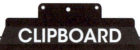

Welcome to IMG Academy

Touted as a "sports utopia," IMG Academy in Bradenton, Florida, is a private sport training institute for youth, high school, collegiate, and professional athletes. It features eight sport programs (tennis, golf, soccer, baseball, basketball, American football, lacrosse, and track and field or cross-country) as well as athletic and personal development programs that focus on the total development of participants (see figure 1.1). IMG also offers a fully accredited pre-K to 12 school that includes postgraduate courses. With nearly 500 acres, IMG facilities include 52 tennis courts (hard, clay, indoor, outdoor), 13 soccer fields, 3 full-size baseball fields and 4 practice diamonds, 12 indoor and outdoor batting cage stations, 15 practice pitching mounds, 18-hole golf course with multiple practice areas and ranges, 2 lacrosse fields, 2 football fields, 4 basketball courts, 4-lane track, covered turf practice field, and a 10,000 square foot weight room. A new residence hall and multiuse sports stadium opened in 2013. One of three Gatorade Sports Science Institute labs is located on IMG's campus, providing expertise in human performance and nutrition for all academy athletes.

Children as young as 11 are eligible to board at IMG—that is, to live there during the typical 10-month academic school year and train during that time. The admissions process is competitive, yet athletic performance is not the sole determining factor in acceptance. Clearly, money is the most important factor in admission. Examples of 2014-2015 Academy

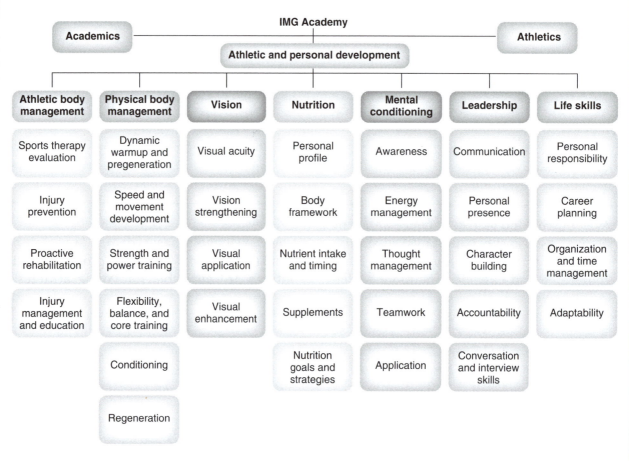

Figure 1.1 IMG Academy model of athletic and personal development.

rates (www.imgacademies.com) were $71,400 for high school tennis and $68,550 for high school team sports, which included private school tuition, sport tuition, and housing and meal options. Upgraded housing and meals were available for another $25,000. Tuition insurance is also recommended and is mandatory for those on the payment plan, which would be another $2,650. Private lessons and other add-ons such as media training can push total costs to close to $100,000 per year (Farrey, 2008). Obviously, most families cannot afford between $70,000 and $100,000 per year for their child's sport training.

IMG markets an impressive success rate. Between 2009 and 2012, 326 IMG graduates (60%) committed to National Collegiate Athletic Association (NCAA) Division I universities (less than 6% of student-athletes nationally go on to play collegiate sport). Also during this time period, IMG reported an average of $1.2 million of total scholarships for the first year of college (compared to less than 2% of student-athletes nationally earning a college scholarship). It's clear that IMG Academy offers outstanding training to young athletes and enables them to achieve academic and athletic success that typically leads to college. However, parents should not buy into the illusion that IMG is a young athlete's ticket into the "bigs" (professional sport). A baseball coach at IMG stated, "Creating professional players is not the standard I set for success." (He admits that it is a rarity for any of his players to get drafted into professional baseball despite the hours and money devoted to the sport at IMG.) "Every now and then you get a kid with great genetics, a real quick kid or a big, exceptionally strong kid. But those are the exceptions. We take what we're given here and work with it" (Sockolove, 2008, p. 200).

Overall, IMG Academy is a very impressive sport training enterprise, and its holistic approach to developing athletic, academic, and life skills in young athletes provides an enticing experience for those youth who have the commitment (and financial means) to pursue their dreams. However, attendance at IMG or any other sport academy is no guarantee of achieving elite sport status or even a college scholarship.

youth development organizations such as the YMCA and Boys and Girls Clubs. The objectives of these programs are to have fun, be physically active, experience social development, and gain confidence and competence in basic sport and physical skills.

Sport-specific nonschool camps have proliferated and have become more professionalized and specialized. These range from local camps that children attend daily to boarding camps where young athletes stay and train for several days or a week. Examples include U.S. Sport Camps, Elite Sports Camps Ltd. (England), Soccer Camps International (Europe), and Australian Sports Camps. All of these camp programs offer multiple camps in locations throughout the respective countries.

PATTERNS OF PARTICIPATION IN YOUTH SPORT

Now you have a basic idea of how youth sport is structured and what programs and options are available for young athletes. So how is it working? Where do most kids participate, and what activities are most popular around the world? In this section, we'll offer an overview of what youth sport looks like in the United States, as well as in other countries, in terms of patterns of participation in various types of youth sport. (With the exception of China and a few European nations, the countries highlighted in this section are English-speaking, which facilitated our efforts to access information about youth sport in those countries. We acknowledge that there are many examples of youth sport around the world not included in this review.)

Youth Sport in the United States

Over 40 million American kids participate in organized youth sport. Across all ages, boys outrank girls in sport participation; and for those kids aged 5 to 18, 66% of boys play organized sport compared to 52% of girls (Athletic Footwear Association, 2012). One-third of American kids play on three or more teams, with boys more likely to be highly involved in multiple sports than girls. American youth sport programs are found in school and nonschool settings.

School-Based Youth Sport

Younger children play more in recreation department and community-organized programs, typically because interscholastic and intramural sports are not available to elementary school children. However, there is a big increase in school-based sport participation in grades 6 to 8 (12- to 14-year-olds). The 10 most popular competitive sport programs for boys and girls in American high schools are shown in the following list.[1] Basketball and track and field are the two most popular sports for boys and girls in high school, followed by volleyball and softball for girls and baseball and football for boys (National Federation of State High School Associations, 2014). Sport participation in American high schools has increased every year since 1989.

Top Ten Sports in American High Schools

Girls

1. Basketball
2. Track and field
3. Volleyball
4. Softball
5. Cross-country (running)
6. Soccer
7. Tennis
8. Golf
9. Swimming, diving
10. Competitive spirit squads

Boys

1. Basketball
2. Track and field
3. Baseball
4. Football
5. Cross-country (running)
6. Golf
7. Soccer
8. Wrestling
9. Tennis
10. Swimming, diving

Adapted, by permission, from National Federation of State High School Associations, *2013-14 High School Athletics Participation Survey*, pg. 55.

[1] These are the most popular high school sports in terms of numbers of programs offered at schools. These rankings do not reflect actual numbers of participants, because school sports differ widely in the number of athletes in programs (e.g., football and track and field typically have larger numbers of participants than basketball and volleyball).

Physical education historically has been a significant source of physical activity for U.S. children, but in recent decades many schools have stopped requiring physical education or have cut back on programs. One in five U.S. schools do not offer physical education at all, and daily physical education is very sparse (less than 4% at the elementary and middle school levels) (Sabo & Veliz, 2008). Physical education participation and opportunities decrease from elementary to high school.

Nonschool Youth Sport

Nonschool youth sport has flourished in the United States based on the many organizations that offer these programs. Sixty percent of kids surveyed in 2012 played sports outside of school (some of whom participated in both school and nonschool programs) (Athletic Footwear Association, 2012). Table 1.1 shows the most popular sports for U.S. youth participation overall, categorized by sex and age range.[2] Noticeable participation trends include an increase in volleyball and decrease in soccer participation for girls as they move into middle school (12-14 years), and the increase in basketball and football participation and decrease in soccer and baseball participation for boys as they age and move into middle school. The data also show that overall participation declines as youth move into middle school (12-14 years), particularly among girls.

Emerging Trends in American Youth Sport

A few trends in American youth sport seem important to highlight. First, due to economic difficulties, a recent trend in school-based sport is the "pay to play" requirement. Historically, school sports were free to participants as part of a school's extracurricular program offerings. Many American schools can afford to field teams and competitions only if they charge students a participation fee, popularly called pay to play. Seventy

Table 1.1 Most Popular U.S. Youth Sport Activities

GIRLS	
7-11 years	**12-17 years**
1. Soccer	1. Volleyball
2. Basketball	2. Basketball
3. Gymnastics	3. Soccer
4. Softball	4. Softball
BOYS	
7-11 years	**12-17 years**
1. Basketball	1. Basketball
2. Baseball	2. Football
3. Soccer	3. Baseball
4. Football	4. Soccer

Adapted from National Sporting Goods Association 2012.

percent of parents recently surveyed paid more than $100 for their children to participate in school sports (Sports and Fitness Industry Association, 2013).

Second, although the traditional American sports of basketball, baseball and softball, and football still show large numbers of participants, several nontraditional sport activities have increased in popularity for kids. These include the so-called extreme sports, such as skateboarding, in-line skating, snowboarding, and bicycle motocross (BMX). Extreme sports are rarely sanctioned by schools but are attractive to kids due to the constant activity and "cool" marketing of these events, such as the X Games sponsored by ESPN television (Rinehart, 2008). Other emerging alternative youth sports in the United States are lacrosse, rugby, and Ultimate Frisbee (Woods, 2011).

A third trend is the drastic decrease in free sport play, or games and physical activities without adult guidance, by American children in the past two decades. A research study found that children 6 to 12 years spent an average of 30 minutes per week outdoors engaged in unstructured play, and that fewer than one in five children spent any unstructured time at all playing outdoors (Hofferth & Sandberg, 2001). These researchers partly explain this phenomenon as the overscheduling of children, with parents eager to nurture achieving children by enrolling them into multiple organized, supervised, adult-led activities such as organized sport, music lessons, and leadership and self-development programs. Of course, another contributing factor is the abundance of electronic entertainment for kids, including

[2] For this survey, participants were youth 7 to 17 years who participated in the listed sports more than once per year. These participation numbers may reflect school and nonschool as well as adult-organized sports and more youth-organized pickup activities. Participation was high in several activities that we did not report here, such as swimming, bicycle riding, bowling, and exercise walking or hiking. We chose to report activities that are representative of more structured competitive youth sports as opposed to swimming and bicycling, which kids typically do as leisure or play activities.

multiple television channels, computers and Internet access, and video games. American children between the ages of 8 and 18 years spend an average of 7 hours a day on screen activities such as these (Rideout, Foehr, & Roberts, 2010).

Lack of National Coordination in American Youth Sport

Unlike what is seen in many other countries, youth sport in the United States has not been organized or coordinated by the government. As shown on pages 12 and 13, the organization of American youth sport is diverse, with many types of organizations and without any national coordination. The United States Olympic Committee and the NGBs of the various Olympic sports offer one sort of central governing body, but these organizations govern only a very small percentage of youth sport programs, most of them elite. This lack of a national ministry of sport or central governing body for youth sport hampers initiatives like national youth sport policy development, systematic DAP participation guidelines and strategies, a national coaching education and certification requirement for youth coaches, and funding and resources for grassroots youth sport development.

Youth Sport in Canada

Similar to the situation in the United States, youth sport in Canada is conducted in both school- and community-based (nonschool) programs. The most popular high school sports in Canada are basketball, soccer, volleyball, track and field, and cross-country (Camire, 2014). Soccer has the most youth sport participants and is the fastest-growing sport in the country. An estimated 44% of Canadian youth participate in soccer ("Garnier-Ombrelle," 2013), with the overall soccer participation rate being 58% for males and 42% for females ("Soccer Still," 2008).

Interestingly, youth sport participation in ice hockey has decreased since 2010, with just 10% of Canadian boys aged 5 to 19 years registered to play organized hockey (Mirtle, 2012). What makes this significant is that ice hockey is popularly considered the national sport of Canada. However, parents cite rising costs and concerns about concussions as reasons for the recent decline in youth hockey participation in Canada. Sport participation tends to peak in the early teenage years, but remains the likely choice for out-of-school activities for children between 10 and 13 years, particularly for boys. A notable feature of Canadian sport is the developmentally appropriate National Coaching Certification Program (NCCP), which was initiated in 1974 by the Coaching Association of Canada (discussed further in chapter 14).

Youth Sport in Europe

Traditionally, youth sport in Europe has mainly focused on sport clubs that serve entire communities. This is what is often termed a **grassroots sport** approach, meaning that sport is organized and conducted locally and is open to all people in the community (as opposed to being exclusive). The most popular sport in Europe, for youth and adults, is soccer (or football as it is termed everywhere except in the United States and Canada). Youth sport has great social relevance in Europe, because the sport club system has always emphasized community and cultural identity and a sense of belonging to that community or culture.

Youth Sport in the United Kingdom

The youth sport system in the United Kingdom is similar to the American model because schools there do offer physical education, intramural sport, and interscholastic sport for youth. About one-half of children under age 12 and one-third of children 12 to 18 participate in extracurricular school-based sport (either intramural or interscholastic) on a weekly basis in the United Kingdom, boys participating more than girls (Green, 2010). Participation in school-based sport and sport clubs declines from age 10 to 16, and female sport participation decreases drastically in all youth sport types around age 14. Girls are more likely to be offered fitness activities such as dance, gymnastics, and yoga, whereas boys get more opportunities to play cricket, basketball, and rugby (Vasagar, 2010).

Overall, considering all types of youth sport, 39% of children in the United Kingdom regularly participate in competitive youth sport. Soccer is by far the most popular youth sport in the United Kingdom, with many football (soccer) clubs available. Unlike what is seen in mainland Europe, most sport clubs in the United Kingdom are dedicated to a single sport, with soccer, cricket, dance, rugby, swimming, athletics (track and field), and tennis as the most common types of clubs (Quick, Simon, & Thornton, 2011). Sport England has instituted the new Youth Sport Strategy, investing millions of national lottery monies to increase youth sport participation. Strategies to do this include creating 6,000 new school–sport club links, upgrading facilities, and establishing the new School Games program, which is a year-round schedule of 30 sports competing at the intra- and inter-school levels and culminating in regional and national events.

Youth Sport in Other European Countries

Sport and physical activities are very popular across almost all of the European Union member states. For example, around 70% of Irish youth participate in some form of extracurricular sport on a weekly basis (Woods, Moyna, Quinlan, Tannehill, & Walsh, 2010), and youth sport participation has increased in the past few decades in

Sweden, Finland, and Iceland. Surveys also show sport and physical activity to be the most popular leisure activity for youth in Belgium, Estonia, Germany, Hungary, and the Czech Republic. A trend in European youth activity is the increase in participation rates in lifestyle sport and activities, such as cycling, swimming, and running, which have served to broaden and diversify the number of sport and physical activity opportunities beyond traditional team competitive sports (Green, 2010).

Sport clubs are so popular in Germany that it has been called the "country of clubs," and most Germans participate in sport via at least one sport club within a national network. These clubs are often state supported, with their facilities available to the public for a nominal fee. They offer sport competition for people of all ages in a variety of sports. Germany has also received much global attention for its national youth training programs for soccer, considered that country's national sport (discussed in more detail in chapter 10).

Youth sport in Russia has changed from the strong government control and support of programs since the demise of the Soviet Union. Yet, President Putin pledged increased funding of programs and infrastructure for youth sport and children's physical education in a 2013 address from the Kremlin ("Opening Remarks," 2013). He stated that sport has rightly returned to being a state policy priority and that major national changes are needed to enhance mass sport, particularly sport for children. Russia has received international attention for its youth training of tennis and ice hockey players, with multiple stars in these professional sports. Youth hockey in Russia is club driven, with the clubs owned and administered by professional hockey teams and governed by the Russian Hockey Federation. Hockey coaches are paid professionals and are required to have extensive education and sport-specific training.

Youth Sport in Australia

Australia is often cited in the news as a "proud sporting nation," so it is clear that participation in youth sport is highly valued by Australians. Approximately 63% of children aged 5 to 14 participate in at least one organized sport outside of school hours (Australia Bureau of Statistics, 2011). As in other countries, sport participation is higher among boys (70%) than girls (56%). Popular organized sports for children are swimming, soccer, Australian rules football, netball, rugby, cricket, and basketball. Australia is known as a strong swimming nation with the majority of Australians living close to the seacoast, so it makes sense that swimming is the most popular youth sport. Surf lifesaving and surfing are also immensely popular. Amazingly, there are 47 Olympic-sized 50-meter pools in Sydney alone (Light, 2011). Netball (similar to basketball, but with seven players on a team and a basket with no backboard) is the most popular team sport for girls in Australia, with Australian women having won 9 of the 12 world championships held in netball since 1963.

Sport clubs have historically been a big part of Australian culture and of youth experiences in growing up. However, youth sport is also provided through interscholastic, intramural, and physical education opportunities in Australian schools. Young athletes who have a strong interest in a sport typically play it during the week in school; they also play for their clubs on the weekend in the same sport or different sports. Australia is known for its systematic talent identification and development program for youth athletes (discussed in chapter 10). The Australian Institute of Sport directs the national elite sport program along with satellite government academies in different states.

Youth Sport in New Zealand

In New Zealand, a Commonwealth country (of British colonial heritage) like Australia, popular sports for children include rugby, cricket, netball (for girls), soccer, athletics (track and field), and swimming (Sport New Zealand, 2012b). Rugby union is the national sport of New Zealand, with the national rugby team, the All Blacks, a key part of national identity. Cricket is the national summer sport, and netball is the most popular girls' and women's sport, as in Australia. These sports are played in both club and school settings, similar to the Australian and U.K. models. Sixty percent of boys and 50% of girls belonged to a sport club in 2011, and 50% of both boys and girls participated on school sport teams. Participation in club and school sport teams was highest for 11- to 14-year-olds. Similar to what occurs in other countries, participation drops off in the teenage years, particularly for girls. KiwiSport is a government funding initiative to promote sport for school-aged children. The program is an example of DAP, divided into developmentally progressive programs and resources for youth 0 to 5 years, 5 to 12 years, and 13 to 18 years.

Youth Sport in China

Our final country to discuss in relation to youth sport is unique and of particular interest based on several cultural factors. China has the largest population in the world at 1.3 billion, and it has the largest economy in the developing world. China is a communist state, with its central government controlling all policies related to youth sport. And finally, China is fast becoming a world power in sport, having led the gold medal count at the 2008 Beijing Olympic Games and trailing only the United States in gold and total medals at the 2012 London Olympic Games.

Between 1988 and 2008, China increased its total Olympic medal production 400% and its gold medal production 1,000% (Miller, 2009). This achievement is attributed to the youth sport development system sponsored by the Chinese government. Therefore, the youth sport system in China has come under particular scrutiny and is of global interest.

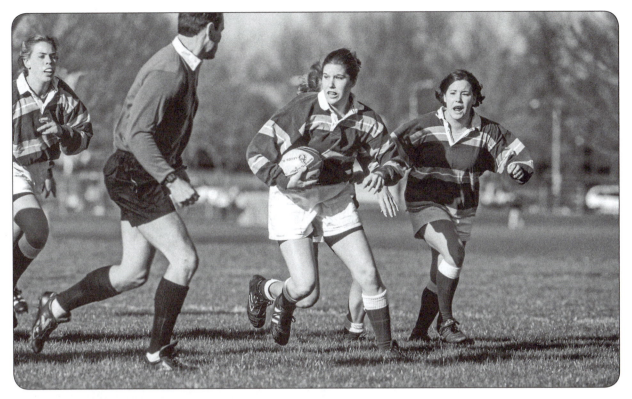

Rugby is a popular sport in New Zealand and Australia.

Traditional Chinese culture highly values physical fitness, and children are assessed in relation to national standards of physical fitness. Most Chinese children, with or without sport talent, participate in physical education and intramural sports in primary and secondary schools. Physical education is compulsory for all students from primary school through the first two years of university. As in other countries, critics state that elite athlete development is overemphasized at the expense of mass sport opportunities for all youth (Liang, Housner, Walls, & Yan, 2013).

Another tension has to do with the emphasis on educational attainment in China, with the many classroom learning hours precluding youth sport or fitness development. Although fitness is viewed as important, Chinese parents for the most part do not wish for their children to seek professional sport careers, stating that "only the brainless people will use 'body skill' to earn money" (Bennett, 2011, p. 2). They see sport as a

risk (which it is, without subsequent education), and young athletes must then choose between continuing their sports or studying at universities.

Overall, it is a tremendous challenge for China to provide quality physical education and youth sport programs to such a large number of people. China's success in the past three summer Olympic Games demonstrated its focus on elite athlete training, but this success has not led to the revival of physical education and youth sport opportunities for all Chinese youth (Liang et al., 2013).

So what about China's vaunted youth sport elite talent training? It starts with the "spare-time sport schools" around the country that offer specialist coaching for young athletes selected for their abilities and potential. The regional and national sport schools (sport academies as discussed in this chapter) select the best athletes from spare-time sport schools, and students then live and train together at this site (with schooling provided either on- or off-site). Students in these schools are provided the best training facilities and instruction from high-quality coaches, and typically train 6 to 8 hours per day. Many athletes are selected from poor families and are sent to a sport school that best fits their athletic potential. For example, table tennis is a national obsession, and the Luneng Table Tennis School provides a gymnasium set up with 80 tables. State-sponsored sport schools (academies) are available in many sports, with traditional success shown in badminton, diving, and gymnastics, among others. In 2011, the National Basketball Association opened the Chinese Basketball Association's Congguan Basketball School, a training center for elite players aged 12 to 17. Basketball is becoming very popular in China.

China commits a great many resources to talent development in youth sport. It uses a "gold-medal strategy" of placing youth in sports that offer the most Olympic medals (e.g., fencing offers 10 gold medals, kayaking offers 16). Also of interest, young girls' and women's programs are strongly funded. However, there are criticisms of the Chinese elite sport system. It is argued that these child and teenage athletes are not permitted to be children and have been denied normal family and social lives, and that those who don't achieve international success experience difficulty in finding jobs outside their sport areas because of a lack of formal education (Hong, 2008; Hong & Zhouxiang, 2013).

BARRIERS TO YOUTH SPORT PARTICIPATION

Youth sport is widely accepted across the globe as an important activity that serves to enhance the physical, psychological, and social development of children. But do all children have access to youth sport? What factors influence kids' opportunities to participate in youth sport? And what factors block their participation? **Youth sport barriers** are situations or conditions that obstruct kids' opportunities to participate fully in sport. In this section, we identify seven categories of barriers that influence youth sport opportunities for kids:

1. Gender and type of community
2. Race and ethnicity
3. Family factors
4. Disabilities
5. Maturational status and critical period skill development
6. Adult leaders and cultural stereotypes
7. Psychological and personality factors

Personal Plug-In

My Personal Youth Sport Story

Think about your personal experiences in youth sport. What types of youth sports did you participate in (school, nonschool, community recreation, select, sport club)? What specific sports did you engage in? Consider the reasons for your personal participation pattern. Why was this your youth sport experience? Now consider any barriers you faced that affected your participation in youth sport. That is, what factors may have prevented you from participating in certain youth sport types, levels, or activities? Consider not only your immediate family and community barriers but also broader cultural barriers that you faced.

Gender and Type of Community

Boys are more likely than girls to be involved in sport at every age and more likely to play multiple sports. However, this gender gap differs by community. In U.S. suburban communities, participation rates between boys and girls are comparable. But in rural and urban communities, girls are less involved in sport (Sabo & Veliz, 2008).

Girls (7.4 years) tend to join sports later in life than boys (6.8 years), and girls drop out sooner and in greater numbers. Also, 84% of urban and 68% of rural girls have no physical education classes at all in the 11th and 12th grades, compared with the 48% of suburban girls who do not participate in physical education. Schools with greater economic resources provided more sport participation opportunities for both boys and girls, as higher community income levels were related to higher levels of participation among boys and girls in grades 3 to 8 (Sabo & Veliz, 2008). Yet, overall, boys were afforded more sport participation opportunities than girls regardless of the economic viability of the school (Women's Sports Foundation, 2011).

Water Break

To Saudi Arabia: Let the Girls Play!

In May 2013, the Saudi Press Agency announced that female students enrolled in private girls' schools could take part in sports so long as they wear "decent clothing" and are supervised by female instructors (Reuters, 2013). Earlier in 2013, the Saudi government stated it would begin to license women's sport clubs for the first time ever. These were two small steps toward, but a long way away from, establishing the rights of girls to participate in youth sport in that country.

Although two women competed for Saudi Arabia in the 2012 Olympic Games (the first ever allowed to do so), girls and women are not free in that country to participate in sports. Girls in public schools are banned from sport and physical activity, including physical education. Girls and women have also been denied participation in gyms and sport clubs (of 153 youth ministry-supported sport clubs, none have women's teams), and the National Olympic Committee of Saudi Arabia has no programs for women athletes. This lack of equity in sport participation is part of systematic Saudi discrimination against girls and women as they are forbidden from traveling, conducting official business, driving, and undergoing certain medical procedures or marrying without permission of male guardians. A spokesperson for Human Rights Watch states, "The world cheered when Saudi women shared the Olympic spotlight, but millions of girls and women in Saudi Arabia are still stuck on the sidelines. This is a moment for the global sporting community to press Saudi Arabia to allow sports for women and girls, once and for all" (Human Rights Watch, 2012).

Race and Ethnicity

Youth sports in the United States are racially and ethnically diverse, but inequities exist. Fewer girls of color are sport participants as compared to white girls, and girls of color are much more likely than their male counterparts to be nonathletes. Interestingly, the largest discrepancy between boys' (35%) and girls' (9%) sport participation has been shown to be among Asians. For both girls and boys, children of color entered sport at a later age than did white girls and boys, particularly in urban communities (Sabo & Veliz, 2008). Again, the issue of urban living as a barrier to sport participation emerges, perhaps due to fewer sport resources, options, and opportunities (e.g., public parks, sport facilities, community programs).

Family Factors

The socioeconomic status (SES) of families clearly influences young people's sport opportunities. Socioeconomic status is typically assessed as a combination of parents' education level, prestige of parents' occupation, and household income. Children and adolescents from lower SES families in the United States, Australia, and Canada participated less frequently in organized youth sport both in and out of schools (Bengoechea, Sabiston, Ahmed, & Farnoush, 2010; Dyck, 2012; Sabo & Veliz, 2008). Children in wealthier families enter sport at earlier ages and are more highly involved athletes compared to those from less wealthy families. Children with a parent holding a graduate or professional degree (60%) were more likely to participate in sports than children of parents with a high school education (42%) or less (22%) (Clark, 2008). Along with the basic economic barrier of lack of financial resources for equipment and entry fees, the barriers of time and travel to practices and events are difficult for many families to overcome.

Another family factor influencing youth sport participation is the involvement or lack of involvement of parents in sport. Eighty-two percent of kids whose parents were highly involved in sport were youth sport participants, compared to 69% of children whose parents were moderately involved and 24% of those whose parents were not involved in sport in any way (Clark, 2008).

Some evidence exists to suggest that where a person is born can contribute to that individual's likelihood of participating in elite sport. Called the **birthplace effect,** it refers to the overrepresentation of elite athletes born in small towns or moderate-sized cities and the underrepresentation of elite athletes born in large cities (population >500,000). The birthplace effect has been shown in American football, ice hockey, golf, baseball, basketball, cricket, rugby, and swimming (MacDonald, Cheung, Cote, & Abernathy, 2009; MacDonald, King, Cote, & Abernathy, 2009). In a study of participation rates in Canadian youth hockey between 2004 and 2010, players from larger cities (population >500,000) were more likely to drop out, while players from smaller cities were more likely to remain engaged in youth hockey (Imtiaz, Hancock, Vierimaa, & Cote, 2014). Reasons for the birthplace effect are speculative, but they may have to do with greater opportunities to practice, availability of more open play spaces, more supportive relationships, and perceived safer environments to play outside or in community facilities.

Disabilities

Disability refers to biomedical conditions that limit a person's ability to perform specific tasks. Examples of disabilities that challenge youth sport participants include autism, visual impairment, hearing impairment, orthopedic impairment such as the need for wheelchairs, and speech or language impairment. It is important for adult stakeholders to commit to the rights and needs of disabled children to participate in sport. Research indicates that the frequency of physical activity for disabled boys and girls declines more sharply than for participants without disabilities from the elementary to the high school years (Sabo & Veliz, 2008).

For the vast majority of disabled youth, most sport opportunities are offered through special programs and organizations dedicated to disabled sport participants. For example, Disabled Sport USA is a nonprofit community-based chapter network that offers over 40 sports to disabled youth. Its motto is "I Can Do Anything!" and the organization offers scholarships for youth with disabilities and limited financial means to participate in any of its programs across the country. Similarly, the English Federation of Disability Sport (EFDS) is a national organization focused on increasing opportunities and offering sport and physical activity programs for people with disabilities. Other examples of youth programs for athletes with disabilities include the Special Olympics, Wheelchair Sports USA, Just for Kicks (soccer), and Little League Challenger Division.

Maturational Status and Critical Period Skill Development

Because youth sport involves participants in their peak maturational years, several barriers to athlete development can occur based on maturational issues. These are discussed in detail in chapters 4 and 5, but at this point, readers should simply be aware that maturation is a critical determining factor in youth sport success. Maturational status and learning skills during critical periods of development greatly influence children's ability to gain the skill levels needed for select sport participation and high school sport participation. Often, these maturational and skill development barriers lead children to drop out of youth sport as they become discouraged with their lack of skill development in relation to peers.

Adult Leaders and Cultural Stereotypes

Coaches and youth sport directors are critical factors in implementing DAP to allow kids to enjoy sport and develop their skills. It is often non-DAP experiences with coaches or programs that discourage children from continuing participation, or that serve as barriers to skill development, personal improvement, and upward mobility in the sport system. A related barrier is the perpetuation of cultural stereotypes by adult leaders, based on preconceived ideas about physical size, gender appropriateness, and racial advantages or disadvantages. These issues are discussed more fully in chapters 13 and 15.

Psychological and Personality Factors

Although psychological and personality factors are internal to youth athletes, we feel it is important to identify these as barriers to their continued participation, enjoyment, and success. As will be discussed in chapters 6 and 11, personality characteristics such as fear-of-failure orientation, low self-esteem, low perceived competence, and burnout are related to youth sport dropout and decreased motivation to succeed in sport. Our job as adult stakeholders in youth sport is to understand these characteristics as internal barriers to a fully enjoyable and successful youth sport experience. In fact, our job is to understand the multiple barriers that exist and to do what we can to ensure that all children have opportunities for sport involvement and success.

ORGANIZATIONS THAT SUPPORT YOUTH SPORT

Several national service organizations, corporations, and centers support youth sport by providing educational resources and certification programs for directors, coaches, parents, officials, and athletes. Some prominent ones are listed next, and these organizations are explained in more detail in the Resource Guide at the end of the chapter.

- Positive Coaching Alliance (PCA, positivecoach.org)
- National Alliance for Youth Sports (NAYS, nays.org)
- International Alliance for Youth Sports (IAYS, iays.org)
- Human Kinetics Coach Education (former ASEP) (www.HumanKinetics CoachEducationCenter.com)
- Institute for the Study of Youth Sports (ISYS, youthsports.msu.edu)
- Youth Sport Trust (youthsporttrust.org)
- Youth Organisation of the European Non-Governmental Sports Organisation (ENGSO Youth, youth-sport.net)

WRAP-UP

Whew! That *was* a broad overview of youth sport. It's our hope that this breadth of knowledge sets up the rest of the book by helping you understand how youth sport is structured and what it looks like in the United States and other countries. Many innovative developmentally appropriate practices of youth sport are occurring in many different parts of the world. We'll do our best to identify and describe these to you throughout the book.

Two issues raised in the chapter deserve continued discussion, and they will be addressed throughout the book. First, a troubling common trend across countries is the drop-off in participation in sport during the teenage years, particularly for girls. We need to consider the many reasons why this occurs and offer strategies and recommendations that may help to keep young people involved in physical activity into adulthood.

A second issue observed throughout the world is the tension between grassroots youth sport for all and elite sport talent development. This tension is inevitable, yet it is our belief that we can pursue both objectives by implementing developmentally appropriate practice in innovative ways. We believe youth sport can be "all about the kid," whether that kid is the second coming of LeBron James or a kid who lacks the talent to play interscholastic high school sport yet continues to stay active in community recreational sports. So read on—your pursuit of knowledge for practice continues.

LEARNING AIDS

Key Terms

birthplace effect—The overrepresentation of elite athletes born in small towns or in moderate-size cities and an underrepresentation of elite athletes born in large cities.

club sports (in the United States)—Private, nonschool teams or programs in which young athletes are selected for inclusion based on an evaluation of their skills, requiring higher levels of training and competition as compared to recreational teams (also known as travel sport or select sport).

disability—Biomedical condition that limits a person's ability to perform specific tasks.

grassroots sport—Sport programs that are organized and conducted locally and are open to all people in the community (as opposed to being exclusive).

physical activity—Any bodily movement produced by skeletal muscles that results in energy expenditure.

sport—A game-like activity that is governed by specific rules, is competitive, and requires some form of physical exertion.

sport academy—Private or government-funded training centers where young athletes live and focus on sport training, some of which offer academic schooling with the academy itself.

sport clubs (outside the United States)—Membership-based sport programs, usually associated with communities, that offer youth sport participation in several different age-group categories.

youth—Individuals between early childhood and adulthood who are undergoing significant physical and mental development.

youth sport—Programs that provide adult-supervised sport skill development sessions and competitive contests to children in the typical age range of 5 to 18 years.

youth sport barriers—Situations or conditions that obstruct kids' opportunities to participate fully in sport.

Summary Points

1. Youth sport is a unique subculture based on (a) social comparison with peers during a period of rapid developmental change, (b) the involvement of parents and adult leaders, and (c) the fact that sport is a professionalized mega-billion dollar business.

2. School-based youth sport includes interscholastic sport, intramural sport, physical education, and sport camps.

3. Nonschool youth sport includes local service club teams and leagues; national sport organization teams and leagues; national youth development organization programs; community recreation department programs; Olympic NGB national, state, and local programs; club sports; sport academies; and sport camps.

4. Youth sport in the United States offers both school-based and nonschool programs, with observable trends including pay to play, the proliferation of club sport programs, the increasing popularity of alternative and extreme sports (relative to traditional American team sports), and the huge decline in free play or pickup sport in the past two decades.

5. The organization of youth sport in the United States is diverse, with many types of organizations, lacking national coordination or a central governing body as seen in many other countries.

6. The most popular youth sport in Canada is soccer, not ice hockey as would be expected.

7. Youth sport in Europe, Latin America, Australia, and New Zealand is much more sport club–based than in the United States.

8. China commits a large amount of governmental resources to talent development in youth sport, selecting the best athletes suited to specific sports to train in sport academies throughout the country.

9. Barriers to youth sport participation and success include gender, type of community, race and ethnicity, family factors, disabilities, maturational status and critical period skill development, adult leaders and cultural stereotypes, and psychological and personality factors.

10. Multiple national service organizations, corporations, and centers support youth sport by providing educational resources and certification programs for directors, coaches, parents, officials, and athletes.

Study Questions

1. What makes youth sport such a unique subculture? Provide examples of issues that arise in youth sport based on this subcultural uniqueness.

2. What is club sport? Identify several pros and cons of this type of youth sport in the United States, and differentiate between the club sport model in the United States versus the rest of the world.

3. Identify some of the most popular youth sports in the United States, Canada, China, Australia, New Zealand, and the United Kingdom.

4. Discuss the nature of youth sport in the United States, including structural aspects, participation patterns, and emerging trends and issues.

5. Explain the focus on youth sport talent development in China, and how that conflicts with the objective of sport and physical activity for all.

6. Identify the seven youth sport barriers described in the chapter, and provide examples or a description of each barrier.

Reflective Learning Activities

1. Choose one country from around the world (not your own), and search the Internet for an interesting example, occurrence, practice, or structure of youth sport in that country.

2. Create the ideal youth sport structure for a country, in terms of who plans and administers programs, and how this would work at the local, state, regional, and national levels. Anything goes—you have unlimited financial resources for this very important venture.

Resource Guide

Human Kinetics Coach Education (www.HumanKineticsCoachEducationCenter. com). Begun as a coaching education–certification program for youth coaches, this program has expanded to offer educational resources for coaches, officials, sport directors, parents, and athletes. Many online materials, books, and certification courses are available, including sport-specific coaching courses, sport first-aid courses, and youth sport director courses. This program is a for-profit business division of Human Kinetics, the leading international publisher of sport, physical activity, and health resources.

Institute for the Study of Youth Sports (youthsports.msu.edu), or ISYS. The ISYS is an educational outreach center at Michigan State University that provides leadership, research, and outreach programs in youth sport. As a university center, the ISYS is significant in providing an unbiased scientific knowledge base about youth sport so that developmentally appropriate practice can be implemented to enhance youth sport for all participants.

International Alliance for Youth Sports (iays.com), or IAYS. IAYS is a nonprofit corporation created by the National Alliance for Youth Sports to provide educational service for youth sports across the globe. The signature program of IAYS is "Game On! Youth Sports," an educational training and guidance program for community youth sport directors around the world.

National Alliance for Youth Sports (nays.org), or NAYS. NAYS is a national non-profit corporation that offers a variety of programs and services for all stakeholders in youth sports. NAYS offers educational certification programs for volunteer youth coaches, volunteer youth directors, paid youth sport administrators (Academy for Youth Sports Administrators), youth sport officials, and parents. NAYS has extensive partnerships with over 3,000 community-based youth sport programs and offers multiple position statements on a variety of youth sport issues as well as a set of national standards for youth sport.

National Council of Youth Sports (ncys.org), or NCYS. The NCYS was established in 1979 by the Sporting Goods Manufacturers Association to serve as an advocacy and education group for youth sports in the United States. The NCYS publishes reports on trends in youth sports and forges sponsorships and partnerships to promote sport for youth.

National Federation of State High School Associations (nfhs.org), or NFHS. The NFHS sets forth guidelines regarding the rules for athletic associations around the country to follow. Also, the NFHS has sport-specific drills and skill development techniques for coaches to implement in their own practices. The NFHS also has resources available for officials, music directors, and speech and debate teams.

National Intramural-Recreational Sports Association (nirsa.org), or NIRSA. NIRSA is an association of collegiate recreation departments nationwide. NIRSA was founded in 1950 and is one of the largest college recreation organizations in the world. The NIRSA website has a multitude of resources, including preset rules for intramural sports and training materials for student officials.

Positive Coaching Alliance (positivecoach.org), or PCA. The PCA is a national nonprofit corporation with the mission to provide youth athletes with a "positive, character-building youth sport experience." The PCA has chapters throughout the United States and provides extensive educational materials (books, online courses, newsletters, workshops) for coaches, parents, officials, administrators, and athletes.

Special Olympics (specialolympics.org). Special Olympics began in the early 1960s and was spearheaded by Eunice Kennedy Shriver. Her vision was to provide opportunities for people with intellectual disabilities to participate in sports and other activities. In 2012, Special Olympics saw participation of over 4 million individuals with intellectual disabilities from around the world. Special Olympics events take place in North America, but now a World Special Olympics comprises athletes from over 170 countries.

Youth Organisation of the European Non-Governmental Sports Organisation (youth-sport.net), or ENGSO Youth. ENGSO Youth is a nonprofit youth organization of ENGSO, which comprises national umbrella organizations for sport across Europe. ENGSO Youth represents youth sports in 40 countries and actively works on current youth sport issues such as social inclusion, doping, fair play, and participation. Initiatives include the prevention of sexualized violence in sports, standing up against discrimination in sports, and open doors to all abilities in sports.

Youth Sport Trust (youthsportrust.org). The Youth Sport Trust is an independent charity dedicated to enhancing physical education and sport in the United Kingdom. It offers multiple programs in three divisions: Sporting Start (primary), Sporting Chance (inclusion), and Sporting Best (secondary), and is partnered with Sport England along with several other sport organizations.

EVOLUTION OF YOUTH SPORT

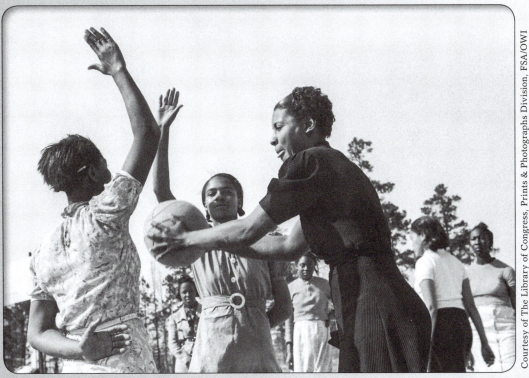

Courtesy of The Library of Congress, Prints & Photographs Division, FSA/OWI Collection, LC-DIG-fsa-8a39951.

CHAPTER PREVIEW

In this chapter, you'll learn

» how youth sport got started in the United States,

» how Title IX changed the landscape of youth sport,

» why nonschool sports became so popular, and

» how the rise of club sports created a major cultural shift in American youth sport.

Here's a scenario that you may have witnessed. A group of 9- to 10-year-old soccer players are waiting for their coach to show up for practice. They each have a soccer ball that was given to them as members of the team. However, instead of dribbling or shooting or even playing a warm-up game, they're standing or sitting around waiting for their coach. When the coach arrives, she asks, "Why aren't you warming up or playing?" The athletes reply, "We didn't know what to do, so we were waiting on you."

This scenario captures the historic sea change in youth sport that has occurred in the past several decades, with adult-organized programs the norm and pickup or sandlot play almost nonexistent. It seems today that kids don't know what to do without adult direction. Perhaps we've conditioned them to think this way, as you'll learn in this chapter. Would you believe that high school football (American) teams in the late 1800s ran their own practices, scheduled their games, and coordinated travel to these games? They actually resisted attempts by school officials to regulate their extracurricular sport (Gems, Borish, & Pfister, 2008).

Our goal in this chapter is to help you understand the most significant historical events in the evolution of youth sport. Why? Because there are clear historical reasons for the youth sport practices that are in vogue today. We want you to understand the evolution of youth sport, or the process of development or progressive change that led up to today's youth sport culture. Our main focus is on the evolution of youth sport in the United States—with apologies to our international readers. Instead of moving through a chronological time line, we thought it would be more interesting to organize the chapter around key questions about the evolution of youth sport. We chose questions that try to get at why youth sport is what it is today. So stay with us—history doesn't have to be boring!

WHEN AND WHY WAS SPORT INTRODUCED INTO SCHOOLS?

Physical education in private schools became part of the effort to enhance the physical fitness of white Protestant American boys of the upper class in the mid-1700s. Yet, in 1810 a children's advice book, titled *Youthful Recreations,* promoted exercise and physical play and argued for poor children's rights to play as well ("they should *at least* play hop scotch!") (as cited in Gems, Borish, & Pfister, 2008). In the 1800s, physical education and sport became part of most school programs in the United States to enhance the fitness and moral education of boys—to help them avoid juvenile delinquency, particularly in the larger cities of the East and Midwest. (Note: Basketball and volleyball were invented during this period in the late 1800s. Basketball was invented to provide a winter activity that would occupy young boys during the interim between football and baseball seasons.)

Interestingly, boys had already been initiating their own interscholastic contests in baseball and football without official sponsorship by school authorities. By 1898, teachers in Chicago high schools formed a board to govern student athletics (standardizing rules, establishing eligibility requirements, prohibiting money prizes). Amusingly, students protested their loss of autonomy and the adult intervention (some students attempted to establish their own league without adult supervision and were expelled from school), but unfortunately, adult-controlled high school sport had begun. By the turn of the 20th century, high school teams traveled throughout the country for regional and national competitions (Gems et al., 2008).

A massive interscholastic sport program (Public School Athletic League, or PSAL) was established for boys in 1903 in New York City. Once again, the impetus for the program was character building and a diversion from delinquency in the overcrowded city. The program included all ages (elementary to high school) and offered three different types of competition: (1) athletic badge tests for physical fitness, (2) interclass competition in track and field (similar to intramurals today), and (3) district and city championships in a number of sports (Wiggins, 2013). A girls' division of the PSAL was created in 1905 with play activities and intramurals but no interscholastic competition. Numerous cities adopted New York's PSAL model, and adults increasingly grew to control youth sport. In 1920, the National Federation of State High School Associations was formed to oversee interscholastic sports in the United States.

Another important milestone for school-based youth sport was the creation of the

Water Break

Sandlots and Playgrounds

The Sandlot is a 1993 American sports comedy film that is a nostalgic, coming-of-age story about a group of youth baseball players during the summer of 1962. This period marked the height of participation in **sandlot,** or kid-organized, games and activities within neighborhoods, which lasted roughly through the 1970s. Have you ever wondered where the term *sandlot* came from?

In 1885, a Massachusetts health agency placed a pile of sand in the yard of a mission in Boston's North End. The pile was called a sand garden, and its purpose was to provide a play area for children (Riess, 1991). It became so popular that several more were created around Boston, and the word *playground* replaced the term sand garden. However, *sandlot* continued to be used to designate any open space for pickup (informal, youth-led) games through the 1990s. Hence the youth sport cult movie titled *The Sandlot*.

It required some forward-thinking social reformers to conceptualize public space for recreation and play in the crowded American cities in the late 1800s and early 1900s. Sand gardens gave way to model playgrounds, with swinging, climbing, and sliding equipment and open spaces for sports and games. As playgrounds proliferated (3,940 in the United States by 1917), cities began to offer recreational programs within the parks and play spaces. The city of Chicago was the first to take the additional step of building field houses for year-round play, gyms, and even swimming pools. The city hired trained park directors, who coordinated the programs that became the community parks and recreation youth sport programs of today. The Playground Association of America (PAA) was formed in 1906 to promote physical activity and develop open playground and park space as a form of recreation for youth.

It all began with a pile of sand and children's natural instinct to play. Today, playgrounds are a multibillion dollar business, with many types of designs. The National Program for Playground Safety offers up-to-date information on all aspects of contemporary playgrounds.

President's Council on Youth Fitness by President Eisenhower in 1956, a program that continues in schools today. The program is now named the President's Council on Fitness, Sports, and Nutrition, and you may remember the Youth Physical Fitness Test required in school physical education classes. We do! So school-based youth sport began to provide fitness training for upper-class kids early on in the United States and evolved to require fitness testing for all youth.

HOW DID NONSCHOOL YOUTH SPORT BECOME SO POPULAR?

Along with school-based youth sport, nonschool programs and facilities for boys were designed and introduced by adults in the late 1800s. The reasons for this included the perceived need for moral development, increased health and vigor, productive leisure and social activity, and skill development, as well as an interest in competition or comparing skills with those of others.

Muscular Christianity

Regarding moral development, a movement known as **Muscular Christianity** promoted sport and physical activity in hand with Christian values and practices (Berryman, 1996). The most important institution in this movement was the Young Men's Christian Association, or YMCA, which offered sport facilities and programs for young boys beginning in 1851. By the late 1800s, many YMCAs offered physical training and sport programs for boys. An important leader of the YMCA movement was Luther Gulick, a professional physical educator at the YMCA Training School in Massachusetts, who also was instrumental in developing the PSAL in New York City as well as the playground movement in the United States. It is significant that Gulick was a professional educator

and sport leader whose expertise allowed him to purposefully structure developmentally appropriate youth sport programs (Wiggins, 2013). A contemporary example of the continuation of the Muscular Christianity idea is the Catholic Youth Organization (CYO) youth sport leagues, which began in 1930 in Chicago.

From these early beginnings in YMCA programs, the 1920s and 1930s were marked by the proliferation of city, regional, and national nonschool youth sport programs. Examples include the establishment of Pop Warner football in 1930 and Little League baseball in 1939. Sport had become extremely popular with the marketing of sport heroes and the belief in its character-building virtues. A 1939 *Life Magazine* article titled "Life Goes to a Kid's Football Game" lauded the virtues of youth sport in terms of character, courage, and nationalism.

Professional Educator Criticisms and Rise of Nonschool Programs

Professional educators in physical education and recreation (including several national governing bodies such as the American Association for Health, Physical Education, and Recreation) became extremely critical of the changes in youth sport that were occurring between 1920 and 1950 (Berryman, 1996; Wiggins, 2013). They felt that these new programs were harmful to kids because of the emphasis on competition and winning, commercialization, and inadequate coaching. These educational groups passed resolutions and issued position statements that contributed to the elimination of most school-based competitive youth sport programs for children under age 12, and the educators refused involvement in terms of leadership and support for the emerging youth sport phenomenon.

So guess what happened? Nonschool programs proliferated, developed and led by people other than the sport and physical education professionals. And guess who ended up smack in the middle of youth sport events, as coaches, officials, and directors? Yes—parents! The upsurge in nonschool youth sports meant that parents were needed to fulfill the leadership and organizational roles previously staffed by professionals, a trend that continues today.

Doesn't this seem silly in retrospect? The proliferation of nonschool sport programs was inevitable based on the rise of sport popularity in the United States and the entrepreneurial nature of American society. There have always been and always will be misguided adults who fail to understand or embrace developmentally appropriate practice in youth sport programs. We don't believe the answer to that is to abolish youth sport. Rather, we believe that the answer is to work doggedly to educate, raise awareness, and develop local and national policies to ensure that kids have developmentally appropriate experiences in youth sport. And, as discussed in chapter 3, competition is an inherent part of sport as a process of socially comparing one's skills to those of others. What is important is how we introduce and structure sport competition for children, and how we help them learn important life lessons from their competitive experiences.

University educators and sport leaders did reemerge in the 1970s to conduct and publish research and large-scale legislative studies, sponsor national conferences, and write books about youth sport. The 1970s and 1980s were also a time when several of the national organizations that support and advocate for youth sport were established, such as the Institute for the Study of Youth Sports and the National Council of Youth Sports.

Thus, youth sport outside the schools, directed by private companies and organizations, flourished starting in the 1930s. Schools continued programs for youth over 12 years of age, but sport competition for preadolescent boys (at that time) became the responsibility of organizations outside the educational network. This legacy continues today given that the majority of youth sport programs are offered by agencies outside the jurisdiction and expertise of schools and professional educators.

Emergence of Club Sport

In the United States, individual sports like swimming, tennis, golf, and gymnastics have historically been offered as club sports for youth. But club sports were not a big part of American youth team sports until the 1990s. As discussed in chapter 1, the club sport (or select or travel sport) model for team sports in the United States involves private, nonschool programs in which young athletes are invited to play or make the teams based on tryouts and selection by adults. Team club sports became popular in the 1990s as a way for youth athletes to continue competing in their sports during the off-season of their school teams, and those who had the financial means chose to participate to enhance their skills and continue playing the sports they most enjoyed. But club sports evolved in the early 2000s into a major industry in American youth sport. Elite club teams began to offer year-round training or competition, to offer travel to tournaments across the country, and to showcase athletes in major competitions for college recruiters.

A trend related to club sport participation starting around 2000 was the decrease in "multiple-sport athletes" in American school sports. Many athletes began to specialize and to focus on one sport (played during the designated high school season and then played during the rest of the year at the club level). The push from adults for youth athletes to specialize in one sport was largely due to the evolution of youth sport from a playful (yet competitive) extracurricular activity to a carefully planned training progression with the goal of collegiate, Olympic, and even professional sport careers.

Facing the rapid rise of elite club sports, the status of school-based sport in the United States is being questioned. It is hard for us to imagine the demise of such traditional events as conference basketball tournaments or Friday night high school football games, which have been central to the identity of and social interactions within communities across the United States for many decades. However, public school sports face economic difficulties, and there are those who question duplicating the effort and offering school sports when clubs sports are available. And although team high school sports at this time remain important for most youth sport participants in the United States, there are athletes today who are choosing to participate in club sports instead of in their high school teams. This is a route chosen by young athletes who wish to pursue a college or elite sport career and who have decided that club sport provides them the best opportunity for that. Time will tell if club sport participation can replace school sport participation in the United States.

HOW DID TITLE IX CHANGE YOUTH SPORT?

In 1972, Title IX of the Education Amendments to the Civil Rights Act became law in the United States. This federal law required equal opportunities for males and females in any school or university that receives federal aid. Title IX states the following:

> No person in the United States shall, on the basis of sex, be excluded from participation in, be denied the benefits of, or be subjected to discrimination under any educational program or activity receiving Federal financial assistance (U.S. Department of Labor, 1972).

Why was Title IX necessary and how did it change youth sport? A quick historical review should answer these questions and frame Title IX as the most significant legislative influence on youth sport to date. Early in the United States, young girls enjoyed some of the same physical play and recreational games as boys, but as girls aged, their play diminished while boys continued to pursue physically rigorous sports and games. At this early point, gender identity in sport was created as a prerogative of boys. What a legacy it has been to live down!

As discussed previously, the Public School Athletic League (PSAL), started in 1903 in New York City, gave boys opportunities to participate in fitness, intramural, and interscholastic youth sport. But when the girls' division of the PSAL began in 1905, it was limited to activities like folk dancing and cooperative games, with no interscholastic competitive sport allowed.

Another interesting example has to do with basketball. When basketball was invented in 1891, a "girls' version" of the game with alternative rules was devised by a female instructor at Smith College, in Massachusetts. The court was divided into three zones to restrict strenuous play, and girls were not allowed to cross over zones. Also, no physical contact was allowed, and teams included six players. This form of girls' basketball became extremely popular. Iowa became known as a girls' basketball hotbed; this form of the sport was played there until 1985. The first girls' state basketball tournament was held in 1920; television coverage started in 1951, and interest in the girls' tournament surpassed interest in the boys' (Gems et al., 2008). In her autobiography, eight-time National Collegiate Athletic Association national champion women's basketball coach Pat Summitt (2013) talks of her battle to get the state of Tennessee to change from the limited six-player to the full-court five-player game for girls. Summitt explained that she could not recruit Tennessee high school players to the state university because of the slower pace and the restricted skill development of the six-player game; she

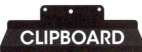

Title IX Q & A

People generally understand the Title IX mandate that outlaws discrimination on the basis of sex in any educational activity (for organizations receiving federal funds), including youth sport. However, many questions arise and myths persist about Title IX, so we've provided some basic questions and answers to help you understand how Title IX should be implemented.

1. What does Title IX require?

Title IX requires *proportional* participation opportunities. The percentage of female athletes in your sport program (numbers of athletes, not numbers of teams) needs to match the percentage of girls in your student body (compared to male athletes and student body members).

2. If we are lacking in terms of proportional numbers, can we do anything else?

You must show that you are gradually adding sports over time to try to expand female participation or that you have accommodated the interest and ability of all girls (no girls want to play another sport in that school). The National Federation of State High School Associations (NFHS) suggests using a sport interest survey every two years to maintain a database of student interest in sport participation.

3. What are some other examples of requirements beyond participation numbers?

- Comparable equipment, uniforms, supplies, practice facilities, and awards and banquets
- Access to weight room and training room
- Equal access to practice and games during prime time
- Same size and quality of locker rooms and competition facilities
- Same quality of coaches and opportunity to play same-quality opponents
- Same support (secretaries, promotion and marketing, cheerleaders, band, pep rallies)

4. If a sport is revenue producing, does that excuse it from being part of the Title IX equation in a school?

No. The educational mission of high school sports does not include revenue production. And, ironically, this argument often falls short at the collegiate level as the vast majority of Division I and Division II colleges and university athletic programs lose money on football (the sport most people use as an example of revenue producing).

5. If girls are allowed to try out for boys' teams (if there is no girls' team for them in the given sport), why don't boys have the right to try out for girls' teams in the same situation?

The law says that any member of the "underrepresented sex" (the sex that has the fewest opportunities) has to have a chance to play on the team of the overrepresented sex if that athlete is not provided with a team of the player's own sex. Since boys have more opportunities than girls (they are members of the overrepresented sex), a boy playing on a girls' team would take away a participation opportunity for the underrepresented sex. Thus, boys are not allowed to take spots on a girls' team even though the reverse is permitted.

6. Hasn't Title IX resulted in the loss of sport opportunities for boys?

Overall, boys' and men's sport opportunities have increased since the passage of Title IX. Schools choose to support, eliminate, or reduce particular sports for males and females based on a number of factors. The government cannot dictate that particular varsity sports be added, retained, or discontinued for males or females.

7. Aren't girls less interested in participating in sports than boys?

The dramatic increase in girls' and women's participation in sport since Title IX was passed demonstrates that it was lack of opportunity—not lack of interest—that kept females out of sport for too many years. The stereotypical idea that females are inherently less interested in playing sport has been repeatedly rejected by the courts. The use of gender-based stereotypes to limit girls' opportunities is illegal (Women's Sports Foundation, 2013).

was told that girls did not have the physical capacity or skills to play the full-court game. Based on Summitt's efforts, Tennessee high schools finally adopted the full-court game for the 1979-1980 season, and Oklahoma and Iowa soon followed.

This legacy of stereotypical and inaccurate perceptions about the physical capabilities and interests of girls in sport historically blocked the vast majority of girls from equal access to youth sport opportunities. The women's rights movement of the early 1970s created the pressure that led to the passage of Title IX in 1972. The law has had an enormous impact on girls' sport participation. Girls' participation in high school sport increased 992% from 1971-1972 (294,015 female participants) to 2011-2012 (3,217,533 female participants). For comparison, boys' participation also increased during this time period: a 22% increase from 1971-1972 (3,666,917 male participants) to 2011-2012 (4,484,987 male participants) (www.nfhs.org).

However, Title IX (and gender equity in general) was fought and challenged in every conceivable way, including multiple lawsuits. Little League baseball notoriously resisted the inclusion of female participants, resulting in several lawsuits filed by girls who were denied the opportunity to play with their local Little League teams. During investigation by the Civil Rights Division in 1973, witnesses for Little League argued that girls were not fit for competitive youth sport due to their weaker bone structure and slower reaction time. Interestingly, the Civil Rights Division expert countered by testifying that bone strength in adolescent girls is actually greater than in boys at that age (Wiggins, 2013). The U.S. Congress went on to amend the Little League's charter in 1974 to permit girls to fully participate. Even then, as now, the codified changes in laws and charters did not remove the cultural stereotype of females as less interested in sport and less competent to participate. This issue is addressed more fully in chapter 13.

HOW DID LITTLE LEAGUE BASEBALL BECOME SO POPULAR?

Little League baseball is perhaps the most historically famous youth sport in the United States. This may be due to the nostalgic period of post–World War II prosperity in which Little League flourished, as well as the clear status of baseball as this country's game during that time. Carl Stotz of Williamsport, Pennsylvania, founded Little League in 1939. His objectives for the program were to give kids the opportunity to play organized baseball while learning important values like fair play and teamwork. He limited rosters to 12 players to promote playing time for everyone.

Personal Plug-In

Reflecting on Title IX

How has Title IX affected you? If you're a female and you're not sure, we urge you to reflect on why you have the opportunities you have as a female athlete. What opportunities have you enjoyed that you may have taken for granted until reading about the mandates from Title IX that created these opportunities for you? If you're a male, and you're not sure, we urge you to talk to female members of your family to learn how their experiences in sport may have influenced you more than you realize. We also urge you to consider the opportunities your daughters will have to participate in sport that they would not have had without the Title IX legislation.

The Cannon Street All-Stars

Along with the institutionalized discrimination against girls so prevalent until later in the 20th century, African American children also faced a lack of opportunity in youth sport. African American boys participated to a limited degree in organized youth sports in the northern United States and participated in a strict, racially segregated manner in the southern United States.

In 1955, South Carolina had its first Little League for black boys—four teams organized by the Cannon Street YMCA in Charleston, South Carolina. At the end of the season, an all-star team was selected from the four league teams to play in the city Little League tournament. However, all the white teams boycotted the tournament. As the default city champion, Cannon Street moved on to the state tournament, but the other 61 white Little League teams withdrew from the South Carolina State Little League tournament to protest the inclusion of the Cannon Street team. The state tournament was canceled, and the Cannon Street All-Stars were state champions by default. The *Charleston News and Courier* published an editorial titled "Agitation and Hate" on August 2, 1955:

The case of the South Carolina Little League could well be cited . . . as an example of why racial relations in the South are becoming increasingly difficult. . . . Some Negro adults, knowing that the colored children weren't wanted in the all-white state league, nevertheless decided to force the colored team into the league. As a result, the entire state league has been disbanded and the colored team has been left in an embarrassing position. . . . The colored team now holds the state Little League championship through the default—the snub—of 61 other teams. . . . The Northern do-gooders who have needled the Southern race agitators into action may have to answer for the consequences (Sapakoff, 1995).

The Cannon Street team was then barred from the Southern Regional Little League championship because they had won their state tournament by forfeiture, and the national Little League office reluctantly held up the ruling. But to try to make amends, the national office invited the Cannon Street All-Stars to be spectators at the Little League World Series in Williamsport. When the team was introduced by the public address announcer in Williamsport, the crowd cheered: "Let them play! Let them play!" Although they were not allowed to participate, they were recognized and appreciated for what they had accomplished and unfortunately had to endure to get there.

As an outgrowth of the Cannon Street All-Stars affair, white adults immediately formed Little Boys Baseball, which was renamed Dixie Youth Baseball in 1958. It was formed for whites only in the southern states with the following official guideline for participation:

The Organizers hereof are of the opinion it is for the best interest of all concerned that this program be on a racially segregated basis; they believe that mixed teams and competition between the races would create regrettable conditions and destroy the harmony and tranquility which now exists (Sapakoff, 1995).

Dixie Youth Baseball amended its charter in 1967 (20 years after Jackie Robinson broke the color barrier in Major League Baseball), deleting the racial segregation participation rule. Dixie Youth Baseball continues today with hundreds of thousands of players across the southern states. Several African American players from Dixie Youth Baseball have gone on to achieve major-league careers. They should thank the Cannon Street All-Stars for helping to pave their way.

But like other youth sports, Little League became bigger, more publicized, and more professionalized. Stotz severed ties with Little League in 1956, disagreeing with the professionalization of the game and stating, "I became utterly disgusted. Originally, I had envisioned baseball for youngsters strictly on the local level without national playoffs and World Series . . ." (Hyman, 2009, p. 12).

By the 1960s, Little League baseball existed in all 50 U.S. states and many countries around the world. Its popularity increased even more when ABC Television broadcast the championship game of the Little League World Series in 1962. In 2012, ABC, ESPN, and ESPN2 combined to present all 32 games of the Little League World Series on television, with great plays highlighted on ESPN's Sports Center. When a youth sport has its own television deal, you know it's popular. Today more than 30 million people play Little League baseball in more than 100 countries, according to Little League. Little League includes divisions for girls and boys aged 5 to 18 in baseball and softball.

WHY DO GRASSROOTS YOUTH SPORT PROGRAMS LACK NATIONAL SUPPORT?

You've already learned about Title IX, a federal policy that has been a significant influence on American youth sport. Another important U.S. federal policy affecting youth sport was the Amateur Sports Act, passed in 1978. This act granted all rights and responsibilities associated with sport and athlete development in this country to the United States Olympic Committee (USOC). But what was particularly significant about the Amateur Sports Act was that it gave responsibility for grassroots youth sport development (along with elite athlete development) to the USOC. However, the USOC's distribution of funds clearly shows its commitment to the development of elite athletes at the expense of grassroots sport development (Sparvero, Chalip, & Green, 2008). This was not what the American government had in mind when passing the Amateur Sports Act and requiring the USOC and its national governing bodies (NGBs) to grow grassroots youth sport.

To be fair, the government does not provide specific funding to the USOC for grassroots youth sport. With limited resources, it is understandable that the USOC focuses on elite athlete programs that lead most directly to Olympic success (medals). And there are NGBs, like USA Wrestling, that do sponsor local grassroots youth developmental programs. But these are in the minority, as most of the USOC and NGB focus is on elite athlete development. The USOC did create the Community Olympic Development Program (CODP) in 1998 to partner with sport communities across the nation to help youth get the best sport development services possible. However, the CODP still focuses on identifying talented youth and then using resources to maximize their potential. This is a noteworthy endeavor, important in giving young athletes with talent the opportunities to maximize that talent. Yet, it still does not address mass sport for all youth in the United States, instead advantaging those kids who have either talent or money. Clearly, the inattention to grassroots youth sport development caused by government inattention and the elite focus of the USOC has created social class barriers to sport participation (Sparvero et al., 2008).

After the Amateur Sports Act of 1978, the Amateur Athletic Union (AAU) stated that it would focus its efforts on providing sport programs for all participants of all ages beginning at the grassroots level. It offers 30 sports, yet there are questions as to whether it truly represents grassroots youth sport participation as opposed to youth sport elite talent development (particularly

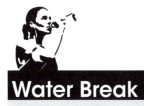

The Gold Mine Effect:
Se Ri Pak and Korean Girls' Golf

A phenomenon known as the gold mine effect occurs when a startling number of elite sport performers emerge from a small geographic location (Ankerson, 2012). There are multiple reasons for the gold mine effect (discussed at more length in chapter 10). But one of the reasons has to do with the influence of a significant historical figure who achieves sport success beyond what was previously viewed as possible. Se Ri Pak is such an individual, and she is largely responsible for the South Korean "gold mine" in women's professional golf.

When Pak came to the Ladies Professional Golf Association (LPGA) tour as a rookie in 1998, she was the only South Korean player on tour. In 2015, 148 of the top 500 (and 38 of the top 100) female players in the world were South Korean (Rolex World Golf Rankings, 2015). What happened to create this amazing gold mine of female Korean golfers? In her rookie year of 1998, Pak won the U.S. Women's Open and the LPGA Championship (both major tournaments for women) and was named LPGA Rookie of the Year. She continued her initial success, winning 25 career titles, including five major championships, and is in the LPGA Hall of Fame. Pak's accomplishments sparked a national obsession with golf and single-handedly influenced thousands of young Korean girls to begin to play golf and to pursue it with a single-minded commitment.

In the late 1980s, Korea had fewer than 200 golfers between the ages of 15 and 18 able to complete a round under par. Today, the country has more than 3,000 young golfers with a handicap of 0 or less. Consider that South Korea has a relatively cold climate, the most expensive green fees in the world, and fewer than 200 eighteen-hole golf courses for a population of 50 million (Florida has more than 1,300 courses) (Ankerson, 2012). Yet, Se Ri Pak awakened the belief among South Korean girls that they could achieve sport success in the same way.

Na Yeon Choi, currently ranked fourth in the world and winner of the 2012 U.S. Women's Open, remembers watching Pak's U.S. Open victory as a 9-year-old in 1998. "It was amazing for all the Korean people. I watched it on TV, and I remember that feeling. I think all the Korean people [thought] that Korea couldn't win. But she did. After she won, I think all the Korean people have a bigger dream than before" (Elliott, 2012). So Yeon Ryu, ranked sixth in the world and winner of the 2011 U.S. Women's Open, states, "Before 1998, golf was not a famous sport in Korea. But after [Pak] won, golf is now a really famous sport, and that's why I am here" (Manoyan, 2012). Pak herself says, "The people respect me. They call me 'The Legend.' I'm happy to hear that. In Korea, they [say that] I am the pioneer" (Ellliot, 2012). Or the developer of a gold mine!

in basketball). Of course, this is a constant tension in many youth sport programs and is a common theme throughout this book.

HOW HAVE CHANGES IN PARENTING INFLUENCED THE EVOLUTION OF YOUTH SPORT?

Although parents and families in relation to youth sport are discussed in chapter 16, a mention of the historical change in parenting styles is important here based on its role in the evolution of youth sport. Before the 1980s, the ideal of creating a "protected" childhood was the parenting norm, so that kids were not pressured and were left to develop their personal autonomy through unstructured social play and activities with their peers (Farrey, 2008). It was not uncommon for kids to be out in their neighborhoods on bikes or in sandlots, woods, or friends' yards all day, without parents knowing exactly where they were. That was the childhood that we experienced growing up in the 1960s and 1970s.

Around 1980, significant changes occurred in what it meant to be a "good parent" (Coakley, 2009; Marano, 2008). The ideal of the "protected" childhood with the goal of raising "normal" kids gave way to the ideal of a "prepared" childhood with the goal of creating "special" kids (Farrey, 2008). To be a good parent meant you knew where your child was 24/7 and that you planned and arranged an array of achievement activities (e.g., music, sports, art classes) to fill your child's schedule. Of course, parents also were concerned for their child's safety, what with sensational media accounts of adult sexual predators and kidnappers. Similarly, organized activities like youth sport were viewed as positive outlets for children, and parents could relax with their children in these programs without worrying about possible mischief and injuries that might occur in unstructured leisure with peers in the neighborhood.

This style of "hothouse parenting" (Marano, 2008) that arose in the United States in the 1980s and continues today has had a major influence on youth sport. Not only have participation numbers increased, but this parenting trend has also led to younger starting ages in youth sport as well as the increase in specialization in specific sports with the intent (often directed by the parents) to pursue elite sport status. And perhaps most importantly, it has contributed to a psychological shift in kids' experiences in playing sport. What once was truly game-like and truly for fun and pleasurable leisure has morphed into a mandatory high-level achievement requirement for community social status and college resume building. Seemingly, the professionalization of parenting has led to the professionalization of youth sport and the decrease in free or child-directed play of past generations.

Research indicates that free play is essential to the cognitive, physical, social, and emotional well-being of youth. Play enhances creativity and healthy brain development. Without play, neural pathways for controlling impulses and emotions fail to develop normally (Ginsburg, 2007). Experimental studies with animals have shown that depriving them of play severely cripples their emotional development (Herman, Paukner, & Suomi, 2011). Undirected play allows children to learn how to work in groups, to share, to negotiate, to resolve conflicts, and to learn self-advocacy skills. When play is child driven, kids engage in decision making and discover their own interests and passions. Most of us cherish the simple joys of play experienced in childhood.

So what is the answer? Should we abandon organized youth sport and leave it to the kids today to direct their own sports and games? We think not. It is fruitless to lament the passing of the romanticized youth and free-play experiences we enjoyed as baby boomers. The world is a different place now; the organized youth sport genie is out of the bottle, and the sandlot is not going to make a comeback to replace FieldTurf. However, we do advocate balance in terms of allowing kids to have time to be kids and engage in free play with each other, as well as directing them to selected organized youth sport activities. In addition, we can be thoughtful in creating developmentally appropriate youth sport experiences within our organized programs that include aspects of free play found to be important to child development (choices and decision making, negotiation and conflict resolution with peers, time for social interaction, and pure joy).

WRAP-UP

Hopefully, you now have a better idea of why youth sport looks the way it does today. It's easier to understand once you consider how youth sport evolved and how it was shaped by the cultural and social forces of different historical times. For those of you who would like to see a chronological progression, we've provided a summary of some key moments in the history of youth sport in table 2.1.

You should also now better understand the example provided at the beginning of the chapter. Why were the kids standing around waiting for their coach instead of playing on their own? We've socialized them to do this by organizing and directing their activities and by curtailing the spontaneity and creativity that is inherent in the free play and games that kids structure on their own. We hope to provide you with ideas throughout the book about how to meet kids' needs for fun, creativity, and autonomy through developmentally appropriate practice within the organized youth sport structure. Yes, we think it can be done.

Table 2.1 Historical Time Line of Events Related to American Youth Sport

1851	Young Men's Christian Association (YMCA) established
1903	Public School Athletic League (PSAL) established in New York City
1905	PSAL program for girls established
1920	National Federation of State High School Associations (NFHS) established
1930	Pop Warner football established
1939	Little League baseball established
1950	Biddy Basketball established
1952	Pony Baseball established
1956	President's Council on Youth Fitness established
1958	Dixie Youth Baseball established
1962	Little League World Series televised for the first time
1964	American Youth Soccer Organization established
1967	Soccer Association for Youth (SAY) established
1972	Title IX of Educational Amendments Act passed
1978	Amateur Sports Act passed
1978	Youth Sport Institute established at Michigan State University
1979	Entertainment and Sports Programming Network (ESPN) established
1979	*Bill of Rights for Young Athletes* published
1981	National Alliance for Youth Sports established
1997	The First Tee Golf program established
1998	Positive Coaching Alliance established
2000	Explosion in popularity of club sports in addition to or as alternative to school sports

We believe it is very important to learn from history—to use the advantage of hindsight to consider how things could have been done better. The discrimination against and exclusion of minorities and girls from youth sport is shameful in retrospect, yet it mirrored broader societal attitudes of the time. We should use this example as motivation to carefully consider youth sport practices of today, which are accepted uncritically or viewed as "just the way it is." Instead of meekly accepting the status quo, we should attempt to use foresight to consider "Is this really the right way to do it?" and to ensure that our programs are developmentally appropriate and inclusive in some form for all kids.

Postscript from the authors: After writing this chapter, we had the pleasure of hearing from our 12-year-old son about how his club basketball team broke into an impromptu, kid-directed game of Capture of the Flag while waiting for their coach to arrive at the gym for practice (using a kid's baseball cap as the flag). We laughed at how this contradicted our story in the first paragraph of this chapter about how kids wait around for adults to tell them what to do. A few weeks later we observed the players launching into an impromptu game of dodgeball while once again waiting for the coach to arrive and start practice. Great stuff, and perhaps we stand corrected.

LEARNING AIDS

Key Terms

Muscular Christianity—A movement starting in the late 1800s to promote Christian values and practices within sport and physical activities.

sandlot—An open space or field used for informal, youth-led pickup games or sport activities.

Summary Points

1. Sport was introduced into American schools to enhance physical fitness and moral development and to combat juvenile delinquency.

2. The Public School Athletic League (PSAL) in New York City began in 1903 for boys, offering intramural and interscholastic sport from elementary to high school ages.

3. A girls' division of the PSAL was established in 1905 with play activities and intramurals, but no interscholastic sport.

4. The popular term *sandlot* came from the use of sand gardens in the late 1800s, which were the precursors to modern playgrounds.

5. The Muscular Christianity movement led to the development of YMCAs throughout the United States.

6. Professional educators in physical education denounced youth sport programs due to their increasing competitiveness and professionalization, leading to the elimination of many school-based youth sport programs in the 1930s.

7. From 1920 to 1970, a large number of city, regional, and national nonschool youth sport programs were established, such as Pop Warner football in 1930 and Little League baseball in 1939.

8. Private nonschool club sport exploded in popularity in the late 1990s and early 2000s and led to the increased professionalization of youth sport in terms of year-round participation and specialization in single sports.

9. Title IX was the most influential piece of legislation in the history of youth sport, finally requiring American society to provide equal access to youth sport for females.

10. Little League is probably the most famous youth sport in history, based on its development during the nostalgic period after World War II, when baseball was considered the national pastime, as well as its Little League World Series, which is televised each August on ESPN.

11. The Amateur Sports Act of 1978 gave all responsibility for sport development in this country to the United States Olympic Committee, which has prioritized elite athlete development over grassroots sport opportunities for all children.

12. Parenting practices shifted in the 1980s to focus more on scheduling children's time extensively in achievement activities, including youth sport.

13. Free play enhances creativity, healthy brain development, social skills like conflict resolution and self-advocacy, and emotional well-being.

Study Questions

1. Describe the establishment of the Public School Athletic League in New York City, including why it was developed and what types of activities it provided.

2. How did nonschool sport become so popular, and how did the exodus of professional school educators influence this movement?

3. Where did the term *sandlot* come from, and how did this relate to the development of playgrounds in the United States?

4. Why is free play important for children, and what is the place of free play today in relation to organized youth sports?

5. When and how did the club sport phenomenon influence youth sport?

6. What did Title IX mandate and what effect did it have on youth sport participation?

7. Why do grassroots youth sport programs lack national organization and support?

8. How did changes in parenting philosophy and practice influence the evolution of youth sport?

Reflective Learning Activities

1. Write a position paper about your opinion on the club sport phenomenon in the United States. Include your suggestions as to how club and school sports should coexist, if you think they should.

2. Besides Se Ri Pak, can you identify any nationally or internationally known athletes who have sparked a youth movement of interest in a sport? This doesn't have to be a total gold mine effect as with Se Ri Pak, but rather key performances in particular historical situations that influenced youth sport in some way.

3. Pick a historical event or issue in which you are interested, and research the event or issue to further your understanding. Examples could be lawsuits and obstacles to Title IX implementation, a history of Little League, the All-American Soap Box Derby, the Public School Athletic League in New York, segregation and integration of youth sport in the United States, a history of high school football (or any other sport), the state of Iowa's girls' basketball tournament history, or the Amateur Sports Act of 1978. Or choose a topic not discussed is this chapter to add to your understanding of the evolution of youth sport.

Resource Guide

SHAPE America (shapeamerica.org). SHAPE America is an organization advancing professional practice in areas related to sport and physical activity. It is one of the oldest sport advocacy groups in the United States.

Women's Sports Foundation (www.womenssportsfoundation.org/ home/advocate/ title-ix-and-issues).

chapter 3

PHILOSOPHY AND OBJECTIVES OF YOUTH SPORT

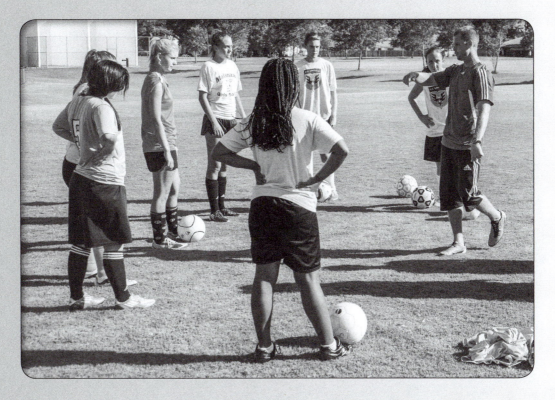

CHAPTER PREVIEW

In this chapter, you'll learn

» how to create a developmentally appropriate POPP sequence,

» the key tension points surrounding youth sport philosophy and objectives,

» how to select a youth sport program for your child, and

» about a substitute for the pyramid model of sport.

Our daughter's 8th-grade volleyball team was playing their rival Jefferson Middle School in the finals of the conference tournament. Ruchelle, our daughter's coach, followed the lineup she had typically used all season in terms of substitutions so that every player played in the match. The best players started and received more playing time, but every person on the team got to play. However, the Jefferson coach left her subs on the bench for the entire championship match, fielding only her top players (along with a few needed strategic substitutions). Jefferson won the match and championship, and it was obvious to all spectators and participants that the different substitution patterns contributed to the outcome of the competition.

What would you have done as the coach in this situation? Would you have followed Ruchelle's philosophy that for an 8th-grade team, the best players will start and play more, but everyone will get in the match and contribute to the team effort—even in a championship contest? Or would you have followed the Jefferson coach's philosophy that even though these are 8th graders, this is a championship match, and the objective of winning at this level supersedes participation by all the players? Your answer reveals your philosophy and how that philosophy drives your decision making in youth sport.

THE POPP SEQUENCE: FROM PHILOSOPHY TO ACTION

Whether one coach is right and the other wrong in our previous example is not for us to say. The decisions the coaches made were based on their philosophies and objectives for their teams. This is what we call the **POPP sequence,** or the ways in which our actions in youth sport are guided by the values and beliefs inherent in our philosophy, objectives, and guiding principles. As shown in figure 3.1, the POPP sequence begins with one's philosophy, which then leads to objectives, principles, and practices (adapted from Martens, 2001). **Philosophy** refers to the basic values and beliefs that people hold. These values and beliefs then lead them through the POPP sequence. They clarify their **objectives,** or the results they wish to accomplish. They determine the **principles** they'll follow, which are predetermined guidelines about how they'll make decisions. And finally, the sequence ends with **practice,** which is what we do and how we do it. As a result of our initial philosophy, and objectives and principles emanating from that philosophy, we make decisions and act.

The coaches in our example arrived at different practices (subbing or not subbing in the championship match) based on their own personal POPP sequences. Ruchelle stated after the match that she was tempted to change her practice of playing every person because it was a championship match. However, upon reflection and after revisiting her philosophy, objectives, and principles, she stuck with what was an important practice for her to follow as a coach of a middle school team. Her predetermined guideline to involve every athlete in the match superseded the decision to play only the better players to win a championship. A tough decision to make! But it is one that is made easier if you have a clear POPP sequence

Philosophy	Objectives	Principles	Practices
Basic values or beliefs	Results you wish to accomplish	Predetermined guidelines about how you will make decisions	What you do and how you do it

Figure 3.1   POPP sequence.

that you believe in and allow to guide you in doing what you feel is right.

When we talked to youth sport directors as background for this book, they told us that the first step for them as managers was to determine the overall purpose of their programs. The next steps were to create a mission statement and specify program objectives that guided everything they did. All the business decisions that followed, such as budgeting and type of activities offered, were based on the purpose, mission, and objectives they had established for their programs. Programs varied in their purpose and mission (e.g., community recreation program vs. club program), but all had POPP sequences that were established to guide their activities.

Youth sport is a context in which a sound philosophy, set of objectives, and predetermined guidelines are critical to engaging in developmentally appropriate practice.

Water Break

Go, Green Death!

Consider the philosophy and objectives espoused by the coach of a 6- to 7-year-old girls' soccer team in the following e-mail he sent to parents. The coach resigned after parents protested to league directors, although some parents supported his approach.

"Team 7 will be called Green Death . . . I fully expect every player and parent to be on board with the team. This is not a team, but a family (some say cult), that you belong to forever. We play fair at all times, but we play tough and physical soccer. . . . I expect 110% at every game and practice. Unless there is an issue concerning the health of my players or inside info on the opposition, you probably don't need to talk to me. . . .

"I believe winning is fun and losing is for losers. . . . While we may not win every game (excuse me, I just got a little nauseated), I expect us to fight for every loose ball and play every shift as if it were the finals of the World Cup. While I spent a good Saturday morning listening to the legal liability BS, which included a 30-minute dissertation on how we need to baby the kids and especially the refs, I was disgusted. The kids will run, they will fall . . . and even bleed a little. Big deal, it's good for them (but I do hope the other team is the one bleeding). If the refs can't handle a little criticism, then they should turn in their whistle. . . . My heckling of the refs is actually helping them develop as people. . . . Second place trophies are nothing to be proud of as they serve only as a reminder that you missed your goal; their only useful purpose is as an inspiration to do that next set of reps. . . . I expect that the ladies be put on a diet of fish, undercooked red meat and lots of veggies. No junk food. Protein shakes are encouraged, and while blood doping and HGH use is frowned upon, there is no testing penalty. . . .

"These are my views and not necessarily the views of the league (but they should be). . . . [I want] girls who will kick ass and take names on the field, off the field, and throughout their lives. Who's with me? Go Green Death!" ("Scituate 'Green Death,'" 2009)

Philosophy and objectives should drive the behavior and the culture, not vice versa. Reversing the POPP sequence (to PPOP, we guess!) is when we begin to do things for the wrong reasons (e.g., winning at any cost, putting our adult needs ahead of the kids' needs) because we lose sight of or fail to consider the developmentally appropriate philosophy, objectives, and principles that we've either forgotten or conveniently discarded in competitive situations.

Consider this example. In a tee ball game for 4- to 6-year-olds, the regular first base player was sick and a less skilled player filled in that position. Because the substitute player was less skilled, the coach instructed the pitcher to run the ball to first base after fielding it instead of throwing it to the substitute player to avoid the possibility of error (Landers & Fine, 1998). The coach clearly emphasized the objective of winning the contest over participation and skill development.

Later in the chapter, we'll provide some examples of POPP sequences used by successful youth sport programs, and get you started in developing your own POPP sequence for your youth sport situation. To help you do that, the next few sections provide some background from the youth sport literature about youth sport philosophies, objectives, and principles.

WHAT SHOULD THE OBJECTIVES OF YOUTH SPORT BE?

What does society want from youth sport programs? Why do we offer these programs? What should the objectives of youth sport be? Overall, the generally accepted objectives of youth sport are the development of sport skills, psychosocial and life skills, and physical health (Cote, Strachan, & Fraser-Thomas, 2008). Most people agree that these are important outcomes to justify youth sport programs.

Developing Sport Skills

The development of basic and advanced sport skills provides the foundation for enjoying sport across the life span and enhancing one's physical health. Kids will be active, and remain active as adults, if they have the skills to competently perform in sport and physical activity. To meet this objective, teachers, coaches, and directors need to understand developmental progressions for skill development. Part II of the book provides information and guidelines about this, including understanding fundamental motor skill development; readiness and prerequisite skills for sports; how sports should be modified for youth to promote skill development; and strategies for teaching sport skills effectively to kids. Having played the sport yourself does not automatically qualify you as a competent teacher or coach, and understanding the hierarchy of motor skill development (chapter 5), as well as how to engage in developmentally appropriate practice for specific age groups, is critical in developing kids' sport skills.

Developing Psychosocial Skills

Providing opportunities for psychosocial development such as self-esteem, emotional management, confidence, cooperation, leadership, and interpersonal skills has always been and should continue to be an important objective for youth sport participation. Positive youth development (PYD) programs have proliferated, many using sport and physical activity to build important psychosocial characteristics in youth (e.g., Camire, 2014; Weiss, Stuntz, Bhalla, Bolter, & Price, 2013). Positive youth development programs focus on developing personal and social skills (assets) rather than on reducing deficits or problem behaviors. Psychosocial outcomes that have been achieved in PYD programs in sport and physical activity are the following:

Academic achievement

Cognitive functioning

Conflict resolution

Cooperation

Decision making

Emotional regulation

Empathy

Goal setting and achievement

Hope

Interpersonal competence

Leadership

Life satisfaction

Positive peer relationships

Self-confidence

Self-worth

Time management

A strategy to remember important PYD outcomes is to think of the five C's: Competence, Character, Connection, Confidence, and Caring/Compassion (Lerner, Fisher, & Weinberg, 2000). Achievement of the five C's leads to the sixth "C" of positive youth development, Contribution, with youth developing into productive citizens within society.

Positive youth development programs have particular potential to promote psychosocial and life skills development in at-risk or low-income youth, who tend to have limited material and social resources, limited access to physical activity and skill learning, lower academic achievement, and greater incidence of health problems. Several PYD programs that have targeted psychosocial skill development in underserved youth along with sport or physical skills development have been successful (Hellison, 2011; Holt, Sehn, Spence, Newton, & Ball, 2012; Ullrich-French & McDonough, 2013).

However, it is imperative to understand that these wonderful psychosocial outcomes occur only when adult stakeholders consciously design and direct youth sport programs with these outcomes in mind. As

discussed further in chapter 16, sport doesn't automatically build character or positive psychosocial skills in kids. Sport, as an attractive activity that kids typically enjoy, has the potential to be a great learning environment for psychosocial growth and PYD. But that occurs only if we, as the adults in charge, set sport up to meet this objective. It doesn't happen magically or by accident. In fact, there are a lot of negative psychosocial outcomes associated with sport participation (aggression, lower moral reasoning, burnout, cheating, violence). If youth sport is to meet its PYD function, then directors, coaches, and teachers have to actively pursue this objective every day, in the same way that they practice physical skills or teach game strategies and tactics every day. Specific examples of how to do this are provided in chapter 16, and we urge you as the adult leader to go beyond lip service and include PYD in intentional and creative ways in your personal POPP sequence.

Developing Physical Health

Improving children's physical health through youth sport participation is an important objective due to the alarming rise of inactivity and obesity in our culture. Besides weight control, sport and physical activity can enhance cardiovascular fitness, muscular strength, muscular endurance, flexibility, and bone health. Perhaps most compelling, persistent participation in youth sport leads to higher levels of physical activity in adulthood (Telama, Yang, Hirvensalo, & Raitakari, 2006), thus helping to protect against problems in later life such as heart disease, obesity, diabetes, stroke, depression, and cancer. As discussed previously, youth sport leaders must keep this objective in mind when designing and conducting youth practices and training activities. Poorly planned training sessions in which kids are inactive for long periods or an overemphasis on tactics to the detriment of kids' activity levels are developmentally inappropriate practices that prevent achievement of the important objective of developing kids' physical health.

Ensuring the Rights of Youth Athletes

Along with the three main objectives of developing (a) sport skills, (b) psychosocial skills, and (c) physical health, youth sport leaders should also ensure the basic rights of youth sport participants as shown in figure 3.2. This Bill of Rights for Youth Athletes (Martens & Seefeldt, 1979) is patterned after the first 10 amendments to the U.S. Constitution (the Bill of Rights) that confirm the fundamental rights of American citizens (e.g., freedom of speech, press, assembly, religion).

As seen in figure 3.2, youth athletes have fundamental rights such as the right to participate, to have developmentally appropriate experiences, to have qualified coaches, to have fun in sports, and to be treated with dignity. Consider the ways in which these rights are or may be denied to youth athletes. We recommend that all youth sport coaches be given a copy of these rights, and that organizations and program leaders ensure that these rights are upheld in youth sport.

TENSION POINTS IN YOUTH SPORT PHILOSOPHIES AND OBJECTIVES

Not many people would dispute the three objectives identified for youth sport in the preceding section. If youth sport serves to

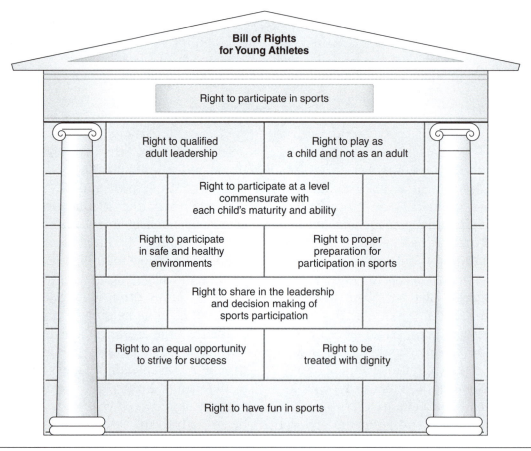

Figure 3.2 Bill of Rights for Youth Athletes.

Guidelines for children's sports, 1979, reprinted with permission from the National Association for Sport and Physical Education (NASPE), 1900 Association Drive, Reston, VA, 20191-1599.

teach kids sport-specific skills and techniques, enhance their psychosocial development, and boost their physical health, isn't that a terrific contribution to our society? So why all the controversy? Where do the pressure on kids and bad behavior from adults come from, if we generally agree on these as important objectives for youth sport? The answer lies in four tension points that elicit disagreement and controversy regarding youth sport philosophies and objectives:

a. The "dueling objectives" of talent development for elite performance versus providing physical, psychological, and social developmental benefits to all participants

b. The nature and place of competition in youth sport

c. Where fun and enjoyment fit into youth sport

d. A unidimensional specialized focus on one sport compared to a more multidimensional approach for young athletes

The Dueling Objectives

Although the previously identified three objectives of youth sports are generally accepted by most people, disagreement and tension arise based on who should be the focus of these objectives. Should youth sport be about identifying and focusing on the most talented young athletes, so they can go on to represent high schools, universities, and countries in elite levels of competition? Or should youth sport be about providing physical, psychological, and social developmental benefits to all participants? These are the dueling objectives of youth sport.

Rationally, it makes sense that both of these objectives—talent development for elite sport and participation and skill development for all—can be a part of youth sport. Certainly, youth sport should provide systems to identify talented young athletes and offer high-level sport training to help them

compete at the highest levels possible. And youth sport should also provide mass participation opportunities for kids to enjoy sport and develop their physical and psychosocial skills. This mass participation objective is important to get kids "hooked" on physical activity to create a lifelong commitment to physical activity and thus improved health. Of the approximately 40 million kids between the ages of 5 and 18 participating in youth sport in the United States, around 3% will go on to be college athletes. So although developing athletic talent for elite performance is a worthy objective, equally, if not more, important are the physical and psychosocial benefits provided to the 97% of the youth sport population that will not go on to be college athletes.

The best-case scenario is to offer many different types of youth sport (as discussed in chapter 1) so that kids with different needs, interests, and talents can find the best fit for themselves. However, this best case relies on youth sport directors, coaches, and parents understanding developmentally appropriate practice, such as how and when to focus on identifying and developing talent. It also requires organizations to carefully consider and be explicit about their objectives so that young athletes and parents are clearly informed.

Competition and Youth Sport

A second tension point related to philosophies and objectives in youth sport is the place of competition. Competition is generally fun and often stimulates focus and effort. From a family game of Knock-Out (a competitive basketball shooting game) in the driveway, to relay races at the end of practice, to competing for a high school conference championship, we can easily observe that kids typically get psyched up to compete. However, negative outcomes can be associated with competition, which are particularly troubling in youth sport.

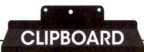

Selecting the Right Youth Sport Program for Your Child

Here are some suggestions parents might use in shopping for and selecting the youth sport program that best fits their child:

1. Very young children (4-8 years) should sample a wide variety of sports and activities. As they move into late childhood and adolescence, they will begin to pare down their activities and choose a select few to focus on.

2. Even if the program philosophy or objectives (or both) are provided, ask questions to clarify the main focus of the program. What are the goals of this program and expectations of athletes in the program? What are the participation rules or guidelines—does everyone play, or is playing time based on ability? Are cuts made, or are all athletes guaranteed to remain on the team?

3. Pay particular attention to skill development. Ask directors or coaches to talk about the place of skill development in this program, and ask for specific examples of the skills that will be developed and how they'll be developed. Ask directors or coaches to explain how much the program emphasizes winning and competition in relation to skill building and athlete development. Ask for specific examples of how the program balances the objectives of winning, athlete development, and enjoyment.

4. Consider the amount of playing time your child will receive by looking at the number of athletes on the team. In our local parks and recreational youth basketball league, the practice is to have only seven players per team to ensure optimal playing time and individual attention for skill building in practice.

That works great. If a recreational basketball team made up of 9- to 10-year-olds with one coach has 10 to 12 players, that's too many. Having this many players will not allow optimal participation time and individualized skill development for all the athletes on the team.

5. Pay attention to the coaches. Talk to the coaches—offer your support and ask questions without being overinvolved or inappropriate. "How are the kids progressing?" or "Can I do anything at home to help Jake's skill development?" are appropriate questions. "Why isn't Jake playing more?" or "I think a different lineup might work better" are inappropriate. Parents usually coach recreational and community-based youth sports, and at this level their warmth, supportiveness, and understanding of children are more important than their technical and tactical knowledge of the sport (Cote, Baker, & Abernathy, 2003). When choosing a club or select program, find out about and consider the coaches' qualifications, including their experience, training, and personality fit for your child.

6. Attend the first few practices, and then casually observe a few practices throughout the season.

7. Talk to your child about the program. Use open-ended questions such as "Tell me what you did in practice today" or "What are some good things you did or new things you learned today in practice?" And, of course, good questions are "Do you like being on the swim team?" and "How's it going on the swim team?"

8. Consider your child's levels of physical, cognitive, and psychological maturation.

Kids the same age often differ widely in their maturation and readiness for different sport experiences. In particular, consider your child's maturation and motivation to move to the club or select level. This is a big developmental step from the "everyone plays and has fun" mentality of entry-level recreational leagues. Our daughter sampled two "select" soccer practices when she was 8, but she was not psychologically ready for the increased commitment, heightened performance expectations, and more intense coaching, so she decided not to continue. She then joined a select team when she was 10, and she had a very positive experience playing select soccer for several years. Carefully consider "Is my child ready for club or select sport?" If not, the child can continue with community-based sport activities or wait until he is ready for club or select sport.

9. Assess your child's prerequisite skills for a particular activity. For example, skating is an important prerequisite for ice hockey, and a learn-to-swim program is a prerequisite for joining a swim team.

10. Identify and carefully consider all the logistics of joining a youth sport program, particularly a travel team or club or select sport. How far is the travel to practices? What is the travel commitment to competitions? What are the practice times, and how often does the team practice? Can your family meet the commitment while fulfilling all the other family needs (siblings, school, parents' work schedules, transportation, family vacations, mealtimes). What are the costs, including participation fees but also the hidden costs of equipment, travel, meals, and uniforms?

11. Ask the parents of athletes who are currently in the program or who have been in the program about the youth sport program you are considering. We've found this to be an excellent source of accurate information about particular youth sport programs.

12. If your child and a program are not a good fit, explain this to the coach or program director in a courteous and respectful manner. Don't buy into the "we have to stick it out because we don't quit" mentality, which too often leads to misery. A negative experience will serve only to dampen your child's enjoyment of sport.

Competition as a Social Evaluation Process

Essentially, **competition** is a social evaluation process (Martens, 1975). It is a process or experience that we all undergo when we perform an activity and are socially and publicly evaluated by others. That's why competition often makes our palms sweaty or gives us butterflies in our stomachs. We feel nervous (some would say excited) because we are aware that others are evaluating our performance.

Now think about how a young child playing in her first youth sport competitive event feels. She is not an adult with a wealth of experience and an established identity. She has joined this tee ball team to be with her friends, have fun, and learn skills. She is learning, but her throwing, catching, and batting skills are not well developed at this stage. She notices that her coach is talking about how important it is that she perform well today, and she notices the long line of lawn chairs with parents and other spectators. She hears her parents cheer for her, and she doesn't want to embarrass herself or let them down. All of a sudden the safe and relatively private experience of learning

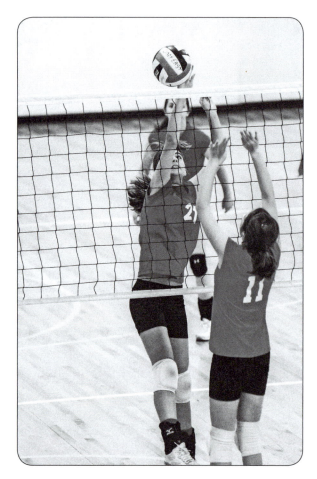

Although competition may be fun and is a big part of sport, it should be introduced in a developmentally appropriate way in youth sport.

to play tee ball is very public and evaluative and creates negative feelings of tension and pressure for this child. Sport psychologist Richard Ginsburg states, "Youth sports aren't meant to be entertainment for adults. The stage is too big for kids so young. A child that age can't differentiate their performance from who they are as a person" (cited in Hyman, 2009, p. 23).

Youth sport is often a child's first experience with competition, or the process of being socially evaluated for one's performance. A big philosophical question regarding youth sport is at what age we should formally introduce competition, such as keeping score, competing with other teams, choosing all-stars, and providing local and even national championships. The Amateur Athletic Union (AAU) stages a national basketball championship for 2nd-grade boys, and Callaway sponsors the 6-and-under Junior World Golf Championship. Is this truly necessary, or even beneficial?

Children's early experiences with competition greatly influence their self-perceptions of competence and their motivation to continue in sport. We must move beyond the glib "competition is good for children" to carefully consider when and how to introduce competition in a developmentally appropriate way. Recommendations for when kids are ready for competition are provided in chapter 5.

Competition and Skill Development or Mastery

Remember our stated youth sport objective—perhaps the most important objective—to help kids develop their physical or technical sport skills. Many adult leaders accept this objective but fail to understand the ways in which competition can hurt skill development and mastery in youth sports. In fact, this might be a second set of dueling objectives, with adult coaches losing sight of the key objective of skill development in their feverish zeal to compete and win. The objective of skill development and mastery should never be superseded by the objective of winning in youth sports before high school.

Think of the many examples of how competition can harm skill development. Our previous example of telling the tee ball pitcher to run the ball to first base as opposed to throwing to the first base player who is not great at catching the ball is one example. Another example would be relegating smaller or less skilled athletes to less central positions in team sports to "hide" them so they won't hurt the team's chances of winning. A short boy is told to take several pitches to try to earn a walk to get on base for the team, as opposed to using his skills

Your First Competition

Reflect back on your first competitive experience in youth sport. Were you aware of the heightened social evaluation, and how did you respond to it? How do you think your early experiences with competition influenced your personality and the way you think about and respond to sport competition today?

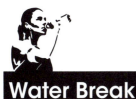

Water Break

Fourteen Grand Slams Later . . .

Pete Sampras won 14 Grand Slam tournaments in his illustrious professional tennis career and is considered one of the greatest tennis players of all time. In his autobiography, Sampras (2008) says that a pivotal moment in his development came as a 14-year-old, when his coach convinced him to switch from a two-handed to a one-handed backhand. His coach felt that this change would pay off in the long term and allow Sampras to play at a higher level on the fast grass and hard courts of the pro circuit. However, it was a risky move for a 14-year-old junior tennis phenom who was consistently winning while playing up an age group.

Sampras admits that after the switch, he struggled for two years and was beaten repeatedly by players who would not have beaten him if he hadn't changed his technique. People began to doubt his talent and question the change. But Sampras was committed to developing his skill for the long term, as opposed to focusing on short-term results of winning junior tennis matches. He states, "It was always about playing the right way, trying to develop a game that would hold up throughout my career" (p. 24). What a great lesson about valuing skill development over winning! Sampras' ability to forego the quick glory of winning to hone his skills made him into the great champion that he became.

to actually swing the bat and try to get a hit. A common practice we've observed in youth basketball is designating the best player to be the point guard and setting up clear-out or pick plays for her to go one-on-one to score points for the team (as opposed to involving teammates in the offense).

Youth sport directors should consider how best to structure sport programs with skill development as the most important objective. Our Soccer Association for Youth entry-level program (5- to 6-year-olds) has two events per week, with both of them focused on skill development through fun games and enjoyable drills. There is no interteam competition; rather, teams play 3 on 3 or 4 on 4, often with no goalie. Tee ball is an American institution and seems like a good lead-up game with players batting off a stationary tee. However, after a few weeks of practice, players spend much more time in competitive games against other teams than they do learning to throw, catch, field, and bat. It is our observation that not much skill development occurs in tee ball. Overall, research demonstrates quite conclusively that humans learn better in cooperative, as opposed to competitive, situations (Johnson & Johnson, 2003). Once people have developed some basic skills, competition provides them the opportunity to test their skills and evaluate themselves.

Competition Versus Decompetition

There are people who argue that youth sport has become too competitive and that youth sport should be about cooperative games and learning. Although we just argued for an emphasis on skill development over competition and winning, by no means are we advocating the discontinuation of competition in youth sport. Competition can be fun, exciting, and motivational for kids, as long as it is introduced and conducted in a developmentally appropriate manner. The essence of sport is to test oneself by using the informative feedback gained from competing against others at the given level.

So what about the argument that competition breeds aggression, anger, intimidation, and cheating? It's true. Research on competition indicates that these negative outcomes are often the result of the very nature of competition, in which the main goal is to block your opponents from achieving their goals (Deutsch, 2000; Shields & Bredemeier, 2009). This blocking of goals is frustrating and often creates antagonistic relationships between competitors. So how can we argue for competition, especially for children, when it has repeatedly been shown to elicit negative behaviors from coaches, athletes, and parents?

We advocate using youth sport as a developmental "laboratory" where children are gradually introduced to competition so they can gain experience in social evaluation and emotional regulation. Young athletes should also be taught the true meaning of competition: To compete is "to strive together" (from the Latin *competere*). Shields and Bredemeier (2009) call this true competition, in which each party pursues excellence by attempting to meet the challenge presented by the opponent's best effort. These authors coined the term **decompetition,** the opposite of true competition, which fails to include the cooperation and mutual respect that is needed to strive together in a competitive event. In youth sport, competition turns to decompetition when officials are abused by coaches, when players are allowed to taunt and disrespect opponents, or when competitors cheat to win.

For those who ridicule such a notion, we recommend reading the autobiography of basketball star Bill Russell (Russell & Branch, 1979), who won two national collegiate championships, an Olympic gold medal, and 11 professional National Basketball Association championships in his illustrious career. In his book, Russell states that his greatest pleasure came during competition when both teams were playing at their peak, which in Russell's mind elevated the game to unprecedented levels of excellence. He admitted that on some nights when the caliber of play escalated to this level, he even found himself rooting for the other team to keep up the challenge. Another example is the principle known as Honoring the Game within the philosophy of the Positive Coaching Alliance, a nationally recognized youth sport resource center. According to the philosophy of the PCA, Honoring the Game means getting to the ROOTS of true competition by demonstrating respect for **R**ules, **O**pponents, **O**fficials, **T**eammates, and one's **S**elf.

Summary on Competition

Keeping perspective and managing emotions is a challenge in competition. It requires educating young athletes, parents, and coaches about the true nature of competition and challenging them to be respectful competitors using the ROOTS principle of Honoring the Game. It also requires developmentally appropriate philosophies, with the goal to provide competition for enjoyment and skill evaluation, but not at the expense of skill development. Youth coaches should teach introductory skills in a noncompetitive learning environment free from intense social evaluation so kids can gain some competency and confidence before being thrust into a public community competition. Lead-up games and small-sided competitions in practice help young athletes learn how to use their skills in game-like situations and prepare them for later inter-team competitions.

What About Fun?

A third tension point involves debate about where fun and enjoyment should fit into the philosophy and objectives of youth sport. Jim Thompson (2003), director of the Positive Coaching Alliance and youth sport book author, advocates that we keep the "F" word in youth sport. No, not that one—FUN! Multiple research studies over the past three decades have repeatedly shown that "to have fun" is the main reason kids aged 5 to 17 participate in youth sport. However, some people argue that frivolous fun distracts from the focus and effort needed to develop skills and practice team strategies. Both sides are right, if we consider the difference between fun and enjoyment.

Fun, as a light-hearted experience of pleasure, certainly has a place in youth sport. But sometimes it is emphasized too much (Shields & Bredemeier, 2009), and kids get the wrong idea that they should be experiencing "yahoo" fun every moment. This reminds us of our son, who woke up the morning after a fun-filled yet exhausting day at a big amusement park, to ask "What are we gonna do fun today?" It seemed like an addiction, and perhaps it is.

The goal of continuous fun is impossible and unhealthy and is not a good objective for youth sport. We agree with other youth sport experts who state that enjoyment and love of sport is a better objective. Youth sport coaches should build in a few drills and activities that are fun, along with activities that require the focused effort and concentration essential in learning and skill development. As former college basketball players, we loved our sport and enjoyed the pursuit of personal and team goals. But not every moment, such as running stadium stairs during two-a-day practices, was fun. As young athletes mature, they will experience the enjoyment that is part of putting forth great effort to accomplish meaningful goals (Shields & Bredemeier, 2009). So, keep the "F" word in youth sport, but make your objective about nurturing enjoyment and a love of the game.

Personal Plug-In

The Place of Fun

Identify the differences you felt as a youth athlete in terms of fun, enjoyment, and love of your sport. Can you think of examples of when fun was used creatively and had positive outcomes, as well as when fun distracted from your sport experience?

The Importance of Multidimensionality

The final tension point in youth sport involves the debate about whether specializing in one sport is better than diversifying and sampling multiple activities. As discussed in chapter 2, youth sport has evolved from sandlot play and participation in multiple sports to a professionalized model in which kids choose (or are forced to choose) to specialize and focus their attention on one sport. This is discussed at length in chapter 10, but we note it here as a key philosophical difference between those who advocate diversification and those who advocate specialization.

As you'll learn in chapter 10, specialization is not necessarily a bad thing and is certainly appropriate in some sports, for some kids, and at certain ages. But childhood should be a smorgasbord, not a feeding tube. Research shows that the positive developmental outcomes associated with sport participation are stronger for kids who spend time in multiple activities (Zarrett, Fay, Li, Carrano, Phelps, & Lerner, 2009). Children should sample a variety of activities, and then, of course, narrow in and focus on their signature skills and interests as they mature. The adage about not putting all your eggs in one basket is wise advice. Multidimensionality protects kids, gives them lots of pieces in their personal identity pie, and helps them rebound from setbacks and disappointments that they will naturally encounter in sport and other activities.

Summary of Philosophical Tension Points in Youth Sport

Although most people embrace developmentally appropriate objectives for youth sport, the larger sport culture often seduces us to lose sight of these objectives. This seduction usually occurs at the tension points of (a) talent development versus skill development for all, (b) the place of competition in youth sport, (c) the place of fun in youth sport, and (d) multidimensionality versus early specialization in youth sport. Keep these tension points in mind, as they are possible pitfalls waiting to wreck your developmentally appropriate POPP sequence and good intentions.

One idea to clarify these tension points is the development of a national categorization of youth sport programs by philosophy and objectives that parents and athletes could easily recognize when considering programs. Wiersma (2005) was the first to suggest such a system, and he compared it to the film rating categories of the Motion Picture Association of America. We thought this was a great idea that could serve a useful function in clarifying the nature of youth sport programs. We expanded Wiersma's (2005) four categories into five levels that differ in their objectives and characteristics (see table 3.1). It is our hope that youth sport leaders and organizations consider sponsoring such a categorization for youth sports to clarify their focus and objectives.

CONSEQUENCES OF DEVELOPMENTALLY INAPPROPRIATE PHILOSOPHIES AND OBJECTIVES

We've identified the main objectives for youth sport as well as some contentious areas where philosophy and objectives are popularly debated. So what happens when adults adopt developmentally inappropriate philosophies and objectives? Well, kids drop out, burn out, sustain serious injuries, use illegal performance-enhancing drugs, develop eating disorders, and engage in cheating and violence. These negative outcomes are well publicized. However, in this section, we focus on two outcomes of

Table 3.1 Proposed Categorization of Youth Sport Programs by Philosophy and Objectives

Level	Philosophy, mindset	Objectives	Characteristics
1.	"This is fun and I can do it."	Develop interest, excitement	No competition (other than fun activities in practice)
		Sampling of activity	Creative modification to fit athletes' needs
		Develop fundamental skills	Open to all; no travel; common location
		Meet other kids	Minimal time and money; no scoring or standings
2.	"I want to be active and play sport."	Basic skill development	Open to all; community based at common location
		Very basic tactics	Low-level competition; no leagues or standings
		What it means to compete	No tournament or all-stars; creative modification
		Meet other kids	Minimal time and money; everyone plays equally
		How to be a good teammate	
3.	"I want to get better and learn to compete."	Skill building, improvement	Open to all; playing time for all
		Begin focusing on physical training	Common location or local travel
		Goal setting and monitoring	Leagues and standings
		Emotional regulation	Tournament and championships
		Leadership and responsibility	Moderate time and money
4.	"I'm an athlete."	Advanced skill development	Selected, accepted, or invited (not open to all)
		Higher-level competitive experience	Regional travel; extensive time; more money
		Mental skill development	More qualified coaches; playing time earned
		Physical training requirement	Higher performance expectations
5.	"I want to push it to see how good I can be."	Advanced, refined technical training	Selected or accepted based on talent or performance
		Elite performance	Year-round commitment to training, competing, or both
		Intense physical training	Significant time and money investment
		Mental toughness	Restriction of other activities (sacrifice)
		Advanced tactics	Highly trained, qualified coaches; only the best play

Based on Wiersma 2005.

inappropriate philosophies and objectives that are more subtle and less well understood or noticed. We think these outcomes occur with great regularity in youth sport; even adult leaders who have kids' best interests in mind can fail to see how the culture dupes us into these negative consequences.

Identifying "Who's Good" in Youth Sport Before Maturation

Earlier in the chapter, we discussed the problem of placing competition and winning ahead of skill development in sport. We strongly

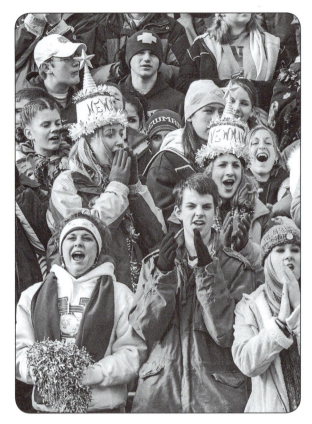

The pyramid model of sport ensures the systematic exclusion of young athletes and influences them to become spectators and discontinue their own participation.

advocate that coaches and directors actively pursue the objective of skill development for *all* their athletes. We emphasize all athletes, because a common pitfall in youth sport is to pay more attention to the athletes who are more physically mature or who have better skills. At the elite level, coaches identify the most talented athletes, and those athletes receive the most attention because they will help their teams win. But the objectives of youth sport differ from those of elite sport, and we tend to forget that. Kids are not miniature adults—they are continuously growing, maturing, and developing. Our objective should be to develop every child's talent, instead of attempting to prematurely identify "talented" children who then receive more attention from coaches and better learning opportunities (discussed more fully in chapter 10).

This emphasis on talent development for all is based on former president Kennedy's point that "not every child has an equal talent . . . but they should have the equal right to develop their talent." That is a great objective for youth sport. All youth sport participants should be afforded the opportunity to develop their skills, even if they lack ability and are not strong contributors to the team goal of winning at that time. Even though youth sport looks the same as adult sport, its philosophy and objectives are very different. Let's not lose sight of who it's all about—the kids! All kids, not just the budding first-round draft choices.

Creation of the Spectator Ethos by the Pyramid Model of Sport

A second negative, yet inherent, consequence of the current youth sport culture is the creation of the spectator ethos by the pyramid model of sport. As shown in figure 3.3, the pyramid model begins with a broad base of many participants in school physical education, intramurals, recreational sport, and community-sponsored youth sport. However, the numbers of participants decrease according to an "up or out" mentality based on the idea that athletes have to make the cut of higher and higher levels of performance or else discontinue participation. The pyramid model is particularly evident in American sport and has been noted in the United Kingdom as well (Bailey, Collins, Ford, MacNamara, Toms, & Pearce, 2010).

The pyramid model ensures the systematic exclusion of participants as they move through the youth sport system. Although ability is the main factor needed to move up the pyramid, other factors such as socioeconomic status, opportunity, coaches, and parents influence young athletes' movement up or dropping off of the pyramid. As discussed in the previous section, the pyramid model of up or out subverts the talent development of all individuals, particularly late-maturing kids or those who enter sport later than others.

The pyramid model also influences kids to move from a **participation ethos** to a **spectator ethos** (Murphy, 1999). Large numbers of kids participate when they're young, but by the age of 9 or 10, the push begins for selecting out the "best" athletes to continue playing with better coaches, more training, and stronger competition. Those who drop off of the pyramid become spectators, watching the higher-skilled athletes perform. Clearly, a culture that spends hundreds of millions on professional sport arenas, yet allows community recreation centers to shut down because of lack of funding, strongly encourages the spectator ethos.

Don't get us wrong—we understand that advancement in sport via the pyramid model is inevitable and often warranted. Athletes with greater skill and higher levels of motivation and commitment should be admired for their movement up the pyramid. We're not so naïve as to believe that all youth athletes should play club (select), college, and elite sport. We also understand that many kids sample sport at the bottom of the

pyramid and many choose other activities (music, art, debate teams, academic and social clubs) instead of continuing in sport. And finally, we're all for spectating, watching highly skilled athletes perform amazing feats, and rooting for the home team.

The problem is the complete discontinuation of sport participation and physical activity by most of those who drop off of the pyramid. Actually, the pyramid model greatly contributes to our sedentary lifestyles and the health problems that result from those lifestyles. The problem is the "up or out." Why can't it be "up or over" to another sport venue? At a women's professional basketball game in Australia, I (first author) had a conversation with the mother of one of the Australian pro players. She had played professional ball in Australia, and when I told her that I had played college basketball in the United States, she asked, "Where do you play now?" I admitted that I did not play at all. She replied, "You Americans! You think if you're not the best, then you should not play." She had continued playing on a club team for women her age in Australia, and she could not believe that I no longer played the game that I loved. She had a good point.

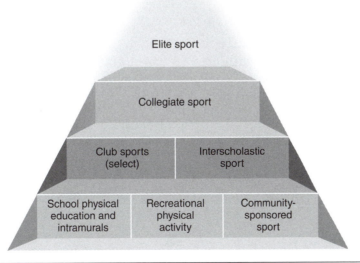

Figure 3.3   Pyramid model of sport participation.

So although the pyramid model is inevitable in selecting and training athletes for elite sport, the common default to the spectator ethos (and death of the participation ethos) in youth is troubling. We need to find ways to change this shifting cultural ethos so that young people have many alternatives to participate in sport and physical activity beyond the pyramid.

PALM COMMUNITY MODEL OF YOUTH SPORT

As an alternative to the pyramid model, we offer the palm community model of sport (see figure 3.4). This is not a picture of a standing (vertical) palm tree, but rather a flat palm tree–shaped community structure built as an archipelago into the sea. These human-made archipelago communities were developed in Dubai of the United Arab Emirates to increase the amount of viable coastline for people to live on. We think the palm community serves as a useful metaphor for a more inclusive, open opportunity for sport participation as opposed to the more exclusive pyramid model.

The model begins with kids' entry into sport participation and includes an extensive variety of options for different types of sport participation. And although there still may be a progression from basic to advanced forms of sport, the flat palm community symbolizes a culture where people move in and out and up and down through many different types of sports across their lifetime. The pyramidal up or out idea is replaced by the community "in and remain in" idea of moving back and forth between many different types of sport activities.

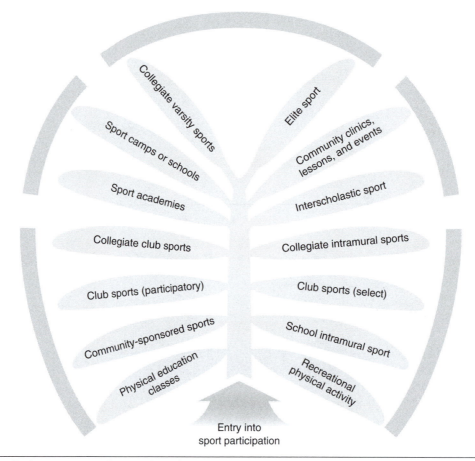

Figure 3.4   Palm community model of sport participation.

You might argue that these various types of sports are available now, and you're correct. But what needs to change is the ethos, or the spirit of or assumptions about the sport culture. The pyramid idea of up or out is ingrained and moves kids away from the participation ethos to the spectator ethos. Simply suggesting a new model won't change the ethos overnight, but we hope it will spur youth sport leaders and society toward thinking and talking about sport differently, as well as finding ways to market and offer sport programs to support our goal of lifetime physical activity participation. Toward this end, note the breakwater barriers provided around the palm community to protect inhabitants from tidal surges. In our portrayal of the palm community model for sport, these breakwater barriers represent us—adult directors, coaches, teachers, and parents who can nurture and preserve a participation ethos and an inclusive sport culture.

EXAMPLES OF YOUTH SPORT PHILOSOPHIES AND POPP SEQUENCES

You've digested a lot of information about youth sport philosophy and objectives. Now let's take a look at some popular youth sport programs to see how they put this knowledge into practice, in terms of their specific philosophies and objectives.

Positive Coaching Alliance

The Positive Coaching Alliance (positivecoach.org) provides manuals for coaches (Thompson, 2010b), parents (Thompson, 2009, 2010a), and youth athletes (Thompson, 2011) to pursue their mission to "transform youth sports so sports can transform youth" (Thompson, 2010b, p. 7). PCA's objectives are to transform

- coaches into "Double-Goal Coaches," who prepare athletes to win and learn life lessons through sport;

- athletes into "Triple-Impact Competitors," who make themselves, teammates, and the game better; and

- parents into "Second Goal Parents," who concentrate on the child's character development while letting athletes and coaches focus on the first goal of winning.

Following the POPP sequence, PCA's philosophy and objectives lead to three key principles of positive coaching:

1. Honoring the Game, by getting to the ROOTS of positive play (respect for **R**ules, **O**pponents, **O**fficials, Teammates, **S**elf)

2. Redefining "winner" by emphasizing the ELM tree of Mastery (**E**ffort, **L**earning, bouncing back from **M**istakes)

3. Filling Emotional Tanks with encouragement and praise

The PCA continues its POPP sequence by suggesting many specific practices for coaches, athletes, and parents to follow, such as these:

- Using a behavioral Mistake Ritual to help young athletes move beyond their mistakes

- Giving targeted Symbolic Rewards (small, creative awards for specific accomplishments)

- Using the Two-Minute Drill to inject positive energy into a training session

Human Kinetics Coach Education

A sample POPP sequence from the Coaching Principles course (Martens, 2012) of the Human Kinetics Coach Education (www.HumanKineticsCoachEducationCenter.com) is as follows:

Philosophy: "Athletes first, winning second"

Objectives: Teaches coaches how to balance the three objectives of youth sport, which are (a) striving to win; (b) having fun; and (3) helping young athletes develop physically, psychologically, and socially

Principles (examples): Coach for character; adopt a cooperative coaching style; the coach as a strong communicator; the coach as a master teacher; use logical consequences for rules violations; catch athletes doing well

Practices (examples): Productive team meetings with athlete participation; encouragement outweighs criticism; performance and effort are rewarded when earned; athletes receive feedback high in information

A catchy phrase that captures the essence of your philosophy is a great starting point for your POPP sequence. "Athletes first, winning second" really sets the tone for the program emphasis on athlete development as the most important objective. We find that athletes and parents remember and buy into program philosophies when they are creative and memorable.

Our Philosophy and Objectives

Our philosophy, "It's all about the kid," emphasizes our foundational belief in child-centered youth sport. It reminds us of what we're doing in youth sport when our competitive juices start flowing and we want to beat a rival coach's team or impress our adult friends with our coaching expertise.

The objectives espoused in this book for youth sport leaders are to understand and engage in developmentally appropriate practice to

1. provide physical, psychological, and social benefits to all participants;

2. develop athletic talent; and

3. nurture an interest in and commitment to physical activity across the life span.

The rest of the book is designed to provide you with our ideas of principles and practices that make it all about the kid and help you pursue these objectives. In addition, we invite you to develop your own POPP sequence, following the directions on page 64 in Reflective Learning Activities. Although your personal POPP sequence will evolve and even change for different youth sport contexts, it's a good idea to begin considering the philosophy and objectives that resonate most deeply within you.

WRAP-UP

Philosophy. It sounds boring and impractical. It isn't. Objectives. People think they're just administrative jargon, that they sound good but don't really matter. They do. One of the biggest needs in youth sport is the careful consideration and adoption of a developmentally appropriate philosophy and set of objectives. They guide us every day in making the right decisions. They clarify the nature and focus of youth sport programs for parents and athletes. They help all involved find their right "fit," in terms of the myriad programs that are available to kids with different skills and interests. They ensure that youth sport is all about the kid.

So much media attention is directed toward the sensational negative happenings in youth sport. Many writers state that youth sport is a broken system with overzealous parents and morally corrupt coaches. We don't agree. There are adults who exploit children in all areas of society, but according to our observations, these adults are a minority. We see examples of terrific coaches, supportive parents, and engaged kids every day. But what is required are thoughtful attention and an explicit commitment to child-centered youth sport that meets the developmental needs of children. We *can* shape the culture, instead of being shaped by it, if we continually clarify what we're doing, why we're doing it, and who we're doing it for.

LEARNING AIDS

Key Terms

competition—A social evaluation process, or the process that we experience when we perform an activity and are socially and publicly evaluated by others.

decompetition—The failure to engage in the cooperation and mutual respect needed to strive together in a competitive event.

objectives—Results you wish to accomplish in your program.

participation ethos—The mindset and commitment in a culture to engage and remain engaged in sport or physical activity at any level.

philosophy—Basic values and beliefs that people hold.

POPP sequence—The ways in which our actions in youth sport are guided by the values and beliefs inherent in our philosophy, objectives, and guiding principles.

principles—Predetermined guidelines about how you'll make decisions.

practice—What you do and how you do it; the behaviors you engage in within your program.

spectator ethos—The mindset and commitment in a culture to watch others (typically at a higher skill level) engage in sport.

Summary Points

1. The POPP sequence involves developing a philosophy, which then guides the development of objectives, principles, and (developmentally appropriate) practice.

2. The generally accepted objectives of youth sport are the development of sport skills, psychosocial and life skills, and physical health.

3. Positive youth development (PYD) programs often use sport or physical activity to develop personal and social skills (such as the five C's) in children.

4. Positive youth development occurs only when adult stakeholders consciously design and direct youth sport programs with this objective in mind.

5. The dueling objectives of youth sport are talent development for elite performance versus providing developmental benefits to all participants.

6. Competition, as a public social evaluation process, should be introduced gradually in youth sport.

7. The objective of skills development and mastery should never be superseded by the objective of winning in youth sports before high school.

8. Although fun is the biggest reason kids play sports and should be included in youth sport, the goal of continuous, frivolous fun is not a good objective for youth sport.

9. The pyramid model of sport ensures the systematic exclusion of participants as they move through the youth sport system.

10. The palm community model of youth sport strives to create a culture in which people remain in sport throughout their lives by sampling many different types of activities.

Study Questions

1. What is the POPP sequence? Define each part of the sequence and provide a real-life example of each part. How can the POPP sequence benefit adult leaders in youth sport?

2. What are the three broad objectives of youth sport? Explain why each objective is important.

3. What are the dueling objectives of youth sport?

4. Describe the issues surrounding competition in youth sport. When is it problematic and when is it useful?

5. Explain the difference between fun and enjoyment in youth sport.

6. Explain the pyramid and the palm community models of youth sport, and identify pros and cons of each model.

Reflective Learning Activities

1. This activity will help you begin conceptualizing a POPP sequence that represents your vision for a specific youth sport program. You can revisit the examples provided in the chapter to help get you started. Remember that the most important criterion for your POPP sequence is that it be developmentally appropriate for the age and level of athletes in your program.

   a. Identify the specific youth sport program you have in mind for this activity and POPP sequence.

   b. Come up with a short phrase to represent your philosophy.

   c. Go to appendix A, on page 366, and complete the 100-Points Exercise (adapted from Thompson, 2009). This will help you clarify what objectives are most important to you.

   d. Write out at least three objectives for your program based on what you learned from the 100-Points Exercise.

   e. Identify three or four principles or predetermined guidelines about how you'll make decisions. Several examples of key issues from which your principles will be based are listed in appendix B, on page 367. Read over these key youth sport issues, which may help you identify your significant personal principles.

   f. To complete your POPP sequence, list four or five practices or specific things you'll do in your program that logically extend from your philosophy, objectives, and principles.

   Congratulations! You've taken an important step in clarifying the philosophy and objectives that will drive your program and your behavior in youth sport.

2. Develop a flyer for or a letter to parents to educate them about the philosophy and objectives of your program. Make sure you pick a specific sport and age group, such as 6- to 7-year-old boys' or girls' soccer, 11- to 12-year-old boys' ice hockey, or high school girls' tennis. Make your flyer or letter interesting and informational.

3. Identify specific behaviors and activities for each statement in the Bill of Rights for Young Athletes to ensure that that right is protected in youth sport.

4. Search for and identify a positive youth development program that uses sport or physical activity to teach positive values to kids. Describe the program, including its philosophy and objectives, as well as any positive outcomes that have been documented as the result of this program. Provide your assessment of or opinion about the effectiveness of the program.

Resource Guide

Positive Coaching Alliance, www.positivecoach.org.

Maturation and Readiness for Youth Sport Participation

Welcome to part II of *Best Practice for Youth Sport,* which broadly addresses the concepts of maturation and readiness. Here's a sampling of things you'll learn in the next five chapters:

- How kids physically grow and mature, and how this affects their readiness for youth sport
- How kids learn motor skills, and when they are ready to use those skills to compete

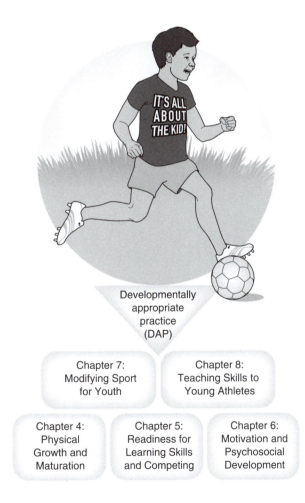

Developmentally appropriate practice (DAP)

| Chapter 7: Modifying Sport for Youth | Chapter 8: Teaching Skills to Young Athletes |

| Chapter 4: Physical Growth and Maturation | Chapter 5: Readiness for Learning Skills and Competing | Chapter 6: Motivation and Psychosocial Development |

- How motivation works in kids and how they mature psychosocially
- How to modify youth sports to fit kids' needs
- How to teach skills using developmentally appropriate progressions

Part II is the heart of the book, exploring how and why youth sport is different from adult sport. Picture yourself in your daily job routine: attempting to complete assigned tasks, taking feedback from your boss, negotiating with coworkers . . . and you're 9 years old. That would be absurd, right? It's equally absurd to expect that kids are ready to participate in adult forms of sport and to think that they are motivated to learn and compete in the same way as adults. They're not. Let's make it all about them and shape the youth sport culture to meet their unique maturational needs.

chapter 4

PHYSICAL GROWTH AND MATURATION

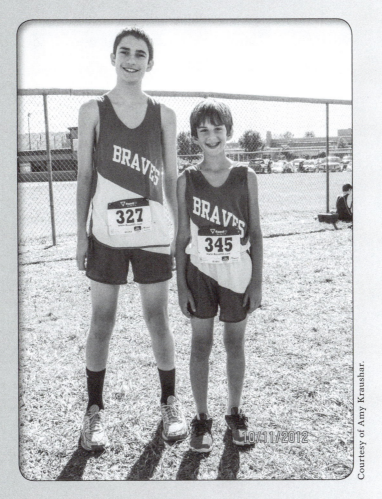

Courtesy of Amy Kraushar.

CHAPTER PREVIEW

In this chapter, you'll learn

- » how children physically grow and mature,
- » the difference between biological and chronological age,
- » how to assess maturation in children, and
- » how the relative age effect influences youth sport athletes.

The two boys in the photograph are 13-year-old cross-country teammates who are exactly the same age (their birthdays are two days apart). Obviously, they differ considerably in maturation. The boy on the left, Jackson, has undergone his adolescent growth spurt, while the boy on the right, David, has not yet begun his growth spurt. So although these boys are the same age in terms of birth dates, they are at very different maturational points in their progress toward adulthood. The size difference between Jackson and David seems incredible, yet it is quite common among 13-year-old boys.

Consider how such maturational discrepancies influence youth sport athletes. How might adult coaches assess kids' suitability for specific sports by looking at their sizes and shapes? What positions would they be assigned, and what skills would they be taught based on these positions? How are their abilities to understand and perform sport skills influenced by their maturational status? How do they feel about their bodies in relation to the size and shape of their teammates and friends?

To determine children's readiness to learn and perform motor (movement) skills, we must consider their maturational levels and not just their ages. Attempting to teach children motor skills before they are physically ready is frustrating and counterproductive to their learning and motivation. It is critical for youth sport leaders to understand how children grow and mature and then to use that understanding to engage in developmentally appropriate practice (DAP).

Development in this sense refers to all the physical and psychological changes that humans undergo over a lifetime (Bukato & Daehler, 2012). In this book, we're interested in how kids change and how to best fit the youth sport experience to them. This chapter focuses on physical growth and maturation, which are part of development. Development is a broader concept, including the biological aspects of development discussed in this chapter as well as the behavioral

aspects of development discussed in other chapters of the book. Unlike physical growth and maturation, development doesn't stop at a particular age but continues throughout life. Children's entry into youth sport, and subsequent sport experiences throughout adolescence, are important developmental transitions for them. We want these developmental transitions to be successful, and they will be if we, as adult leaders, understand growth, maturation, and development—and the key needs of kids at different developmental stages.

GROWTH

When people talk about "growing up," their phrasing is correct. The most noticeable way we grow is "up," as we grow in height. **Growth** refers to an increase in body size, either as a whole or as attained by specific parts of the body. As children grow, they become taller and heavier, their lean and fat tissue increases, and their organs increase in size (Malina, Bouchard, & Bar-Or, 2004).

Some General Principles of Growth

1. **Growth proceeds at different rates during different stages.** Children experience periods of rapid and slow growth, and different parts of the body may grow at different times. A girl who is 20 inches (50 centimeters) at birth and stops growing at age 18 at 70 inches (178 centimeters) does not increase in height equally each year from birth to 18 years. She experiences periods of both rapid and slow growth until she reaches her full height.

The pattern of human growth is usually S-shaped (called a sigmoid curve, after the Greek letter for s). As shown in figure 4.1 (adapted from Scammon, 1930), human growth generally (1) is rapid during infancy, (2) is slower yet steady during early and middle childhood, (3) is rapid during adolescence, and (4) slows down and finally stops after adolescence.

2. **Human growth follows a cephalocaudal pattern, which means that growth proceeds from the head downward (to the feet).** Although the body as a whole generally follows the sigmoid growth pattern, the differential growth rates of different body parts result in changes in the body's appearance across ages. As shown in figure 4.2, the head is one-fourth of the total height at birth but only one-eighth of adult height (Timiras, 1972, as cited in Haywood & Getchell, 2009). The legs are about three-eighths of the height at birth but almost half the adult height. Notice how the red line representing center of gravity moves down with age, as kids become less top-heavy. Think about how toddlers walk—they sort of stumble along with their upper body tilted forward due to their high center of gravity. Balance is much more difficult for young children as compared to adults, as evidenced by the early-childhood way of descending stairs—one step at a time using both feet. Motor skills such as skating or bicycling are challenging for very young children due to their higher center of gravity.

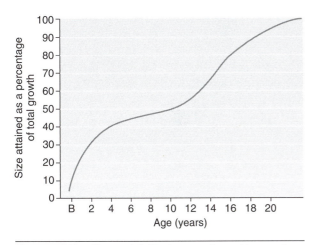

Figure 4.1 Sigmoid (S-shaped) pattern of human growth.

3. **Human growth is proximodistal, meaning from the center outward.** The

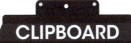

How Tall Will My Child Be at Adulthood?

Parents and coaches often speculate on how tall a youth athlete will be as an adult. Research scientists and physicians can use radiographs (x-rays) of the hand and wrist bones to assess the amount of skeletal maturity, from which they can estimate adult height, or stature. There are also anthropometric formulas that include parents' heights and the child's current height, weight, and age to predict adult stature. Check out the website http://children.webmd.com/healthtool-kids-height-predictor. Type in parents' heights, and the site performs some simple calculations to estimate a child's adult height. The error inherent in the process makes the result plus or minus 4 inches (10 centimeters), so it isn't exact.

Or you can compute the estimation of adult height yourself:

1. Find the average of the parents' height by adding together the mother's and father's heights (in either inches or centimeters) and dividing by 2.

2. To calculate the height of a boy, add 2.5 inches (6.5 centimeters) to the average of the parents' height. To calculate the height of a girl, subtract 2.5 inches from the average of the parents' height.

3. The resulting number is the midparental height for girls and boys. The child's adult height can be expected to fall within a range of 4 inches (10 centimeters) more or less than the midparental height.

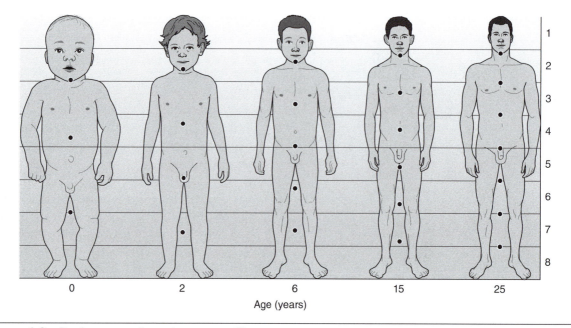

Figure 4.2 Body proportion changes with age.

term *proximodistal* describes fetal growth from inside out and also the development of motor skills as an inside-out process. Babies and toddlers gain control over the center of their bodies (head, neck, shoulders, torso) before they develop dexterity in the distal parts of their bodies (limbs). Finger and toe muscles (used for fine motor skills) are the last to develop.

General Stages and Patterns of Growth

Although people differ in their growth patterns, there are generally recognized stages and patterns of growth (see table 4.1; Horn & Butt, 2014). Prenatally and in infancy (conception to 2 years), growth is very fast, with the head and trunk growing faster than the legs. Based on the cephalocaudal principle just discussed, infants and toddlers are very top-heavy. Early (2 to 6 years) and middle (6 to 10 years) childhood are characterized by slower but very steady growth rates. Notice that in early childhood the legs are growing faster; and by age 6, children are generally increasing bone and muscle mass more than

they are fat. This increased development of the muscular and skeletal systems provides the 6-year-old with better motor skill abilities (Horn & Butt, 2014).

Late childhood to early adolescence (10-15 years) is another period of very fast growth, but generally girls and boys differ in the timing of this growth spurt (Horn & Butt, 2014; Malina, 2014). Girls' growth spurts typically range from 10 to 13 years, during which time they may grow 8 to 9 inches (20 to 23 centimeters) in height and gain 30 to 35 pounds (14 to 16 kilograms) in body weight. Boys' growth spurts typically range from 12 to 15 years, during which time they may grow 9 to 12 inches (23 to 30 centimeters) and gain 35 to 45 pounds (16 to 20 kilograms) in body weight. So it is common for girls to be taller than boys between 10 and 13 years of age. Typically, this growth begins in the hands and feet and then proceeds to the legs and finally the trunk (Horn & Butt, 2014). Sexual maturation also begins in this growth stage, along with changes in body shape and composition.

The final growth stage is middle to late adolescence (15-20 years). Growth rate slows, yet sexual maturation and changes in body shape

Table 4.1 Stages and Patterns of Physical Growth

Growth stage	Approximate age range	Growth patterns
Prenatal	Conception to birth	• Very fast growth. • Head and trunk grow faster than legs (sitting height at birth is 85% of total body height).
Infancy	Birth to 2 years	• Very fast growth (especially in early months of infancy). • Head and trunk still growing comparatively faster.
Early childhood	2 to 6 years	• Slower growth rate. • Lower legs grow faster than head and trunk (sitting height at 6 years is 55% of total body height).
Middle childhood	6 to 10 years	• Slower growth rate, but some children exhibit a midgrowth spurt between 6.5 and 8.5 years.
Late childhood through early adolescence	10 to 15 years	• Very fast growth rate. • Sexual maturation begins. • Body shape and composition change.
Middle to late adolescence	15 to 20 years	• Slower growth rate. • Continuation of sexual maturation. • Continuation of body shape and composition changes.

From: Developmental perspectives on sport and physical activity participation, T.S. Horn and J. Butt, *Routledge companion to sport and exercise psychology: Global perspectives and fundamental concepts,* edited by A. Papaioannou and D. Hackfort, Copyright 2014, Taylor and Francis, reproduced by permission of Taylor & Francis Books UK.

and composition continue. Most of adult height has been attained at age 17 for girls and age 21 for boys (Payne & Isaacs, 2008).

Overall, the adolescent growth spurt in height occurs before the growth spurt in body weight. This general rule gives youth sport practitioners an idea where children are in their individual growth patterns. However, remember that the general stages and patterns of physical growth presented in table 4.1 are averages based on large samples of children, and that there is considerable individual variability in growth patterns. Some kids begin their growth spurts earlier, some later; some spend a longer time in their growth spurts, and some grow faster and cease growth earlier.

MATURATION

Maturation refers to progress toward the biologically mature state (Malina, 2013), or the process one undergoes to reach full adult status in terms of physical, cognitive, and emotional functioning. Maturation varies with different biological systems. **Sexual maturity** occurs when people have fully functional reproductive capabilities. **Skeletal maturity** occurs when people have fully ossified (hardened bone) adult skeletons.

As shown in the photo at the beginning of the chapter, maturation is an innate, individual process. You've probably heard the term *biological clock,* the common metaphor for maturation. Individuals have unique biological clocks, with variations in the timing and tempo of their maturation (Malina, 2014). With regard to timing, people achieve maturational milestones (e.g., onset of puberty, beginning of growth spurt) earlier or later than others their age as the result of their personal biological clocks. The tempo difference in people's biological clocks is the length of time people spend in certain maturational phases (e.g., duration of puberty, length of growth spurt). Our individual biological clocks are largely innately

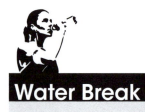

Is There Such a Thing as Adolescent Awkwardness?

A popular assumption is that the rapid growth in height during adolescence can cause kids to temporarily lose some motor coordination, or to be awkward. This temporary disruption in motor abilities during adolescence is discussed in many child development texts, where adolescents are described as "clumsy, awkward, and poorly coordinated" (Lambert, Rothschild, Altland, & Green, 1972, p. 114), or where a "slight adolescent lag in motor ability" is noted (Eckert, 1987, p. 317).

This idea stems from the concept of **peak height velocity, or PHV,** which is the time at which kids are growing the fastest during their adolescent growth spurt. In adolescence, the rate of growth in height increases until it reaches a peak or maximum (the PHV, which on average occurs at age 12 for girls and at age 14 years for boys). Growth then gradually decreases and eventually ceases as adult height is reached. This rapid growth during the PHV, particularly among boys, has led people to speculate that boys' increases in height may "outgrow" their muscular strength. This is partly true, as adolescents generally achieve their height spurt first, followed by their weight spurt. However, a generalized decrease in motor abilities and coordination has not been substantiated by research.

The "awkwardness" idea was specifically tested in a study that examined performance and coordination across a range of motor tasks in prepubescent, pubescent, and postpubescent individuals (Davies & Rose, 2000). These tasks included walking on a balance beam, one-leg balance, throwing, running, standing long jump, arm movement accuracy, head movement control, riding a scooter board, obstacle course, and cup displacement (a combination of gross and fine motor tasks requiring coordinated movements and bilateral motor control).

What did the researchers find? There was no evidence for impaired coordination, or adolescent awkwardness, for boys or girls—a particularly strong finding because the skills that were tested were specifically selected to be sensitive to adolescent awkwardness. Instead, they found that kids performed better at each successive stage—from prepuberty to puberty to postpuberty. Interestingly, there were more performance differences between prepubertal and pubertal participants than between pubertal and postpubertal participants. This suggests that there are more changes in the development of motor skills before puberty.

Some individual kids have been shown to decline on certain motor tasks during adolescence (Beunen et al., 1988), and it may be that rapid growth that occurs in the feet can temporarily disrupt agility and coordination (Horn & Butt, 2014). But this is uncommon and transitory, as no general period of adolescent awkwardness or decrease in motor coordination is supported by research evidence. The idea that kids need to relearn skills after their growth spurt is a myth, as they will quickly learn to adapt to their growing dimensions.

hardwired, although obesity, nutrition, stress, and environmental chemicals have been implicated in influencing early maturation in some children (discussed later).

A person's maturation does not proceed in unison with her chronological age. **Chronological age** is how old people are based on their particular dates of birth. **Biological age** is how close people are to their fully mature state (also called maturational age). Children of the same chronological age can differ in maturation by as much as five years, based on their own personal biological clocks. Two athletes may both be 12 years old (chronological age), but one may be 10 and the other 14 in terms of maturational age. Youth sport leagues, teams, and events are organized by chronological age, so differences in maturational age give certain kids advantages, disadvantage others, and also influence the perceptions of coaches and teachers when working with kids of different maturational ages.

How Do We Assess Maturation in Youth Sport?

Youth sports are organized by chronological age, because that's the most practical way to divide kids. And that's okay, as long as youth sport leaders are aware of maturational differences within age groups. Maturation is a process that cannot be directly measured, but we can use certain indicators to infer maturational levels. Three common maturational assessments are radiology to assess skeletal maturation, markers of sexual maturation, and tracking growth and weight gains.

Radiology to Assess Skeletal Age

The best method for assessing maturational age is the use of radiology, or x-ray analysis, to assess the skeletal maturity of a growing child. All children start with a skeleton of cartilage prenatally and have a fully developed skeleton of bone in early adulthood.

This process of skeletal development from cartilage to bone allows us to observe a child's maturity level by examining radiographs, or x-rays, of their bones. Typically, the bones of the hand and wrist are used to assess skeletal maturity (see figure 4.3), although other sites may be used. Although skeletal assessment is the most reliable method, most youth sport leaders and parents do not have the access and expertise to assess maturation in this way.

Markers of Sexual Maturity

A more practical way for youth sport practitioners to assess maturation in kids is to observe markers of sexual maturity. As shown in table 4.1, sexual maturation with changes in physical features of the body occurs in late childhood and through adolescence (approximately 10-20 years of age). **Puberty** is the transitional period between childhood and adulthood; it includes the appearance of secondary sex characteristics, maturation of the reproductive system, and the adolescent growth spurt (Malina, Bouchard, & Bar-Or, 2004). Puberty is a phase, not a point in time. Girls usually begin puberty between 9 and 14 years, and boys usually begin between 10 and 16 years (boys are typically one to two years behind girls). Puberty typically lasts two to five years, but it can be much longer. It is the time of the greatest variability among individuals in both physical characteristics and motor abilities. (**Adolescence** is a similar term used to describe the transitional period between childhood and adulthood, but adolescence is viewed as broader than puberty and includes physical, psychological, and social transitions. The word *adolescere* in Latin means "to grow up.")

The assessment of sexual maturity is based on markers that become apparent during puberty. These are known as **secondary sex characteristics,** which are features that distinguish the two sexes but that are not directly a part of the reproductive system.

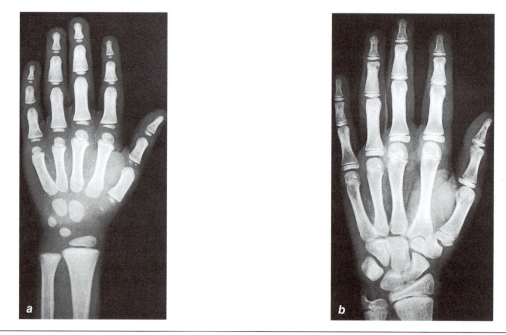

Figure 4.3 X-rays of hand and wrist bones to assess maturation. These images are from an anatomical atlas, with (a) showing the standard for girls 37 months old and boys 48 months old, and (b) showing the standard for girls 128 months old and boys 156 months old. Note that in the image in b, representing older children, there is much more ossification (hardening of the bones), which appears whiter on the image.

Reprinted, by permission, from Bolton Brush Growth Study Center. Copyright Bolton—Brush Growth Study—B.H. Broadbent D.D.S.

(Primary sex characteristics are body structures directly concerned with reproduction [penis, testes, ovaries]). Secondary sex characteristics observed in boys are facial and body hair; deepening voice; and an increase in muscle mass, body weight, and shoulder girth. For females, breast development and increased weight are markers of sexual development. The hormones that increase during puberty can cause acne on kids' faces and bodies and also increase sweating and body odor. Of course, such markers as pubic hair for both girls and boys, as well as time of **menarche** (first menstrual period) for girls, are characteristics of maturation, but it is too invasive for youth sport practitioners to use these indicators.

Tracking Growth and Weight Gains

The third way to assess biological or maturational age is to track growth and weight gains for individual children. On average, children grow 2.5 inches (6 centimeters) a year and gain about 5 pounds (2.3 kilograms) a year until they hit their growth spurt. The average "takeoff" point, or starting time, for the adolescent growth spurt is 9 to 10 years for girls and 11 to 12 years for boys (Malina et al., 2004). The average PHV, or fastest growing period, is at 12 years for girls and 14 years for boys. However, these are averages, as we know that kids mature in very individual ways.

Therefore, it is helpful to track a child's growth in stature along with his sexual maturation and changes in body composition. For girls, breast budding occurs around the time the growth spurt begins. Girls then reach their PHV and achieve menarche (generally one year after PHV). Changes in body composition for girls (some muscle mass and a large increase in fat mass) then follow the PHV. Similarly for boys, the PHV is accompanied by the development of secondary

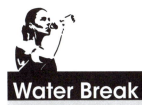

Why Are Girls Starting Puberty Earlier?

Today in the United States, about 16% of girls enter puberty (defined by breast development) by age 7 and about 30% by age 8 (Fuhrman, 2011). Another fact is the decreasing age of menarche, or first menstrual period. In Europe in 1830, the average age of menarche was 17. In the United States in 1900, the average age of menarche was 14.2. By the 1920s, the average age of menarche in the United States had fallen to 13.3; by 2002, it had reached 12.34 (although the decline slowed in the 1960s) (McDowell, Brody, & Hughes, 2007).

Researchers point to several factors that seem to be contributing to the decline in age of entering puberty (Walvoord, 2010). First, increasing rates of childhood overweight and obesity have been associated with earlier puberty in girls. Excess body fat alters hormones that regulate pubertal timing. Second, increased animal protein intake in children has been associated with earlier menarche. Meat and dairy consumption also involves the ingestion of environmental endocrine-disrupting chemicals (EDCs) and bovine growth hormone that have accumulated in animal tissues. Third, EDCs in the environment such as bisphenol A, or BPA (found in plastic cups, water bottles, and food storage containers) can mimic, inhibit, or alter natural hormones. Fourth, significant family stress and conflict have been linked to early puberty. And finally, some cases of early puberty are caused by medical conditions that influence premature hormone release. This is sometimes referred to as **precocious puberty**, or when the bodily changes of puberty happen earlier than normal (before age 8 in girls and age 9 in boys) (Berberoglu, 2009).

Why is early puberty an issue? It has been linked to breast cancer, obesity, lower self-esteem, eating disorders, depression, anxiety, and shorter stature (early closure of growth plates in bones) (Walvoord, 2010). Girls who mature early are also more likely to take part in risky behaviors, including smoking, alcohol use, and sexual activity. Girls who are 7 or 8 years old are not emotionally and psychologically equipped to navigate puberty.

What should families of early bloomers do? Visit a pediatric physician to rule out any treatable medical conditions. Focus on helping girls stay physically active and at a healthy body weight. Treat them as children the age they are, not the age they look. Defend them against a culture that attempts to sexualize young girls at an early age (more on this in chapter 13), and support and educate them about making good choices to avoid risky behaviors. Involve them in youth sport, and support them to continue participation when their bodies change as the result of puberty.

sex characteristics; then muscle mass and weight increase about a year after the PHV. Growth in the feet often is an indicator that the growth spurt is about to occur.

Overall, observe this pattern of maturation: height spurt, development of secondary sex characteristics, and weight spurt (muscle and fat). Tracking basic growth at least four times a year (quarterly) may provide an estimation of children's maturity status in relation to their chronological age. These systematic measures of growth can be charted, which will make the PHV very apparent (Balyi & Way, 2011).

How Maturation Influences Sport Participation for Boys and Girls

Kids can be categorized into three maturity groups according to how quickly they are growing and reaching maturation. **Early maturers** are those whose maturational ages are one year greater than their chronological ages. **Late maturers** are those whose maturational ages are one year less than their chronological ages. **Average maturers** are those whose maturational age is within one year of their chronological age. Youth sport leaders should pay particular attention to early- and late-maturing girls and boys, because these maturational groups have distinct characteristics that advantage or disadvantage them as young athletes. The following descriptions are generalizations based on typical maturational patterns, as all adolescents do not follow these categorizations exactly.

Early-Maturing Boys

Compared to their peers, early-maturing boys are taller and heavier, with more muscle mass and greater shoulder girth. This advantages them in activities that require strength and power. For example, early-maturing adolescent boys (12-17 years) were better at a static strength arm

pull, the shuttle run for speed and agility, and explosive strength in the vertical jump when compared to average- and late-maturing boys (Malina et al., 2004). So, for maturational reasons, these boys are often able to outperform their peers in many youth sport activities. Because of this early success, early-maturing boys receive a lot of recognition, which fuels their confidence, self-esteem, and motivation to continue in sport (Fairclough & Ridgers, 2010).

But often, early-maturing boys are "caught" as the later-maturing boys catch up in biological maturation, and it is frequently hard for the early maturers to understand that the biological advantage they once had is now gone. Youth sport coaches and parents should be aware of this catch-up phenomenon and counsel and support early-maturing boys during this time. Because early-maturing boys are stronger and bigger, they may fail to learn fundamental skills that are needed for more advanced skill development later in their athletic careers. Coaches should emphasize a personal mastery approach with individual performance goals for these boys, and not allow them to rely on their short-term biological advantage (which they will lose in time). Early maturers could also play up a level so they are competing against boys similar to them in maturational age. Coaches should avoid pigeonholing prepubescent athletes into certain sport positions, because the athletes' postpubescent heights and builds may not fit the position they were forced into when they were younger. For example, it would be detrimental for youth basketball coaches to designate early-maturing boys as post players and not teach them perimeter shooting or dribbling skills.

Ironically, early-maturing boys (and girls) tend to end up as shorter adults. Early maturers stop growing in stature first, and children in the other two maturity categories continue to grow for a longer period of time (Malina et al., 2004). In addition, early-maturing boys (and girls) have, on

Are Teenage Brains Different From Adult Brains?

We, like other parents of teenagers, despair over our teens' rude, moody, disorganized, risk-taking, impulsive behaviors. Recent studies in brain development have revealed a maturational explanation for such prototypical teenage behavior. The brain's prefrontal cortex is not fully developed in teenagers as compared to adults and typically does not fully mature until the mid-20s (Giedd et al., 1999). This part of the brain helps to inhibit impulses, to understand consequences of action, and to plan and organize behavior.

So while adults can use rational processes when facing emotional decisions, teenagers are not as biologically equipped to think through things in the same way. Research shows that when processing emotions, adults have greater activity in their frontal lobes than teenagers. In addition, adults have lower activity in their amygdala than teenagers. The amygdala of the brain is the emotional center and is involved in instinctive (gut) reactions, including the fight-or-flight response of humans. Part of the maturation of teenagers is shifting from the amygdala to the frontal lobes in making decisions, moderating behavior, and processing emotions. Teens' brains also have highly active reward centers, which make them more interested in seeking short-term rewards, entering uncertain situations, and taking risks.

Our brains mature as axons (the long nerve fibers that allow our neurons to connect) are encased in a fatty substance called myelin. Myelin insulates the axon, allowing more rapid transmission of nerve signals down the axon and across the synaptic junctions (Sowell, Thompson, Tessner, & Toga, 2001). The better myelinated our axons

are, the faster and more efficiently we can think. Another process that speeds up in the frontal lobes during the teenage years is synaptic pruning, whereby synapses that are frequently used strengthen and those that are rarely used lapse. In early childhood, myelination and synaptic pruning are concentrated in the posterior brain areas. Brain maturation occurs from back to front, with the frontal lobes last.

Understanding that teenagers' impulsive, emotional, and irrational behaviors are related to the biological maturation of their brains may help adult coaches and parents cope. Although annoying and exasperating at times, the situation is temporary.

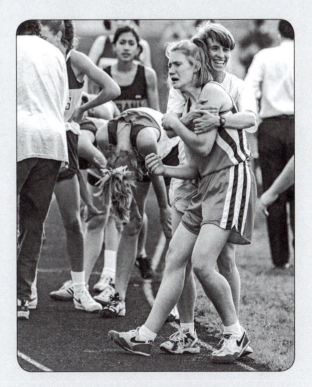

Teenagers' impulsive and emotional behaviors are related to the delayed maturational development of their brains.

average, greater body weights and greater weight-for-height as adults than the other two maturity groups, with physiques called **mesomorphic** (muscular) or **endomorphic** (round and heavy).

Late-Maturing Boys

Late-maturing boys are more linear in build, with physiques called **ectomorphic.** These boys are typically not as successful in early youth sport experiences because they are not as physically strong or mature and are thus at a biological disadvantage in sport activities that require strength and power. They may be successful in such sports as cross-country and diving at a young age. Often, late-maturing boys are teased due to their lack of a prototypical male "sport body" and their lack of success in popular team sports, and they may become discouraged and look to drop out of sport. It is imperative

that youth sport coaches continue to provide competent instruction and skill development for late maturers and not to assume that they're "not as good" as early-maturing boys. They are behind in maturation, and their physical performance disadvantage is temporary.

A legal duty of coaches is to match athletes appropriately in terms of age, size, maturity, and skill. Coaches would breach this duty if they matched a smaller late-maturing boy with a much larger and more muscular early-maturing boy in a contact drill (e.g., football or ice hockey). If the late-maturing boy were injured as a result of this mismatch, the coach could be found negligent in court and suffer legal consequences from this negligence. Matching athletes by maturational levels and modifying practice structures when mismatches are apparent are recommended coaching practices to protect smaller, late-maturing athletes from injury.

Water Break

The Amazing Growth Spurt of Anthony Davis

A famous example of late maturation in boys is Anthony Davis, who was the number-one draft pick in the 2012 National Basketball Association (NBA) draft and is now a star for the New Orleans Pelicans. Beginning his junior year of high school, Davis was a 6-foot, 2-inch (188 centimeters) guard known for his ball handling and slashing moves to the basket from the perimeter. By his senior year, he had grown an astounding 8 inches (20 centimeters) into a 6-foot, 10-inch (208 centimeters) skyscraping shot blocker and rebounder. But because he had developed his

dribbling and shooting skills before his growth spurt, he was a complete player by his senior year who could play in the post as well as handle the ball and shoot 3-pointers from the perimeter. Davis' late growth spurt helped make him the "total package" college recruit (he played one year for the University of Kentucky, and the team won a National Collegiate Athletic Association championship) and top NBA draft choice. Had he achieved his growth much earlier, chances are that he would not have developed such a complete repertoire of basketball skills.

Late-maturing boys tend to be taller as adults. Research has shown that motor performance in late-maturing boys improved from 18 to 30 years of age, whereas early and average maturers showed little change or a decline (Lefevre, Beunen, Steens, Claessens, & Renson, 1990). This research emphasizes the continued maturation and enhanced motor performance of late-maturing boys beyond the typical age limits of adolescence. Our challenge as youth sport leaders is to educate coaches, parents, and young athletes about maturation so that late-maturing boys will hang in there during the difficult early-adolescent phase when they are maturationally behind.

Early- and Late-Maturing Girls

Like boys, early-maturing girls tend to be more mesomorphic (muscular) or endomorphic (round), while late-maturing girls are more ectomorphic (thin, linear) in physique. However, the influence of maturation on the motor performance of girls is not as clear as with boys. Yes, early-maturing females are taller, bigger, and stronger than late-maturing girls; but female adolescence adds more fat weight than muscle weight (opposite of boys). Thus, the strength advantage is in gross strength due to larger body size (e.g., holding position in basketball against an opponent, throwing a discus), but not always in relative strength (in relation to one's own body, as in pull-ups, push-ups, or jumping).

In addition, our culture may socialize endomorphic early-maturing girls to drop out of sport; and early-maturing girls have been shown to have lower self-esteem, more dissatisfied body image, and higher levels of social physique anxiety compared to later maturers (Negriff & Susman, 2011). Coaches may alter expectations based on the changes in body shapes of early maturers. In particular, maturation affects female athletes in gymnastics, diving, and skating, where smaller body sizes are advantageous. Kristie Phillips was the top American gymnast at the age of 14 when she appeared on the cover of *Sports Illustrated* and was identified as the favorite Olympic medal prospect for the 1988 Games in Seoul. She had won every American competition from 1985 through 1987. However, the onset of puberty and subsequent growth spurt in 1987 hindered her ability to perform at the highest level, and she failed to make the 1988 Olympic team despite her years of training and early success.

Similar to boys, late-maturing girls have a longer period of steady leg growth than early maturers, and generally are taller adults. Early maturers tend to be shorter adults, and early maturation is associated with overweight and obesity in females.

Late-maturing boys and early-maturing girls seem most at risk for discontinuing sport participation for the wrong reasons. Be on the lookout for these individuals, and use your knowledge about maturation to support and encourage their continued sport involvement. Provide them with examples of accomplished athletes who had to negotiate maturational issues but went on to experience success and enjoyment in their sport participation.

Personal Plug-In

Describe Your Maturational Timing

Think back to your adolescence. Were you early, average, or late in maturation as compared to your peers? How did that affect your sport participation in terms of performance and the sport activities that you chose? How did your maturational timing influence your feelings about your body and your overall confidence and self-esteem?

PHYSICAL GROWTH AND MATURATIONAL INFLUENCES ON SPORT OPPORTUNITIES AND PERFORMANCE

Young athletes' physical growth features and maturational status play a big role in their sport performance and opportunities in sport.

Maturational Trends in Sport Types and Positions

Maturational status often predicts who plays which types of sports as well as positions within sports. In youth baseball, players who participated in the Little League World Series and on elite teams were maturationally advanced in height, weight, and skeletal age (French, Spurgeon, & Nevett, 2007; Hale, 1956; Krogman, 1959). In particular, pitchers, shortstops, and first basemen were postpubescent and exhibited larger body sizes than children who played other positions. Turn on ESPN in mid-August and you can observe the advanced maturation of youth baseball players, particularly by position, in the televised Little League World Series.

Similar results were found for junior rugby league players, who were all taller, heavier, and more mature than the normal population (Till, Cobley, O'Hara, Chapman, & Cooke, 2010). Maturational differences were also found between positions, with larger physical attributes and advanced maturation evident among the forwards, whose performance required physical collisions and tackles. In a study of 13- to 15-year-old male Portuguese soccer players, body mass and maturity were predictive of sprinting speed and vertical jump performance (Malina et al., 2004).

An opposite maturational trend in sport participation was shown in figure skating, as late maturation is viewed as advantageous for the smallness and physical linearity needed in subjectively judged sports, where aesthetic appeal is important (Monsma, 2008). Eighty percent of the pre-elite and elite figure skating participants were found to be average or late maturers.

So maturational status often influences the types of sports young athletes choose, the positions they are assigned to in these sports, and their performance abilities. That's fine, as long as all athletes, regardless of maturational level, are provided opportunities to develop their individual talents. Remember that early maturers end up as smaller adults, and premature exclusive sport choices and position assignments may undermine their overall talent development.

Physical Talent Identification

Physical growth and maturational characteristics are often assessed as part of systematic talent identification programs. **Talent identification** is the process of distinguishing (and often selecting) children and youth who demonstrate potential for expertise in a particular sport. For example, Australia and China have systematic talent identification programs for youth sport (discussed in chapter 10). Children are tested and then selected for training in certain sports based on their physical characteristics, which make them most likely to benefit from intensive training in particular sports. Examples include height, body mass, arm span, and hand and foot size.

The idea is to attempt to guide children into sports for which they are physically suited. Because talent identification is not widely practiced, it is often by chance that certain young athletes choose sports that best fit their physical attributes. Michael Phelps was not identified through any systematic program, but consider his physical attributes in relation to the performance demands of swimming (Hadhazy, 2008). He is 6 feet, 4 inches in height (193 centimeters) with a 6-foot, 8-inch arm span (203 centimeters). This height and the extra reach provide an important physical advantage in swimming. He has huge hands and size 14 feet, which can bend 15° farther at the ankle than in most other swimmers, making his feet into virtual flippers. Phelps is the most decorated Olympic swimming champion of all time (18 gold and 22 overall medals). Missy Franklin, another American Olympic and world champion swimmer in multiple events, has similar physical features that enhance her swimming ability. She is 6 feet, 1 inch in height (185 centimeters), with a 6-foot, 4-inch arm span (193 centimeters), and has size 13 feet. Of course, Phelps and Franklin have other characteristics that influence their success as swimmers, including the commitment to training needed to compete at such an elite level. But physically, you could say that they are built for swimming.

There are many popular examples of physical attributes possessed by highly successful athletes. Hall of Fame baseball catcher Johnny Bench could hold seven baseballs in one hand . Height is a prerequisite for elite professional basketball careers, as is physical size in sports like soccer, ice hockey, rugby, and American football. Shorter stature and smaller body size is related to success in gymnastics, diving, and figure skating. Apart from size, such characteristics as muscle fiber type predominance and aerobic capacity are important factors in success in certain types of sports. Overall, talent identification is becoming more sophisticated so that coaches and directors in many sports are prescribing the physical characteristics and body types that are facilitative for skill development in the given sport. The pros and cons of talent identification in youth sport are explored more fully in chapter 10.

The Relative Age Effect

A common practice in youth sport is to group athletes into one-year (11-year-olds) and sometimes two-year (e.g., 11- and 12-year-olds) age groups for teams and leagues. The intent in chronological-age groupings is to provide developmentally appropriate instruction, fair competition, and equal opportunity. However, differences in age between individuals born in the same calendar year, termed **relative age** (Barnsley, Thompson, & Barnsley, 1985), have been shown to have a major effect on the success that kids achieve in sport.

What Is the RAE?

If a youth ice hockey league age eligibility year is January 1 through December 31, a team could have a player born on January 1 (relatively older) and a player born on December 31 (relatively younger). The cutoff date for age eligibility is December 31, and athletes born later in the year (closer to the cutoff date) are relatively younger than athletes born early in the eligibility year. So the potential age difference within any given year grouping is anywhere up to 364 days. Other eligibility years would follow the same pattern, such as a typical youth soccer eligibility year of September 1 to August 31 (August 31 being the cutoff date for age eligibility that year).

These age discrepancies create what is called the **relative age effect (RAE)**, in which athletes born early in an eligibility year (relatively older athletes) are overrepresented on sport teams compared to those athletes born later in the eligibility year (relatively younger athletes). This phenomenon was noticed first in elite ice hockey, where significantly more athletes in the National Hockey League, as well as three elite male junior leagues, were born in the first part of the year (January-March) and significantly fewer were born in the last quarter of the year (October-December) (Barnsley et al., 1985). The RAE has also been found in Canadian women's ice hockey (Weir, Smith, Paterson, & Horton, 2010) and has been shown in Canadian youth ice hockey with players as young as 5 to 8 years old (Hancock, Ste-Marie, & Young, 2013).

The RAE is a worldwide phenomenon and has been seen in soccer, basketball, cricket, rugby, baseball, tennis, volleyball, and swimming (Cobley, Baker, Wattie, & McKenna, 2009; O'Connor, 2011). These are a few examples of the RAE in youth sport:

1. American male elite youth soccer players born in January are over five times as likely to be selected for the national player pool as are boys born in December (Glamser & Vincent, 2004).

2. Seventy-four percent of female Brazilian volleyball players under the age of 14 participating in a national elite tournament were born in the first six months of the eligibility year (Okazaki, Keller, Fontana, & Gallagher, 2011).

3. The birth date distribution of elite male youth soccer athletes in Spain significantly decreased from early in the eligibility year (January-March) to the end of the year (September-December) (Del Campo, Vicedo, Villora, & Jordan, 2010). The RAE was evident for different ages (see figure 4.4), as well as for different positions across ages (see figure 4.5). As with other RAE studies, this distribution differed significantly from the birth date distribution of the general Spanish population. This means that the RAE is an effect above and beyond the typical distribution of births across months of the year.

Why Does the RAE Occur?

Clearly, the RAE is a problem in youth sport. It impedes the personal development of relatively younger athletes and the overall talent development of a community and nation. It creates a structural inequality that benefits or hampers children based on the chance occurrence of the month in which they are born. Why does it occur? We view it as a domino effect.

The first domino in the RAE chain is physical and cognitive maturation. Older kids are bigger, stronger, and faster and have more experience in movement skills and playing the game. This initial advantage turns into an accumulative advantage as subsequent dominoes fall in response to the early-maturational advantage. The older athletes experience more success in their sport, and they receive more attention from coaches and more

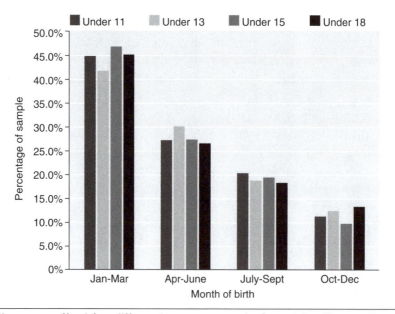

Figure 4.4   Relative age effect for different age groups in Spanish elite youth soccer.

Adapted, by permission, from D.G.D. Del Campo et al., 2010, "The relative age effect in youth soccer players from Spain," *Journal of Sports Science and Medicine* 9: 190-198.

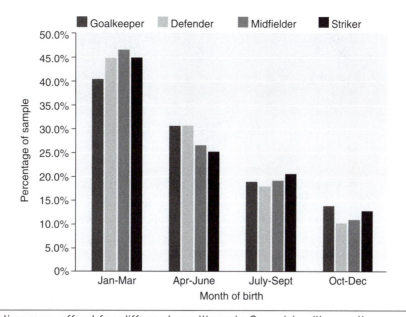

Figure 4.5 Relative age effect for different positions in Spanish elite youth soccer.

Adapted, by permission, from D.G.D. Del Campo et al., 2010, "The relative age effect in youth soccer players from Spain," *Journal of Sports Science and Medicine*, 9: 190-198.

playing time (particularly at key positions). This allows them to qualify for more select teams with stronger competition and better instruction. Based on this early success, older athletes develop greater confidence, perceive that they are more competent, have higher self-esteem, and experience greater motivation than the younger athletes who have fallen farther and farther behind. Consider the double whammy of a young boy who is relatively younger *and* a late maturer—he doesn't have a chance in most sports. Relatively younger athletes, like late-maturing boys, are prime candidates to become discouraged and drop out of youth sport.

How Can We Combat the Unfair RAE?

The RAE is difficult to overcome. In an alternative to chronological-age eligibility cutoffs, athletes could be classified in youth sports based on biological age using some of the assessments discussed previously in the chapter. However, this is largely impractical for youth sport directors and might be unpopular among kids who want to be with their age-group friends.

In large cities with many participants, two or three leagues could be set up, divided by month of birth to lessen the range of age differences. However, this is not feasible in smaller towns and communities where there are not enough youth athletes to be subdivided by relative age. Youth sport directors could rotate cutoff dates from year to year to provide different groups with the relative age advantage. At the very least, different sports should use different eligibility years and cutoff dates to ensure that relative age changes across sports.

The most practical and most important way to combat the unfair RAE is education and awareness. Coaches and teachers must fully understand the possible effects of relative age in youth sport and incorporate this understanding into their philosophies and objectives. This requires the objective of helping each athlete develop her unique abilities, regardless of skill or maturation, to supersede the objective of playing only the better, relatively older kids to ensure winning. Coaches who give players equal time and rotate positions at the youth level are more likely to minimize the RAE on their teams.

Committing to developmentally appropriate practice means understanding the RAE and other maturational influences on kids' participation in youth sport. Not only is it all about the kid—it's all about *each* kid. That includes the late-maturing boys, early-maturing girls, relatively younger athletes, and kids with less developed physical attributes.

WRAP-UP

There's a lot of technical information in this chapter, and you may feel overwhelmed in trying to understand the intricacies of physical growth and maturation. Don't worry about it. Some of the chapter material can be used as a reference if you wish to look back at it later. For now, we want you to have a basic understanding of some important ways in which growth and maturation influence kids in sport and physical activity.

When do kids typically grow the fastest? How does their maturity status influence their abilities to perform in sport, as well as how they feel about themselves? How can you estimate where a kid is in his maturational process? How can you help the early and late maturers in your sport programs, and what kind of help and encouragement do they need? How will you work to combat the inequality of the RAE for younger athletes?

If you can give basic answers to these questions, then you're definitely driving on DAP Avenue. You realize how different youth sport should be from adult sport and consistently use developmentally appropriate practice as a result of your understanding. We hope that's so—and good luck!

LEARNING AIDS

Key Terms

adolescence—The physical, psychological, and social transition from childhood to adulthood.

average maturer—A person whose maturational age is within one year of his chronological age.

biological age—How close people are to their fully mature state (also called maturational age).

chronological age—How old people are based on their particular dates of birth.

development—All the physical and psychological changes that humans undergo over a lifetime.

early maturer—Person whose maturational age is one year greater than her chronological age.

ectomorphic—Referring to a lean and linear physique, or body shape.

endomorphic—Referring to a large and round physique, or body shape.

growth—An increase in size, either of the body as a whole or of specific parts of the body.

late maturer—Person whose maturational age is one year less than his chronological age.

maturation—Progress toward the biologically mature state, or the process one undergoes to reach full adult status in terms of physical, cognitive, and emotional functioning.

menarche—Time of first menstrual period in girls.

mesomorphic—Referring to a muscular physique, or body shape.

peak height velocity (PHV)—The time at which kids are growing the fastest during their adolescent growth spurt.

precocious puberty—When the bodily changes of puberty happen earlier than normal.

puberty—Transitional period between childhood and adulthood; includes the appearance of secondary sex characteristics, maturation of the reproductive system, and the adolescent growth spurt.

relative age—Differences in ages between individuals born in the same calendar year.

relative age effect (RAE)—A phenomenon in which athletes born early in an eligibility year (relatively older athletes) are overrepresented on sport teams compared to those born later in the eligibility year (relatively younger athletes).

secondary sex characteristics—Features that distinguish the two sexes but that are not directly a part of the reproductive system.

sexual maturity—Period during which people have fully functional reproductive capabilities.

skeletal maturity—State achieved when people have fully ossified (hardened bone) adult skeletons.

talent identification—The process of distinguishing (and often selecting) children and youth who demonstrate potential for expertise in a particular sport.

Summary Points

1. Unlike physical growth and maturation, development doesn't stop at a particular age, but continues throughout life.

2. Human growth is S-shaped; the two fastest growing periods are infancy and adolescence.

3. Balance is difficult for very young children due to their high centers of gravity.

4. Research does not support a general decline in coordination, or adolescent awkwardness.

5. Children of the same chronological age can differ in maturation by as much as five years.

6. Maturation may be assessed using x-rays to determine skeletal age, by observation of secondary sex characteristics, and by tracking growth.

7. Puberty is occurring earlier in girls due to obesity, ingestion of animal protein, ingestion of environmental endocrine-disrupting chemicals found in plastic, and certain medical conditions.

8. The brain's prefrontal cortex is not fully developed in teenagers, which makes it harder for them to inhibit emotional impulses, plan and organize behavior, and understand consequences of actions.

9. Early-maturing boys are advantaged in youth sports that rely on strength, speed, and power.

10. Late-maturing boys and girls typically end up as taller adults because they are in the growth period for a longer period of time.

11. Female athletes tend to be late maturers, while early-maturing girls often are more dissatisfied with their body image and may tend to drop out of sport.

12. Maturational status influences who participates in different types of sports as well as positions within sports.

13. The relative age effect creates inequality in youth sport, as relatively older athletes are more physically mature, are more experienced, gain more attention and better instruction from adults, and develop more positive self-perceptions than relatively younger athletes.

Study Questions

1. Explain the differences between development, growth, and maturation.

2. Identify and explain three general principles of physical growth.

3. Identify and explain the general stages and patterns of physical growth.

4. Explain the difference between chronological and biological age.

5. Explain three ways in which biological maturation can be assessed in children and adolescents.

6. Explain the anatomic reasons why teenagers' brains are different from those of adults and how this affects their reasoning and behavior.

7. Describe the physical, psychological, and behavioral characteristics of early- and late-maturing girls and boys. Provide examples of how adults can help these individuals deal with their maturational experiences.

8. Explain what the relative age effect (RAE) is and provide some examples of the RAE in sport. Why does the RAE occur, and what can we do to combat this phenomenon in youth sports?

Reflective Learning Activities

1. Research the relative age effect (RAE) in a specific sport. Develop a brochure or fact sheet for coaches in this sport to educate them about the RAE and to provide them with specific tips on how to overcome the RAE in their teams.

2. Read the four case studies provided in appendix C. For each case description,

   a. identify the child as an early, late, or average maturer;

   b. estimate the child's current biological age;

   c. estimate how tall the child will be as an adult; and

   d. provide some suggestions for how adults might help this child understand his or her unique maturational pattern.

Resource Guide

USA Swimming articles: Patterns of Physical Growth, A Young Athlete's Physical Growth and Development, Sport Participation and Maturation (www.usaswimming.org).

chapter 5

READINESS FOR LEARNING SKILLS AND COMPETING

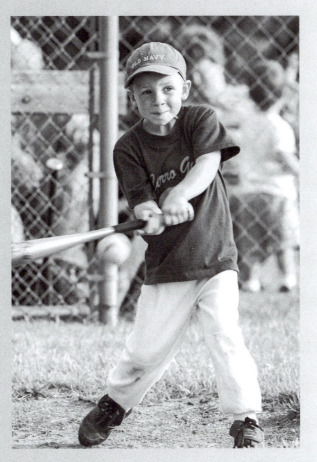

CHAPTER PREVIEW

In this chapter, you'll learn

» about the mountain of motor skill development,

» strategies to build fundamental motor skills in children,

» when and how children should begin learning sport skills, and

» how and when children should begin sport competition.

Tiger Woods, age 20, exploded on the Professional Golfers' Association (PGA) tour in 1996, winning two of his first seven professional tournaments (a very difficult feat on the PGA tour). This came on the heels of six straight national amateur titles as well as the 1996 National Collegiate Athletic Association title. He won the prestigious Masters tournament in 1997, and continued on to win more major golf championships than any other golfer in history except for the legendary Jack Nicklaus. Woods is often described as one of the greatest of all time in the game.

How did Tiger Woods get started in golf? He would hit balls at the driving range at the age of 18 months and afterward fall asleep in his stroller (McCormick & Begley, 1996). Instead of playing in sandboxes, he practiced chipping out of them. He shot a 48 over nine holes (a respectable score for an adult amateur) at age 3. He was a golf prodigy who began practicing as an infant . . . and that is the problem.

Oh, we don't have a problem with Tiger Woods. As golfers ourselves, we have observed his exploits on golf courses around the world with amazement and admiration. The problem is that millions of parents around the world believe that their children can be the next Tiger Woods (or Sidney Crosby or Serena Williams or LeBron James) simply by following the "Tiger formula." That is, start as early and train as hard as possible.

Unfortunately, this formula doesn't fit everyone, or even most kids. Not every child is ready to begin sport at such a young age. Tiger Woods' parents describe how he was infatuated with golf even as a baby. He would sit and watch from his highchair as his father took practice swings in their garage. He began swinging on his own at 10 months, and throughout infancy and early childhood he would beg his father to take him to the driving range. This is uncommon motivation, which cannot be taught or forced. Woods' father, Earl, admits in his book titled *Training a Tiger* (Woods, 1997)

that "arbitrary imposition of the game is guaranteed to bring about negative results (p. 17)," and that "sometimes no matter how good your intentions, your child might show no interest in [a sport]" (p. 19). Karrie Webb, Ladies Professional Golf Association Hall of Fame member, started playing at age 8, and Greg Norman (another World Golf Hall of Famer) didn't hit a golf ball until age 15. Norman is an exception in terms of lateness to the game, as is Woods in terms of his exceptionally early start.

When should children begin sport participation? When are they ready to learn sport skills? And when are they ready to use these skills in competition? Although there is no one formula to follow, our intent in this chapter is to provide you with information that you can use to answer these questions. You'll understand that each kid has her own unique "formula" to consider in terms of when she is ready for youth sport.

WHAT IS READINESS?

Readiness is the state of being prepared for something. In youth sport, **readiness** is a developmental point at which a child has the capacity to successfully learn or engage in a certain activity. That activity might be a specific sport skill—for example, when a child is ready to learn to ice-skate. But readiness also applies to the following questions. When is he ready to skate with a hockey stick and puck? Can he skate backward as well as forward? Can he control the puck well enough to succeed in certain drills and activities? Is he ready to play hockey in competition, with opponents and tactical strategies and with spectators watching? Should he join a select club or stay at the recreational level? We need to not only assess youth athletes' readiness when they begin sport participation, but also continue to assess their readiness for different challenges and types of activities as they move through youth sport.

Three factors need to be considered to determine when a child is ready to engage in an activity: maturation, prerequisite skills, and motivation (Magill & Anderson, 1996). As illustrated in figure 5.1, the three components are like the wheels on a tricycle—all three are necessary to ensure that a child is ready for a given activity.

Maturation

Children are smaller and shorter than adults, with less strength, power, and coordination. They may not be physically mature enough to pitch a softball with speed and accuracy, shoot a basketball at a 10-foot (3-meter) rim, or kick a soccer ball into the goal from beyond the penalty box. In addition, children's cognitive (mental) processes are maturing. A child may be physically mature enough to hit and throw a ball but not cognitively mature enough to understand the tactics and strategy of tee ball. As former tee ball coaches, we know this all too well. Many children would run over first base into right field, have no idea where to go when they rounded first base, or have no idea

what to do with the ball when they fielded it on defense.

Parents, teachers, coaches, and youth sport directors should carefully consider the maturational demands of different motor or sport activities, and attempt to introduce these activities at the most optimal times. Motor skill competency is gained through repeated practice of a skill that is initially not well learned, and errors naturally occur in the learning process. However, adults must distinguish between errors that are part of learning from errors that result from children's lack of maturational abilities to perform a skill. It's okay to try an activity, only to observe that children are not ready, and then reintroduce the activity later when they are more mature. We were excited to take our kids ice-skating when they were 4 and 6 years old. They couldn't stand up without falling, hated it, and cried about being sopping wet from falling on the ice. Not a particularly good assessment of their readiness! However, we tried it again a year later, and they did fine and loved it. They were ready when they were ready, and not before.

Prerequisite Skills

Maturation is important, but by itself it's not enough to ensure readiness. It may be that a 12-year-old girl has the physical and cognitive maturation to play softball, but her lack of throwing ability and catching and striking skills are major obstacles to her successful participation in this sport. All sports have prerequisite skills that young athletes have to master to be good at that sport. **Prerequisite** means "required beforehand." Ice hockey players must be good skaters, golfers need good eye–hand coordination, and divers must have good posture and balance—all these skills are required before they can become proficient at those sports. Our job as parents and youth sport leaders is to design programs so that kids develop the prerequisite skills to be successful in sport. That means spending time on developing

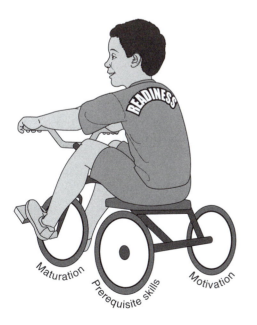

Figure 5.1   The three essential wheels of readiness.

skills, as opposed to rushing children into competitive situations before they have the skills needed to compete (see "The Spartak Tennis Way").

A limitation of youth soccer in the United States is the focus on competition, team play, and winning over early individual skill development (Farrey, 2008). A youth development coach explains, "The key period in development is at an early age when their acquisition of skills is so important. But in this country that is not emphasized at the appropriate age or time in development. What's appropriate for kids is not winning

Water Break

The Spartak Tennis Way

Russia has become a hotbed for producing world-class tennis players, and nowhere is that more evident than at the Spartak Tennis Club in Moscow. Spartak is not a showplace like many sport academies—it is a run-down facility with one indoor court and 15 outdoor clay courts that are frozen half of the year in the winter climate of Russia. No matter. In recent years, the club has produced more top-20 women players than the entire United States has.

The teaching philosophy of Spartak can be summed up in one word: *tekhnika* (technique). The main focus is on learning the prerequisite skills that lead to outstanding tennis. Some examples from the lesson with 5- to 7-year-olds ("Little Group") taught by legendary youth coach Larisa Preobrazhenskaya:

- Warm-up: Fifteen minutes of stretching, calisthenics, agility drills, passing medicine balls, and simple eye–hand drills in which the children bounce the ball and catch it.

- *Imitatsiya* (imitating): Rallying with partners using an imaginary ball; bouncing lightly from foot to foot, turning and swinging, with Preobrazhenskaya roaming the court and

correcting technique (often by grasping the kids' arms and piloting their bodies through the correct stroke). The point is to focus on making the correct swing, which is easier to do when there is no ball to distract the child. Preobrazhenskaya states, "All the motions. It is important to do everything, every practice" (Coyle, 2007, p. 5).

- Slow motion: Practicing the various tennis strokes in slow motion for correct technique.

Students at Spartak are not permitted to play in competition for the first three years in the program. "Technique is everything," states Preobrazhenskaya. "If you begin playing without technique, it is [a] big mistake. Big, big mistake!" (Coyle, 2007, p. 7). Preobrazhenskaya didn't instruct Little Group members on tactics or positioning or offer any psychological tips. All of her focus and energy were directed toward teaching the basic task of hitting the tennis ball cleanly and with pace. Obviously, the "Spartak way" focuses on developing the prerequisite skills that lead to tennis excellence, and the results are impressive.

games and tournaments. Soccer is a skill game, and [that requires] a lot of time on the ball in an environment where an adult really shouldn't be doing much more than cultivating creativity. The ball itself is the best coach there could be" (Schaerlaeckens, 2012). Another outstanding youth soccer coach notes, "It's a mistake to yell at the kids to pass, pass, pass. Young players need to try to dribble. If I get an older player who always wants to dribble, it's not that difficult to encourage or teach him to pass. But it's impossible to teach a player to become a good dribbler who didn't have a chance to dribble when he was young" (Woitalla, 2014).

Professional basketball superstar Kobe Bryant explains the advantage he received by not playing youth basketball in the United States, where competition was emphasized over skill development. He states, "I feel fortunate that I was over in Italy [from ages 6 to 13] when AAU basketball [got big] over here. They stopped teaching kids fundamentals in the United States, but that didn't affect me. Over there, it wasn't about competition and traveling around and being a big deal; it was about fundamentals, footwork, spacing, back cuts – all of those things" (McCollum, 2013, p. 39). Learning the basic, prerequisite skills before emphasizing competition is an important guideline to follow to ensure competent skill development—and more success in subsequent competitive events.

Motivation

The third essential wheel on the readiness tricycle is motivation. It won't matter if children have the maturational readiness and adequate prerequisite skills for an activity unless they have the motivation to do it. **Motivation** is the desire, intent, or drive to do something. Many times, kids get excited to try a sport that they have observed, and they enjoy the activity and wish to continue participating. However, it is unrealistic to assume that young children will know what activities they wish to attempt. Childhood

should be about sampling different activities, to see which fits a child best and which the child prefers. Parents should introduce their children to multiple sport activities. Our experience as parents has been to sometimes even insist that our children try an activity (which they initially resisted and complained about) only to see them fall in love with that sport and develop strong internal motivation to continue participation. Motivation is a complex process and is discussed more fully in chapter 6.

THE MOUNTAIN OF MOTOR SKILL DEVELOPMENT

Children are ready for activities when they (a) are physically and cognitively mature enough to be successful, (b) have the prerequisite skills for the activity, and (c) are motivated to try it. But how do kids acquire sport skills? Are there certain things they should learn first or a certain order to be followed in their development?

Just as there is a pattern to how kids physically grow and mature (discussed in chapter 4), there is also an overall pattern to how kids develop motor skills. Remember that *motor* in this sense means movement. Let's first define terms you'll need to know. **Motor skills** are learned movements that combine to produce smooth, efficient actions to complete particular tasks. For example, walking, eating, writing, throwing, climbing and descending stairs, shooting a basketball, serving a tennis ball, and landing a triple axel in figure skating are all motor skills.

Gross motor skills involve movements of the entire body or major parts of the body—for example, jumping, running, and kicking a soccer ball. **Fine motor skills** require precise movement using smaller muscle groups, such as writing or preparing to release an arrow in archery. Many sports use both gross and fine motor skills (e.g., pitching a baseball, gripping and swinging a golf club, receiving a soccer pass, and dribbling against an opponent).

Motor skills may also be differentiated into locomotor, manipulative, and stability skills. **Locomotor skills** involve moving the body through space, as in walking, running, and jumping. **Manipulative skills** (also called object control skills) involve moving or projecting objects (throwing, dribbling) as well as receiving objects (catching, receiving a soccer ball or hockey puck). **Stability skills** (also called body control skills) involve maintaining body position against forces of gravity, such as holding a position while on a balance beam, in diving, or during figure skating.

So, what is the pattern by which these various types of motor skills are developed, and how does this lead to competence, even expertise, in sport? Think of it as

the **"mountain" of motor skill development** (figure 5.2), where various types of motor skills are developed in a particular order within specific developmental levels (Clark & Metcalf, 2002; Horn & Butt, 2014; Ulrich, 1987). These developmental levels are numbered in figure 5.2 and labeled with approximate ages, although there is overlap between levels and variation among individuals.

Infants, children, and adolescents don't climb the mountain of motor skill development without some help. That is, motor skills don't magically develop and appear based on just maturation. The environment around children has a powerful influence on how they move. Humans are born with preadapted motor behaviors that predispose certain reflexes and basic movements, but these movements are

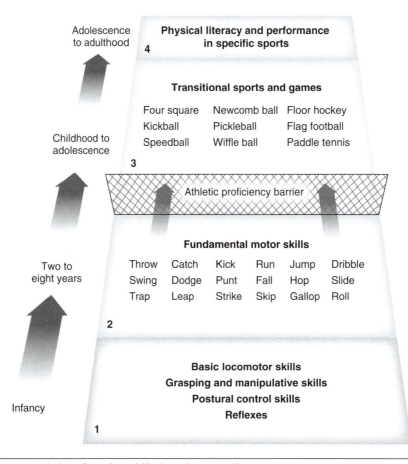

Figure 5.2   The mountain of motor skill development.

Based on Clark and Metcalf 2002; Horn and Butt 2014; Ulrich 1987.

reinforced or modified by the surrounding environment and the learning process (Haibach, Reid, & Collier, 2011). Parents and other adults should be mindful of a child's motor development and provide a variety of developmentally appropriate experiences to support and help children develop a wide variety of motor skills as they move up the mountain.

Level 1: Reflexes and Basic Physical Control Skills

Level 1 of the mountain of motor skill development represents infancy, from birth to about 2 years. This developmental period is characterized by the orderly appearance and subsequent disappearance of numerous **reflexes,** or involuntary movements that infants make in response to specific stimuli (e.g., palmar grasp reflex). The orderly sequencing of these reflexes helps parents and pediatricians assess normal physical development in infants. Postural control skills (e.g., rolling over, sitting up, standing upright) and basic locomotor skills (e.g., creeping, crawling, walking) are important motor milestones observed in all infants as they begin to interact with the environment in goal-directed movements. The other aspect of motor development in level 1 is grasping and manipulative skills, or reaching for, grabbing, and manipulating objects such as toys. Manipulative toys and opportunities and space for the development of basic locomotor skills enhance children's motor development at this stage.

Level 2: Fundamental Motor Skills

At level 2 in our mountain of motor skill development, children should learn to perform a wide variety of basic locomotor, manipulative, and stability skills, called fundamental motor skills. **Fundamental motor skills** are the basic motor movements that are minute parts of all sport skills. They are termed fundamental because they serve as the building blocks for children's learning of more sport-specific skills. Multiple examples of these building blocks are shown in figure 5.2, including throwing, catching, jumping, hopping, and striking. Other fundamental skills important to this phase are fine motor skills; eye–hand coordination; eye–foot coordination; balance; agility (ability to change directions while maintaining balance); and information processing and decision making, such as scanning and selecting the appropriate cues in games and play (Horn & Butt, 2014). These fundamental skills are critical prerequisites for children's sport participation—one of the wheels of the readiness tricycle shown in figure 5.1.

Importance of Reaching the Mature Stage of Fundamental Motor Skills Development

You may have looked at the list of fundamental motor skills in figure 5.2 and thought, "Well, those are easy. Everyone knows how to run, catch, jump, and so on." Yes, we can all do those things, but how well? It is important for children to become proficient at the most mature level in multiple fundamental motor skills. This is like the foundation of a house. If the foundation is not solid and strongly built, the house can be lived in, but it will develop faults and cracks and sag in places. Similarly, children with underdeveloped fundamental motor skills will be able to engage in sport skills as they age; but they will be disadvantaged, and their sport performance will not be solid or as strong as that of others who have proficient, mature levels of fundamental skills.

Children's first attempts at performing fundamental motor skills are, well, not too skilled. In what is called the *initial stage,* kids' first attempts at movements lack proper sequencing and use poor rhythm, with either exaggerated or restricted body movements

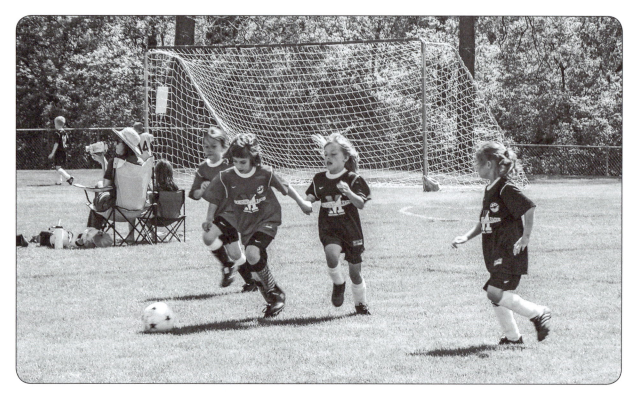

To avoid the athletic proficiency barrier, kids need to develop mature movement patterns in a wide array of fundamental motor skills between the ages of 2 and 10 years.

(Gallahue, Ozmun, & Goodway, 2012). Visualize the high bounces and lack of control of a typical 3-year-old dribbling a basketball in this initial stage compared to a high school basketball player who dribbles with much greater dexterity, control, and smooth movement. Next is the *elementary stage,* in which there is greater control and better rhythmical coordination of fundamental movements (Gallahue et al., 2012). However, patterns of movement in the elementary stage are still restricted or exaggerated. A common example of the elementary stage is seen in children who attempt the overarm throw but fail to rotate their trunk and shoulders (see table 5.1 and figure 5.3). Many individuals, adults and children, fail to get beyond the elementary stage in overarm throwing, as well as in other fundamental motor skills (Gallahue et al., 2012).

The *mature stage* in a fundamental motor skill is characterized by mechanically efficient, coordinated, and controlled

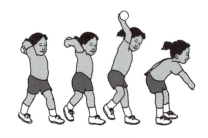

Figure 5.3 A beginning thrower. Note the trunk flexion, rather than rotation, with the throw.

Reprinted from K. Haywood and N. Getchell, 2009, *Life span motor development,* 6th ed. (Champaign, IL: Human Kinetics). Drawn from film tracings taken in the Motor Development and Child Study Laboratory, University of Wisconsin-Madison and now available from the Motor Development Film Collection, Kinesiology Division, Bowling Green State University. © Mary Ann Roberton and Kate R. Barrett.

performance. The previous example of the high school basketball player dribbling with deftness, control, and automaticity is a mature form of dribbling. We've used the example of overarm throwing in table 5.1 to illustrate the different levels of proficiency from the initial to the mature stage (adapted from Haywood & Getchell, 2009).

Table 5.1 Examples of Initial to Mature Stages of Proficiency in Overarm Throwing

TRUNK ACTION	
Initial	No trunk action; only the arm is used in propelling the ball, or the trunk flexes forward at the hips (see figure 5.3 for illustration of this action)
Elementary	Upper trunk rotation or total trunk "block" rotation
Mature	Differentiated rotation; thrower twists away from target line and then starts forward rotation, with pelvis first and upper body following in sequence
ARM BACKSWING	
Initial	No backswing
Elementary	Circular, upward backswing
Mature	Circular, downward backswing
ACTION OF THE FEET WHILE THROWING	
Initial	No step
Elementary	Homolateral step; thrower steps with foot on same side as throwing hand
Mature	Contralateral step; thrower steps with the foot on the opposite side from the throwing hand

Adapted from K.M. Haywood and N. Getchell, 2009, *Life span motor development,* 5th ed. (Champaign, IL: Human Kinetics).

Avoiding the Athletic Proficiency Barrier

It is extremely important that children acquire mature movement patterns in multiple fundamental motor skills during their childhood years. As an example of their importance, a mature pattern of overarm throwing is needed not only to competently play baseball or softball, but also as the foundational movement to serve and hit an overhead smash in tennis, as well as to serve and spike in volleyball (Horn & Butt, 2014).

Developing a broad repertoire of fundamental motor skills provides more options for young athletes when learning skills and training for sport—they become more physically well-rounded with multiple movement capabilities. An Australian women's professional basketball coach states, "Basketball requires a high level of fundamental ball skill development. However, if the players have poor body balance [and] lack agility, explosive power, and lateral quickness, then trying to develop these skills when they are well into their teens makes their progression difficult" (Cooke, 2006). Many motor development experts state that competence in fundamental motor skills is essential if individuals are to remain active over the course of their lives, and we wholeheartedly agree.

However, fundamental motor skill development doesn't occur just through maturation. Children need opportunities for practice, play, instruction, and encouragement to develop these skills. Without such opportunities, children run into the athletic proficiency barrier (Seefeldt, 1980). As shown in figure 5.2, the **athletic proficiency barrier** impedes children's abilities to move from the fundamental motor skill stage and achieve athletic success as they transition into more formal sports and games. Children with undeveloped or even underdeveloped fundamental motor skills will fail to achieve the same levels of athletic proficiency in sports as their peers who have mature patterns of these skills. The black arrows in figure 5.2 represent children's abilities to traverse the proficiency barrier through the development of a wide variety of mature fundamental motor skills. Timing is important in terms of when individuals develop fundamental motor skills. Notice that fundamental motor skill development is recommended from ages 2 to 8. Although this may extend a few years beyond age 8, it is much more difficult to develop mature patterns of these skills after childhood.

Thus, the athletic proficiency barrier occurs when mature patterns of fundamental motor skills are not developed due to a lack of opportunity or practice during the optimal learning time of childhood. Without these skills, kids are unlikely to become involved in sport, and if they do try, they are likely to drop out due to the frustration of not having the prerequisite fundamental skills to be successful. Think of this as the "if you can't, you won't" principle (Balyi, Way, & Higgs, 2013). If you can't run, you won't play soccer, basketball, rugby, or tennis. If you can't throw, you won't play baseball, softball, football, or water polo or go bowling. If you can't swim, you won't participate in surfing, swimming, kayaking, and sailing. The "if you can't, you won't" principle emphasizes the essential nature of fundamental skill development in young children.

Strategies to Help Children Develop Fundamental Motor Skills

Helping children traverse the athletic proficiency barrier requires adults to provide opportunities, encouragement, and instruction for fundamental motor skill development. Here are some specific strategies to follow when children are between the ages of 2 and 10 years:

1. Provide children access to large, open spaces (parks, yards, gyms, pools).
2. Allow children to spend time at active playgrounds with different types of physically challenging equipment.
3. Design fun obstacle courses (indoors and outdoors) so that kids have to run, jump, climb, crawl, creep, hop, roll, walk backward, balance, leap, and use fine motor skills (e.g., moving and replacing bowling pins) to complete the course.
4. Purchase physical activity equipment for play and games at home (balls, hula hoops, bats, goals, Frisbees, bicycles, scooters, skates, and active toys).
5. Play with your child. Wrestle, play tag (and all its variations), play catch, ride bikes, go skating, play kickball and four square. Be creative. We played a lot of balloon volleyball over the coffee table in the living room, as well as beach ball soccer in the basement. Engage in fun physical activities as a family every day, and create an expectation that your family be physically active.
6. Set up play dates with other kids. Host them at your house with planned activities that are fun and physically challenging.
7. Look for instructional motor skill development programs, which differ from organized youth sport teams. These programs are offered by community recreation departments and sometimes by universities. The focus should be on developing skills in a mastery-oriented (not competitive) environment. For example, the National Alliance for Youth Sports (NAYS) sponsors the Start Smart Sports Development Program, which brings parents and children age 3 to 5 years together to learn the fundamental and prerequisite motor skills for the sports of baseball, soccer, basketball, golf, football, and tennis. Youth sport programs can order the different Start Smart programs from NAYS, and at-home programs are also available for parents to purchase (www.nays.org).
8. Guide children to sample or participate in a variety of physical activities at a young age. For example, introductory dance and gymnastics classes are excellent for both girls and boys to develop body control and movement skills.

CLIPBOARD

Strategies to Teach Overarm Throwing to Kids

The four key elements you're looking for are (1) downward-starting backswing, (2) contralateral step, (3) diagonal follow-through, and (4) trunk rotation and derotation. Children need practice; research has shown that not until age 10 were 60% of children able to demonstrate these four key elements in the mature overarm throw (Ulrich, 1985).

One strategy is to use the cue words "nose, toes, show, and throw." The following are good instructions: First, hold the ball in front of you and away from your body (up by your nose). Then bring the ball down by your thigh toward your toes. (This gets the backswing started downward.) Next, bring the ball backward and upward until it's behind your shoulder. Here is where you show the ball to someone behind you, by cocking your wrist. From here, snap your arm forward to throw the ball.

In a variation, you can use these instructions: Start by pointing to the target with your non-throwing hand. Think about a laser beam in your belly button. Open your hips toward your throwing side or turn your laser beam directly to the side (90° from your target line). Bend your elbow on your throwing hand, keeping it as high as your shoulder (think scarecrow). Cock your pistol to hold the ball with a cocked wrist. Bring your throwing arm forward as you close the hips forward and shine your laser beam at your target by stepping forward on your nonthrowing foot. Snap your floppy wrist when letting go of the ball. Follow through with your throwing thumb pointed to the ground outside your front foot.

Other strategies and videos are available on the Internet. Teachers, coaches, and parents should understand that getting to a mature throwing pattern is a developmental process and that it doesn't happen in one session. Continually playing catch with children and providing tips and feedback will help them refine their throwing pattern. But keep it simple and make it fun (throwing rocks in a creek, playing gutter ball at the pool, playing dodgeball), and provide only small amounts of instruction and feedback, so they'll enjoy it and want to continue.

9. Help kids develop fine motor skills using activities such as coloring; building with blocks, Legos, or Tinker Toys; using scissors and paste or glue to make pictures or objects; and self-help activities like putting on socks and shoes as well as buttoning and zipping clothes.

10. Don't make fundamental skill development all about structured, systematic practice. A better strategy is to create the conditions under which young children are drawn to engage in exploratory and enjoyable physical play (Balyi et al., 2013). Think *play, not practice* to keep the right mindset for this stage of development.

Levels 3 and 4: From Transitional Sports and Games to Physical Literacy and Specific Sport Skills

To complete the mountain of motor development (see figure 5.2), it is preferential for children to engage in modified sports and activities to serve as a transition to adult sport participation. Examples, provided in figure 5.2, include lead-up games like four square, kickball, and floor hockey. Most organized youth sports are modified for kids, as they should be in order to match children's maturational and skill development needs (see chapter 7). The fundamental motor skills that were developed for their own sake are now applied to transitional sports and games so that children may continue to develop their skills.

Successfully navigating levels 1 to 3 up the mountain of motor skill development leads to the ability to successfully perform in specific sports and to be physically literate. **Physical literacy** is the physical competence, motivation, confidence, understanding, and knowledge to maintain physical activity at an individually appropriate level throughout life (Whitehead & Murdock, 2006, as cited in Balyi et al., 2013). Physical literacy provides a range of options at level 4 so that individuals can try and succeed in many different sports and activities across their lives.

Parents may look at the mountain of motor skills development and target one specific sport at level 4 for their child to excel at. Clearly, people grow to love certain sports over others and choose to spend time training for those specific sports. But the goal of physical literacy—to have a broad repertoire of fundamental skills and the agility, balance, and coordination to successfully participate in many activities—is the ultimate goal of the mountain of motor skills development. This is the best investment adults can make toward a child's lifelong commitment to physical activity. And as you'll learn in chapter 10, overspecializing at an early age without developing a broad physical literacy can actually hurt athletes' performance in their specialized sports. Youth sport leaders need to be committed to helping each athlete take the next developmental step on his path up the mountain of motor skill development toward the ultimate goal of physical literacy and lifelong opportunities to participate in multiple physical activities.

SENSITIVE PERIODS IN MOTOR SKILL DEVELOPMENT

As portrayed in the mountain of motor development (see figure 5.2), it is advantageous for fundamental motor skills to be learned during early and middle childhood (approximately 2-8 years). This is a **sensitive period,** a limited time period in development when the effect of a specific experience on the brain is particularly strong. A great example of a sensitive period has to do with second-language learning—an earlier start to training results in greater language proficiency later in life. You may know people who grew up speaking a second language in their home as a child, and this language development was much easier for them than trying to acquire a second language in high school or college. The same is true for learning sport skills.

Sensitive Periods as Optimal Readiness Periods

This important time of motor skill development is sometimes referred to as a *critical period.* However, neuroscientists view critical periods as highly restricted time periods when appropriate stimulation and experiences are required for the normal development of the brain and behavior (Knudsen, 2004). *Critical* in this sense means that an important function cannot be acquired outside a specific developmental window. The development of vision is an example of something that occurs during a critical period. Unless an infant sees light during the first six months of life, the nerves leading from the eye to the visual cortex of the brain, which processes these signals, will

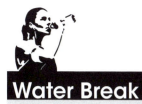

Michael Jordan's Professional Baseball Experiment

In the spring of 1993, Michael Jordan stunned the sports world by announcing his retirement from professional basketball. He had just led the Chicago Bulls to their third straight National Basketball Association (NBA) Championship and had achieved every possible honor in the game of basketball, including multiple MVP awards, scoring titles, All-Star teams, and Olympic gold medals. Even more stunning was Jordan's declaration that he had signed a contract with the Chicago White Sox to play professional baseball.

Playing for Chicago's Double A minor league team, he was an adequate defensive player, and was able to steal bases and leg out infield hits with his speed. However, becoming a professional baseball hitter was beyond the capability of even a great athlete like Jordan. His final batting average was .202, and he struck out 28.4% of the time. What is the reason such a talented and explosive athlete like Michael Jordan could not hit even moderately well in professional baseball? The answer lies in his early brain development.

Harold Klawans, physician and professor of neurology, stated in his book *Why Michael Couldn't Hit* (1996), "The neurologist in me knew he could never make the grade as a major league baseball player.

[He] would not be able to hit a baseball well enough to play competitively at the major league level. His inability to hit would be the direct result of a neurological problem. . . . Hitting successfully is not a pure muscular skill. . . . It is a visual-motor skill, and like all other skills it has to be learned. The brain has to learn how to recognize the spin and speed and direction of the ball as it leaves the pitcher's hand, and then to swing the bat at just the right speed and in precisely the proper location to hit the ball solidly. This is a tall order for anyone's brain. And the sad fact is that at age 31, Michael Jordan's brain was too old to acquire this skill" (pp. 4-5).

Jordan's window of opportunity, or sensitive period, for learning to hit a baseball had closed when he was a child. Oh, he could play recreational softball and be successful, but hitting a major league fastball that travels from the pitcher's hand to the plate in .041 seconds is one of the most difficult visual–motor skills in sport. Jordan's exceptional basketball talents were the result of his practice and play early in life, when he was still developing synaptic networks. Jordan recognized that his sensitive period for learning baseball had passed, and he returned to the NBA, where he promptly won three more NBA championships.

degenerate and die. Most critical periods are under genetic control, as with the development of vision, while sensitive periods have more flexible time frames and are strongly influenced by experience (Penhune, 2011).

Therefore, *sensitive period* is the term most applicable to the importance of developing fundamental motor skills, eye–hand and eye–foot coordination, body control, fine motor skills, and other similar skill-related building blocks during the early and middle childhood years. Sensitive periods of skill development may also be thought of as optimal readiness periods, meaning that children are optimally ready to learn a particular skill (Magill & Anderson, 1996). Skills learned during this time are learned more easily and with less training, which typically leads to greater proficiency in adolescence and adulthood. However, we can't definitively state that motor skills will never be learned if not learned in the sensitive period. Rather, this is just the best, most fertile, easiest time to learn these skills—the time when the window of opportunity is most wide open. It is much harder to develop these skills later. And why is that? The answer lies in how our brains develop.

Neural Wiring and Early Brain Development

Brain development, or learning, is actually the process of creating, strengthening, and discarding synapses, or connections between neurons. Synapses organize the brain by forming pathways connecting parts of the brain that control everything we do. Brain development is activity dependent, meaning that those synapses that are formed and consistently used over time are strengthened, while those that are not used are pruned away by the brain (cells that "fire together, wire together"). This pruning may sound harsh, but it's an essential part of healthy brain development that streamlines children's neural processing and makes the remaining circuits work more quickly

and efficiently. Pruning, or the selection of active neural circuits, takes place throughout life, but it is far more common in early childhood.

Multiple experiences in physical activities and motor skill practice early in children's lives are important to wire their brains in ways that facilitate their athletic development. The main window of opportunity for the development of gross and fine motor skills is from 1 to 9 years, as the general window for most motor functions narrows considerably around age 10 (Chugani, 1998). As discussed earlier, the window does not close completely (as in critical periods), but it does narrow, thus creating a more difficult challenge for developing basic motor skills at a later age.

Beyond synapse development and pruning, another important process that takes place in the developing brain is myelination. **Myelin** is the white fatty tissue that insulates the nerve fibers in the brain to ensure clear transmission across synapses. Young children process information more slowly because their brains lack the myelin necessary for fast, clear nerve impulse transmission. The thicker the myelin gets, the better it insulates and the faster and more accurately the signals that control movement travel. And how do we increase our myelin? Experience and practice. With each repetition, athletes thicken their myelin sheath for an activity. They build more insulation and thus more precision, skill, and speed. Although some myelin is genetically developed, the myelination for motor or sport skills is dependent on activity (Coyle, 2007; Fields, 2005). And although adults retain the ability to produce myelin throughout life, it takes more effort and happens at a slower rate than in children.

Overall, then, the developing brain first creates connections (synapses) that control the execution of motor skills. By actively engaging in different fundamental motor and sport skills, children create a motorically wired brain, so to speak. And through continued sport skill development and repetitive practice, young athletes produce myelin to turbo-charge their motorically wired brains. The optimal time for this wiring and turbo-charging process is in early to middle childhood. Although we retain some brain plasticity throughout our lives, the most sensitive period for developing a brain wired for sport is in childhood.

COGNITIVE READINESS

Cognitive readiness refers to children's abilities to understand the technical and strategic requirements of a sport, particularly their abilities to process relevant information about their performance and the sport environment. Sport performance is a function of motor skill execution (being able to set a volleyball) and cognitive decision making (knowing which sets to deliver to which hitters at what times). So, along with the physical maturation and physical skills prerequisite for sport participation, children's cognitive development influences their readiness for different types of sport activities.

Nonexpert children (those not participating in junior elite sport) differ from older athletes in their cognitive capacities for sport (Haywood & Getchell, 2009). They

- have less "how to do it" knowledge, as well as less strategic knowledge, because they have fewer experiences in sports;
- use considerable mental activity to think about how to do the skill, as opposed to more experienced athletes, who can perform skills automatically;
- are less able to predict and anticipate objects and events;
- are less able to recognize patterns (e.g., the other team's defensive strategies);
- often fail to preplan their responses to specific situations in sport; and
- make slower and less accurate decisions in sport.

Through experience and effective teaching, children become more cognitively proficient, which enhances their performance abilities in sport. Coaches can teach children attentional strategies such as the planning and rehearsal examples in the Water Break study with baseball shortstops. A useful cognitive strategy to teach children is **labeling,** the use of a verbal label or cue to provide a mental image of the correct performance (also known as instructional cues). Earlier in the chapter, we used the "nose, toes, shows, throws" example as a colorful way to remind children of the correct overarm throwing technique. I (first author) remember saying "right, left, right" continuously as I attempted to learn and automate the footwork required for a left-handed layup in basketball. Labels improve learning and performance, and children as young as 5 years can benefit from the use of labels. An effective teaching strategy is to help kids attach simple, colorful labels to sport skills and then use those labels to rehearse the correct technique before practicing the skill.

IS EARLIER BETTER?

The belief that earlier is better is ingrained in popular sport culture; another expression for this is the race to the bottom, referring to the continuing decrease in starting age for youth sport participation (Farrey, 2008). There is considerable debate about this issue, and a simple yes or no answer without qualification is not possible. Here are our three postulates about this issue:

1. Earlier is better for most kids when we are talking about fundamental motor skill development (i.e., it is important to develop these skills in early childhood).

2. What kids do at an early age is more important than when they start.

3. Earlier can be better for some kids (but worse for others) with regard to organized sport participation.

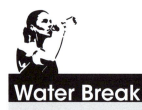

What Do Youth Baseball Shortstops Think About?

An interesting study of cognitive readiness examined what youth baseball shortstops (ages 8, 10, 12, and high school) thought about before the ball was to be pitched to an opposing batter (Nevett & French, 1997). The shortstops talked into a recording device attached to the back of their waists while they were also videotaped. They were instructed to say aloud whatever thoughts were in their heads when playing defense, and they followed this procedure throughout the game.

The high school shortstops (more expert) decided on their defensive plays in advance, chose more high-quality plays, and engaged in more sophisticated mental rehearsal of their plans. In **rehearsal** athletes visualize or talk through a planned movement or strategy either out loud or in their heads prior to executing the skill. The shortstops who were 12 years old and younger did not plan as much in advance, generated weak plans, and did not rehearse or else used less mature forms of rehearsal.

For example, with runners at first and second base, high school shortstops planned and rehearsed like this: "If it's to my right, go to third; if it's up the middle, go to second for the double play." Younger shortstops thought "throw the ball to any base" or "get the out at second." Often, the younger shortstops simply engaged in baseball "chatter" statements (a cultural part of baseball, such as "hey batter, batter"), which was irrelevant to planning their own performance.

Based on these findings, how could coaches help young shortstops plan and focus more effectively? The players could

be taught to monitor the situation (how many outs, how many base runners) and then generate a plan before each pitch. Coaches could teach the players to relax their attention momentarily between pitches, but then, each time before the pitch was to be delivered, to actively rehearse (say out loud or to themselves) what they would do if the ball was hit to them. Simply telling kids to pay attention is not enough. We have to teach them *how* to pay attention or what to pay attention to in different sport situations.

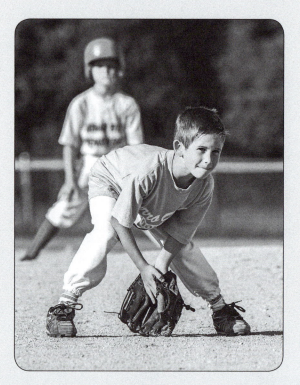

Youth shortstops (12 years and younger) did not plan their defensive plays in advance nor did they mentally rehearse what to do prior to each pitch, while high school shortstops used cognitive planning and mental rehearsal prior to each pitch.

According to the mountain of motor development, early exposure to a wide variety of gross and fine motor skills from birth to late childhood is essential for the motor development that precedes sport skill development and physical literacy. So, in this regard, can it ever be too early to play with your child and introduce him to fun physical activities and develop a wide repertoire of fundamental movement skills? Typically, no. However, remember the readiness formula of maturation + prerequisite skills + motivation = readiness. Some children who are less physically mature may not be ready to roller skate or throw a ball as early as other kids. Some children may not want to try jumping off a diving board as early as other kids due to fear or lack of motivation. That's fine. They're not ready, and they should be given some time to increase their personal readiness.

Additionally, we know that children's brains are most susceptible to motor skill learning in childhood, which also supports the idea of early is better in motor skill development. That is, starting early ensures that children are taking advantage of a short-term window of opportunity in which they are most ripe for learning motor skills. But remember that it is a *window*, or a period of months or even a year, and not a race out of the gate on their second birthday to force them into motor skill activities just because that is when motor development experts say to start.

The problem with the phrase *earlier is better* is that some parents interpret it to mean that the earlier a child joins a competitive youth sport team, the better it is. A youth sport parent experienced this urgency when she attempted to enroll her 7-year-old daughter in a youth softball program. She explained, "When we started our daughter, she didn't play mini-ball, and they basically said, if she didn't play mini-ball, then forget about signing her up. And she was seven. It was like her career was over because she didn't start at age five" (Wiersma & Fifer, 2008, p. 520). The idea that earlier is better in terms of joining a youth sport team and

"learning how to compete" at the youngest age possible is not supported by any research and in fact has been suggested as a obstacle to skill development. Remember the Spartak way of learning tennis and Kobe Bryant's testimony about the importance of learning fundamentals before focusing on competition. Developmentally appropriate practice means that skill learning always trumps competition and winning in youth sport, particularly before adolescence.

However, consider the example of Tiger Woods provided in the opening paragraphs of this chapter. Woods is an example of someone who as a toddler was infatuated with the game of golf. For some children who exhibit a fascination for a sport and develop their skills early, it may be totally appropriate to begin competitive sport participation at a very young age. National Hockey League great Sidney Crosby learned to skate at the age of 3 and by the age of 7 was a hockey phenom in his hometown, playing on teams and in leagues with older players. Another hockey megastar, Wayne Gretzky, had a similar childhood experience of starting competitive hockey play at the age of 6 against older athletes. People read about these famous athletes and assume that they should follow their lead and start as early as possible with their sons or daughters. But most people are not Tiger Woods, Sidney Crosby, or Wayne Gretzky. These are three of the greatest athletes of all time.

Many times in the zeal of getting a child started early in sport, adults forget the critical third wheel of the readiness tricycle—motivation. If motor skill learning is pushed on children before they are motivationally ready, they may view the activity as work as opposed to doing something that they love. A related peril to starting early is burnout, in which young athletes become overwhelmed with expectations and pressure and lose interest in previously enjoyable activities (discussed in chapter 11). Another con to starting early is injuries, with overuse being the number-one predictor of injuries in youth sport.

There are also motor or biomechanical concerns about starting too early in youth sport. If the activity is not modified to fit the maturational needs of the particular age group, bad biomechanical habits can be developed that are difficult to break when the child matures. A tiny 6-year-old boy named Jay used to wow the crowd at halftime of my (first author) high school basketball games with his shooting prowess. However, in heaving an adult-sized basketball at a 10-foot (3-meter) rim, Jay developed a push-shot shooting motion from below his shoulder. He had great difficulty in trying to modify his shooting mechanics after puberty. And finally, it may just be a waste of time to start as early as possible in teaching sport skills to kids when they are not ready (physically, cognitively, motivationally, and in terms of prerequisite skills). This could be frustrating to children and turn them off to the activity. Waiting until a later, more appropriate age often makes the learning easier, less frustrating, and less time-consuming, and yields the same eventual level of performance as would earlier exposure to the skill.

WHEN SHOULD KIDS START ORGANIZED YOUTH SPORTS?

It would be naïve to categorically state exactly when children should start participating in specific youth sports. As you've learned, readiness differs among individuals and across different activities. However, guidelines are available about overall readiness and best practice for kids as they grow and mature.

Long-Term Athlete Development (LTAD) Model

The long-term athlete development (LTAD) model offers a developmentally appropriate, systematic progression of activities for individuals to follow to optimize skill development and physical literacy (Balyi et al., 2013). The LTAD model includes seven stages that prescribe developmentally appropriate goals and activities for individuals in each stage. We briefly review these stages here to help us establish some broad guidelines about the readiness of kids for various youth sport activities.

1. **Active Start.** From birth to age 6, Active Start emphasizes play, exploration, and fun to master basic movement skills. This can be in structured as well as unstructured free play aimed at developing fundamental motor skills, gaining physical confidence, and establishing the joy associated with movement.

2. **FUNdamentals.** From ages 6 to 9 in boys and 6 to 8 in girls, children should continue to develop fundamental motor skills, particularly skills involving agility, balance, and coordination. As the name suggests, the focus is still on fun, and formal competition should be introduced in a minimal way.

3. **Learn to Train.** From the ages of 8 to 11 in girls and 9 to 12 in boys, or until the

---

Personal Plug-In

How Early Did You Start?

When did you start your sport participation? Was this the right time for you? Looking back, would you have preferred to begin your youth sport experience in a different way? What types of things could have happened differently to give you a better start to your sport career?

onset of the growth spurt, this stage involves developing foundational sport skills. However, the emphasis is still on acquiring a wide range of skills, as early specialization at this stage is discouraged. The authors also recommend more time in training (70%) with smaller doses of competition (30%).

4. **Train to Train.** This stage is designed for kids in their growth spurt, which is generally 11 to 15 years for girls and 12 to 16 for boys. This time is ripe for a big increase in training due to kids' physiological responsiveness. They should continue improving their sport-specific skills and acquire more advanced tactical strategies, and also enhance their aerobic base, speed, and strength. Process and improvement are emphasized over results in competition, meaning that more focus should be on skill training and physical development and less on trying to win. Training (60%) should still involve more time than competition (40%).

5. **Train to Compete.** The focus in this stage is optimizing sport skills and learning how to compete. Athletes either can choose to specialize in one sport and focus on developing their talent for that sport or may continue participating at the recreational level and thereby enter the Active for Life stage. At this stage, the focus is more on competition and competition-related training such as scrimmaging (60%) than on training or practice (40%).

6. **Train to Win.** This stage is for elite athletes with identified talent who wish to pursue the most intense training suitable for international competition. Major competition events define the training process in this stage, as winning at the highest level is the focus.

7. **Active for Life.** Young athletes can enter this stage at any age once they become physically literate. This is when they move around in the palm community model of sport introduced in chapter 3. Hopefully, they have the fundamental skills,

confidence, and knowledge to remain active for life in a variety of physical activities.

The LTAD model recognizes both participation- and performance-oriented pathways in sport and physical activity, preceded by the fun- and skill-based development of physical literacy (Balyi et al., 2013). The first three stages emphasize the fundamentals needed for physical literacy, followed by a more serious training commitment to sport or physical activity. The authors provide approximate age ranges, but they caution that moving from one stage to another is based on ability and maturation, not chronological age.

Suggested Age-Readiness Sport-Related Activities

Having looked at the LTAD model, in this section we offer some general guidelines about ages to start and the focus of participation at various levels (see table 5.2). We haven't talked about the issue of kids specializing in one sport because chapter 10 is devoted to this topic. There are sports, such as gymnastics, figure skating, and diving, that are referred to as early-specialization sports (Balyi, Way, & Higgs, 2013; Malina, Bouchard, & Bar-Or.,2004). This is particularly the case for females, with sport-specific training and elite performance typically required before puberty. These sports require a different pathway than the one presented in the LTAD model and in our suggested age-readiness guidelines. Our focus in table 5.2 is on late-specialization sports, with athletes able to participate in several sports at a young age and still choose a "signature" sport in their teens.

We've explained throughout the chapter the emphasis needed for preschool (2- to 5-year-old) children. As summarized in table 5.2, this is a time for multiple activities and free play focused on fundamental motor skill development. Activities like dance, gymnastics, and tumbling are good for this age group to develop body control and balance. Multiple sport or game implements and objects should be manipulated to facilitate the skills of throwing, catching, striking, kicking, and so on.

Ages 6 to 9 are when most kids begin organized youth sport participation. Many coaches and experts cite this as the best time to begin baseball, golf, tennis, soccer, basketball, and hockey (Bigelow, Moroney, & Hall, 2001; Eradi, 1998). In particular, baseball and softball are sports in which early participation pays dividends due to the precise eye–hand skill needed in tracking balls to catch or hit. Batting instructor and former major leaguer Ken Griffey states, "I don't know of anybody who began playing baseball for the first time as a teenager and made it as a successful adult hitter" (Eradi, 1998, p. D6). Griffey's son, Ken Griffey Jr., who became a Major League Baseball superstar, began playing baseball at age 4 and continued until his retirement from professional baseball. His brother Craig Griffey started baseball at the same time but lost interest at age 8. After

playing football in college, Craig tried to pick up again with baseball but struggled as a hitter, and like Michael Jordan could not make the switch to elite baseball.

As shown in table 5.2, we recommend that 6- to 9-year-olds concentrate on skill development instead of competition outcomes, and that sports be modified to small-sided games to maximize touches, skill development, and enjoyment. As you've learned, it is difficult for a child to begin physical activity and join a youth sport team (without extensive free play and prerequisite skill development) after age 9. We estimate that 8- to 9-year-olds are ready for interteam competition, so youth sport directors should consider strategies for ensuring the spread of talent across the teams in the league. One way to do that is to hold player evaluation sessions so that coaches can assess maturation and prerequisite skills leading to a "draft" of players by the coaches (see an example of a letter to parents explaining this process in appendix D).

Competition should be introduced gradually. A developmentally appropriate

Table 5.2 Suggested Age-Readiness Sport-Related Activities

Age	Activities	Focus
2-5 years	Multiple free- or organized-play physical activities with lots of implements and objects; informal competitive games like kickball, wiffle ball, tag, team relays, pickleball, and four square	Exploration, fun, moving body in different ways; fundamental motor skill development, instruction, and practice
6-9 years	Organized youth sport; modified to enhance skill development; small-sided games like 3-on-3 basketball, soccer, or hockey; continuation of informal competitive games and practice of multiple fundamental motor skills in transitional sport activities	Skill development and enjoyment; 6- to 7-year-olds practice and compete within teams; 8- to 9-year-olds compete against other teams without standings or tournaments; emphasis in both age groups is skill mastery and competition used to practice skills in game format
10-13 years	Still modified slightly from adult form of sport; select experiences (school and club) beginning at about age 12; basic tactics and strategy but not at expense of skill development	Skill development, enjoyment, and competition; leagues and standings; more emphasis on skill development and using skills in competition than on competing to win
14-18 years	Adult form of sport; fitness and strength training; advanced tactics and strategy; better coaches for enhanced technique training	More technical skill development and emphasis on skill mastery; competing to win; narrowing of focus from multiple sports to few sports or signature sport

progression might include skill development with enjoyable activities, followed by some intrateam competition to test skills, followed by interteam competition but no league standings or tournaments, followed by interteam competition within leagues with championships and tournament play. Many community swim and dive teams are open to all age groups (5-18), with participants able to compete in meets or just swim in practice to develop skills. These programs offer mock meets in which beginner swimmers get to practice competing before they try interteam competition. Keep in mind that readiness to learn sport skills and readiness to compete using those sport skills are two different things.

The ages of 10 to 13 are when kids have the physical and cognitive maturation to improve their skill execution and focus on tactics and strategies that lead to better performance. We believe that, at this age, kids are ready for league play with standings and tournaments. However, skill development should still be emphasized over competitive outcomes.

By the high school years (age 14-18), adult forms of sport are used, along with more advanced physical and technical training. It is also typical—based on time requirements and the commitment needed at this level—for teenagers to narrow their focus from many activities to a few sports or often a preferred signature sport.

Yes, it's important to begin physical motor skill development early, but what kids do and how they feel about doing it are much more important than starting them as early as possible. Above all, an emphasis on skill development is essential at the younger ages and should continue throughout all levels of youth sport. Do kids a favor, and help them develop the skills to become physically literate athletes and to remain active throughout their lives.

WRAP-UP

A three-step approach to navigating youth sport offered by Ginsburg and colleagues (2006) seems to be a good way to sum up readiness. The three steps are (1) know your child, (2) know the youth sport environment, and (3) know yourself.

1. **Know your child.** Know when your child or a child you coach is ready for youth sport by examining her maturation, prerequisite skills, and motivation. Be sure to account for the unique needs and abilities of that child in particular. Although there are patterns to motor skill development and readiness for sport, there is a great deal of variation among kids within those patterns. A friend of ours named Alex was on his way with his parents to his first interteam swim meet as a 7-year-old. When they reached the competition site, Alex told his parents he felt sick and couldn't swim. His parents, knowing Alex and understanding his anxiety, said it was okay and counseled him to sit in the car for a while until he felt better, so that maybe he could swim in his second event. Alex's parents understood him and the fear he felt about competing for the first time. After going into the pool area and seeing his teammates swim, Alex agreed to swim his second event; he did fine and swam competitively for the rest of the summer and for several years. Knowing your child means understanding and accepting when he is ready to learn and compete.

2. **Know the youth sport environment.** Understand the difference between skill development and competitive programs. Remember that skill development before entering competition is crucial (e.g., the Spartak way). Look around for programs and activities to build fundamental motor skills or sport programs that emphasize skill development. If you're a youth sport director, offer programs for fundamental motor skill development for children age 3 to 5 years,

and provide information to coaches about ways to assess and build prerequisite skills in various sports.

3. **Know yourself.** This third step is particularly crucial for parents. Sometimes kids aren't ready for early sport experiences or motor skill learning when parents or coaches want them to be. Sometimes they're not interested in participating in their parents' favorite sports. Parents' love of certain sports, competitive histories, and desire to provide the best experience for their kids sometimes cloud their abilities to be patient and understanding about their children's optimal readiness states. We understand this, because we've been there—several times. Remind yourself that it's all about the kid, and wait to get children involved when they are most suited to experience success and enjoyment. Good luck!

LEARNING AIDS

Key Terms

athletic proficiency barrier—Obstacle that occurs when children fail to develop mature levels of fundamental motor skills during childhood, which impedes their abilities to achieve high levels of athletic proficiency in sports.

cognitive readiness—Children's abilities to understand the technical and strategic requirements of a sport, particularly their abilities to process relevant information about their performance and the sport environment.

fine motor skills—Use of smaller muscle groups to perform precise movements.

fundamental motor skills—Basic motor movements that are minute parts of all sport skills.

gross motor skills—Movements involving the entire body or major parts of the body.

labeling—A cognitive strategy in which a verbal label or cue is used to provide a mental image of the correct performance.

locomotor skills—Moving the body through space, as in walking, running, and jumping.

manipulative skills—Moving or projecting objects (throwing, dribbling) as well as receiving objects (catching, receiving a soccer ball or hockey puck).

motivation—The desire, intent, or drive to do something.

motor skills—Learned movements that combine to produce smooth, efficient proficiency in a physical task.

mountain of motor skill development—Pattern in which various types of motor skills are developed in an ascending order of specific developmental levels.

myelin—White fatty tissue that insulates the nerve fibers in the brain to ensure clear transmission across synapses.

physical literacy—The physical competence, motivation, confidence, understanding, and knowledge to maintain physical activity at an individually appropriate level throughout life.

prerequisite skill—Basic proficiency that is required before a child can achieve success in a sport skill (proficiency in throwing and catching are prerequisite skills for softball).

readiness—A developmental point at which a child has the capacity to successfully learn or engage in a particular activity.

reflexes—Involuntary movements that infants make in response to specific stimuli.

rehearsal—When athletes visualize or talk through a planned movement or strategy either out loud or in their heads prior to executing the skill.

sensitive period—When the effect of a specific experience on the brain is particularly strong during a limited time period in development.

stability skills—Abilities to maintain body position against forces of gravity, such as holding a position while on a balance beam, in diving, or when figure skating.

Summary Points

1. Readiness is determined through assessment of a child's maturation, prerequisite skills, and motivation.

2. The development of motor, or movement, skills follows a pattern (the mountain of motor skills), in which children develop various types of skills in a sequential order, starting with a base foundation and building to a peak of sport skill and physical literacy.

3. Motor skills can be classified as gross or fine, as well as locomotor, manipulative, and stability types of skills.

4. Reflexes appear and disappear in an orderly sequencing that allows pediatricians to assess normal physical development in infants.

5. Fundamental motor skills are the building blocks for children's learning of more sport-specific skills.

6. The athletic proficiency barrier occurs when mature patterns of fundamental motor skills are not developed due to a lack of opportunity or practice during early and middle childhood (2-8 years).

7. Sensitive periods are optimal readiness periods, or when the effect of a specific experience on the brain is particularly strong during a limited period in development.

8. Multiple experiences in motor skills early in children's lives are important to wire their brains in ways that facilitate their athletic development.

9. The idea that earlier is better in terms of joining a youth sport team and learning how to compete at the youngest age possible is not supported by research and has been suggested as an obstacle to skill development.

10. There are pros and cons to starting early in youth sport, so earlier can be better for some children but not for others.

11. The Long-Term Athlete Development model includes seven stages of developmentally appropriate goals and activities that lead to optimal skill development and physical literacy.

12. Youth sport programs for children aged 6 to 9 years should focus on skill development and enjoyment, using small-sided games and a gradual progression to competition.

Study Questions

1. Identify the three factors that need to be considered to determine when a child is ready to learn a sport skill. Explain why each factor is essential, and provide examples.

2. Describe the different parts of the mountain of motor skill development. Explain the necessary sequential nature of motor development and why each phase is important.

3. Why does the athletic proficiency barrier occur? Identify several specific things that adults can do to help children get past this barrier.

4. What does it mean to reach the mature stage of a motor skill? Using a specific sport skill, describe characteristics of the initial or elementary stage of the skill, as well as characteristics of the mature stage of the skill.

5. Explain sensitive periods, especially in relation to learning motor skills, and explain aspects of brain development to account for why these sensitive periods occur.

6. What are the cognitive differences between nonexpert children and older athletes that influence sport performance? Explain the findings of the cognitive readiness study with baseball shortstops to support your answer.

7. Identify arguments supporting the idea that earlier is better in sport participation, and then identify the possible negative effects of earlier is better.

8. Provide a general overview of when children should begin sport participation and what they should be doing at various developmental levels, based on the LTAD model and material from the chapter.

Reflective Learning Activities

Choose a specific sport that you know well or are interested in learning more about. Create a motor skill development program for that sport. Provide recommendations for when children should start and what they should do at progressive age periods to develop their skills in this sport. Be sure to identify the types of prerequisite skills needed to succeed in this sport (including fundamental motor skills). Also, describe how you will introduce competition into youth skill development. Do not simply reproduce what is currently being done in youth sport. Think innovatively, and offer new and creative ideas based on what you've learned about readiness.

Step 1: Research the developmental sequence for a specific motor skill (e.g., throwing, punting, kicking, catching). You can find this topic online or in a motor development textbook. You will need to identify the stages of development from initial to the most mature pattern of this skill.

Step 2: Choose a child (the best ages would be 3-8 years) to serve as a model for you to observe in performing this skill. Ask the child to repeatedly perform the skill while you observe. Your task is to assess the child's developmental level of proficiency in the skill, or the maturity (from initial to elementary to mature) of the child's skill level on this motor task. Take notes, or check off the child's proficiency in various categories of skill execution on a chart that you have created.

Step 3: Summarize your experience in a written report. Present the developmental sequence for the skill, and describe where your child model (providing age, gender, and sport experience) is in relation to this sequence. Describe your perceptions of the child's skill in relation to the activities that he or she is involved in, and include any other perceptions you have about the assignment and your observations.

Resource Guide

American Academy of Pediatrics, Healthy Children Website (www.healthy-children.org/English/ages-stages/toddler/fitness/Pages/default.aspx). The Healthy Children website has guidelines and time lines for expected growth and attainment of motor skills. The website is governed by the American Academy of Pediatrics and has multiple articles written by physicians regarding age-appropriate sport and physical activity behaviors.

Canadian Coaching Association (YouTube) (www.youtube.com/watch?v=7WS-dUZvE1qs). In this short video, Dr. Colin Higgs discusses the importance of fundamental motor skills. He briefly discusses how they are developed and talks about the importance of these motor skills from a sport and public health perspective.

Kids at Play (http://health.act.gov.au/kids-at-play/active-play-everyday/fundamental-movement-skills). Kids at Play is an Australian organization focused on the overall well-being of young kids. On its website, Kids at Play provides suggestions for active play for kids of all ages. The website has downloadable fact sheets providing information on fundamental movement skills as well as on prerequisite skills.

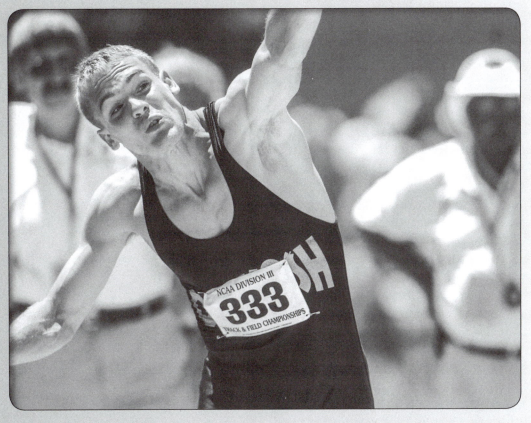

chapter 6

MOTIVATION AND PSYCHOSOCIAL DEVELOPMENT

CHAPTER PREVIEW

In this chapter, you'll learn

» why children participate in youth sport,

» three basic motivational needs of youth athletes,

» practical ideas and strategies to meet these needs, and

» how to create a motivational FEAST for athletes.

If you're reading this book, you probably love sport. You fell in love with your sport because you felt joy when playing with your friends, pride in mastering skills, and exhilaration in competing against others. And you're probably still physically active today, because the love you developed for sport as a child provided you with the skills and interest to continue in physical activity as an adult. That's what we want for kids. An important objective for adults is to help children fall in love with sport. This love is an important part of motivation.

As we defined it in the previous chapter, **motivation** is the desire, intent, or drive to do something. But as you'll learn in this chapter, motivation is complex. It involves multiple interacting internal and external forces that induce people to behave in various ways. What may seem like a good idea to motivate kids can sometimes backfire due to this complexity. Although trophies are popularly viewed as motivational rewards, they sometimes hurt kids' motivation. Likewise, youth coaches think that always being positive and praising athletes helps their motivation, but this can decrease children's motivation.

We typically view motivation as behavior, or something that a person does. We assume that a child is motivated when she chooses to go outside and practice soccer penalty kicks (choice), especially when she does this day after day, practicing for hours (effort). We also infer motivation when she doggedly keeps trying to lift the ball with her foot to hit the high corners of the goal, even though she is unsuccessful at first (persistence). And she appears highly motivated in games as she pursues the ball and opponents with ferocity (intensity). So yes, we can infer motivation from these observable behaviors, but these are just the outward behavioral manifestations of internal motivation. To truly understand motivation, we need to examine how it works inside of kids, in terms of their motivational orientations. **Motivational orientations** are those internal characteristics, such as

beliefs, values, needs, attitudes, goals, and self-perceptions, that predispose people to think and act in certain ways in achievement- or goal-directed activities (like sport). The secret to motivation is not some gimmick, but rather understanding how and why people are motivated.

Kids' motivational orientations develop as part of their overall **psychosocial development.** This means that how individuals come to view themselves is largely influenced by their social experiences—that is, experiences with parents, siblings, peers, teachers, coaches, and even popular media. For example, consider the influence of a parent who is supportive and congratulatory only when his son wins tennis matches, as opposed to another parent who is unconditionally supportive and accepting no matter how well his son performs. Clearly, the motivational orientations, as well as other psychological characteristics, of young athletes are affected by the responses of parents.

The term **motivational climate** is used to refer to the ways in which various social aspects of a situation are conducted, which in turn influence motivation. These social aspects include types of feedback, use of rewards and punishment, performance expectations and evaluation, and overall communication patterns. As you might expect, motivational climates strongly influence youth athletes' motivational orientations and their learning and performance. An important objective of this chapter, and of the book, is to provide you with strategies and ideas about how to create the best motivational climate for your particular youth sport situation.

WHY DO CHILDREN PARTICIPATE IN YOUTH SPORT?

The main reason for playing sports given by children age 5 to 18 years is "to have fun" (Murphy, 1999; Sit & Lindner, 2006). And conversely, "not having fun" is the top

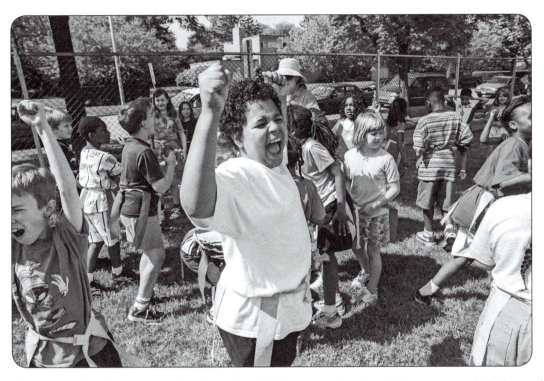

The main reason for playing sports given by children age five to eighteen years is to have fun.

reason given by kids for dropping out of youth sport (Sabo & Veliz, 2008). Along with fun or excitement or challenge, the other two top reasons kids say they play sport are "to learn/improve my skills" and "to be with friends/be part of a team" (Weiss & Williams, 2004).

Although these are the three main reasons children cite for participating in youth sport, there are others. It might be useful to ask a child the reasons she wants to play sport. To help you do this, appendix E provides the Why I Play Sports Survey (adapted from Murphy, 1999). Coaches could use this to understand the motives of youth participants, and parents could use it to consider what types of sport activities would best fit their child's participation motives.

The reasons listed earlier and in appendix E are descriptive, or based on what youth sport participants have stated as their reasons for participating. However, to better understand the motivational orientations of youth athletes, we need to examine their

fundamental psychological needs, which ultimately drive their behavior. Three basic needs have been supported by multiple theories of motivation (e.g., Deci & Ryan, 1985; Harter, 1999; Nicholls, 1989) as ones that are at the core of children's motivation in sport: competence, autonomy, and relatedness. The rest of the chapter focuses on motivation in relation to these needs (see figure 6.1), with an emphasis on competence, which is critical for youth athletes.

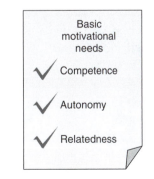

Figure 6.1 Basic motivational needs of children in sport.

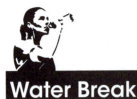

Human Needs and Motivation: The Case of Elena Delle Donne

Have you ever questioned another person's course of action, wondering why the person chose to do something that seemed illogical to you? Most basically, motivation is the desire or intent to reduce a need. The catch is that we may not understand the needs that are most relevant to other people. And although we all struggle at times to sort out our needs and decide what to do, most of us don't have to do this under public scrutiny as Elena Delle Donne did.

Delle Donne is one of the best female basketball players in history. As an 8th grader, she was offered a basketball scholarship to the University of North Carolina. As a 6-foot, 5-inch (196-centimeter) high school player, she demonstrated such impressive all-around skills that the media prophesied that her skill set would alter the game of women's basketball. She led her high school team to three Delaware state championships, scored over 2,000 points, was a high school All-American, and was ranked as the number-one high school recruit in the nation. Delle Donne chose to attend the University of Connecticut, the top women's basketball program in the nation over the preceding decade, which seemed a logical choice. But after two days on the UConn campus, she abruptly left Storrs and dropped out of school, citing "personal issues." She enrolled at the University of Delaware, close to her home, and walked onto . . . its volleyball team? Of course, people were stunned, and Delle Donne's motivation was questioned in the national media.

Delle Donne was very close to her family, particularly to her sister Lizzie, who has cerebral palsy and is blind and deaf. The only way for the sisters to communicate is through touching and hugging. "Lizzie means the world to me," says Delle Donne. "She doesn't know that I'm her sister, she doesn't know that I'm a basketball player . . . but she knows that I'm a really important person in her life" (McGraw, 2013). Once reunited with her sister, and after a season of volleyball, Delle Donne finally said to herself, "What I am doing, not playing basketball" (Wertheim, 2012). She joined the Delaware basketball team and scored over 3,000 points, winning numerous national awards. The second overall draft pick in the Women's National Basketball Association in 2013, Delle Donne was the Rookie of the Year in her first professional season.

Like all of us, Elena Delle Donne has her own personal motivational needs. Her story is powerful because it shows how she struggled to meet her need to be with her family along with her need to fulfill her destiny as an elite basketball player. Realizing how much our personal fulfillment is based on meeting our unique motivational needs is an important lesson to keep in mind when working with youth athletes.

COMPETENCE

Personal competence is at the heart of motivation, and humans' innate (inborn) quest for competence begins in infancy (White, 1959). Infants attempt to physically move in different ways and manipulate objects, striving to have an effect on their environment. Children continue this quest for competence, testing themselves on physical tasks such as jumping off the high diving board, learning to ride a bike, and swimming underwater across a pool. Parents of small children hear "Mom, watch me do this" or "Dad, time me on this" as kids test their competence and seek reinforcement for doing so. **Competence** is having sufficient ability for some purpose, so we can think of **perceived competence** as one's sense of personal ability or skill on a specific task.

Baseball Diamond Model of Competence Motivation

Motivation and competence fuel each other in a continuous cycle, as shown in our baseball diamond model of competence motivation (see figure 6.2, an adaptation of competence motivation theory by Harter, 1978, and White, 1959). Starting at home plate, children's motivation to be competent (A) sends them to first base to try out different skills and activities, called mastery attempts (B). When they succeed at an activity that is challenging to them based on their capabilities (C, at second base), they feel competent, which in turn makes them feel worthy, as well as proud, satisfied, and happy (D, at third base). **Self-worth,** also known as self-esteem, is one's sense of value or worth as a person. There's a lot going on at third base, as these are the important internal feelings and self-perceptions that drive motivation. But if they're achieved, it's a home run! The sense of worthiness, positive feelings, and beliefs that "I can do this!" (perceived competence) send kids in a proud home-run trot down the third base line (back to A) and make them even more motivated to step back up to the plate and try it again (back to B). Or to summarize the model, kids want it, try it, achieve it, feel it, and then want to do it again.

So if kids' at-bats are positive (successful), then, as shown in figure 6.2, they are more motivated and continue in the activity. They

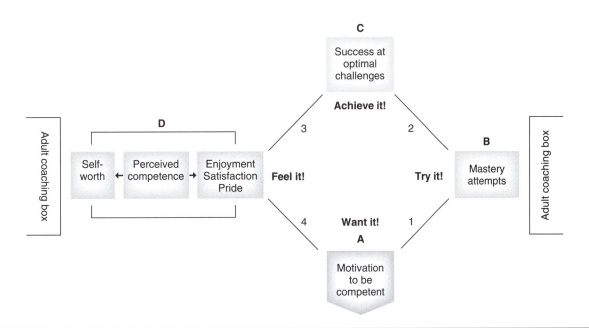

Figure 6.2 Baseball diamond model of competence motivation.

try harder and persevere when they hit obstacles (Whitehead, Andree, & Lee, 2004). However, consider how this cycle can also be negative. A child joins a youth sport team and starts playing (mastery attempts) but is not successful and thus feels incompetent, unworthy, dissatisfied, and even ashamed. This serves to decrease his motivation to continue playing that sport. Kids who don't perceive that they are competent lose interest, effort, and persistence to stay with the sport (Cervello, Escarti, & Guzman, 2007; Whitehead et al., 2004).

There are many places in our baseball diamond model where adults can intervene to help every kid hit a personal home run. In fact, youth sport leaders, coaches, and parents serve as the umpires, managers, and base coaches for all youth sport participants in our competence motivation baseball game—we've noted them in the first and third base adult coaching boxes shown in figure 6.2. Our job is to create and maintain a developmentally appropriate game for all kids who come up to bat. Let's take a look at how we can intervene on each base path (1-4, see figure 6.2) to help kids get around the bases in ways that enhance their motivation and perceived competence.

Dealing With Fear of Failure and Perfectionism (Base Path 1)

Young athletes move from home plate to first base more easily and happily if they are socialized to view youth sport as an exciting challenge and an opportunity to learn and get better, with mistakes viewed as a normal part of that process. This is sometimes difficult, because sport competition is a social evaluation process (as discussed in chapter 3).

Fear of Failure

By focusing on this social evaluation, some children begin to worry about failing. **Fear of failure** is the fear of the consequences of failure, most typically a fear of shame and embarrassment, not being good enough, or letting down others (parents, coaches, teammates) (Conroy, Willow, & Metzler, 2002). Fear of failure is learned, typically between the ages of 5 and 9, as kids become aware of the evaluations and criticisms of others (Sagar, Lavallee, & Spray, 2007). Their focus changes from learning as part of fun-oriented free play to performing in a public social evaluation situation (Martens, 2012).

Failure-oriented kids are threatened by youth sport and often drop out. Some failure-oriented kids who stay in sport try very hard but are devastated when they make mistakes, as opposed to accepting that mistakes are part of any endeavor. Some failure-oriented youth athletes offer minimal effort and fail to persist when obstacles arise, attempting to save face by acting as though they don't care. Not trying hard gives them an easy excuse in case they fail. Although many athletes experience some feelings of fear of failure, most who remain in sport have a much stronger success orientation. Success-oriented athletes understand the negative consequences of failing, but their focus is on the challenge and the possibility of the pride and accomplishment they will feel when they succeed. These athletes seek out challenging situations and persist when faced with setbacks and obstacles. So our goal is to help young athletes focus on the challenge of being successful instead of the negative consequences of failure.

Perfectionism

Similar to fear of failure, perfectionism is another *incompetence-avoidance* motivational orientation (Kaye, Conroy, & Fifer, 2008) that affects the way kids approach mastery attempts in sport. **Perfectionism** is a young athlete's tendency to focus on and strive for flawless performance (Gilman & Ashby, 2006). Some aspects of perfectionism are adaptive, such as having high standards of performance, strong levels of motivation to do one's best, and a preference for organization. However, maladaptive perfectionists are overconcerned with and unable to accept mistakes, are overly critical in evaluating their performances, and unrealistically and irrationally strive for flawless performance. Kids with maladaptive perfectionism might say such things as "I can't make any mistakes today," "Play it safe out there so you don't look stupid," or "I can't believe I missed that shot—I stink." Maladaptive perfectionism has been related to anxiety, excessive anger and aggression, negative body image, reduced confidence, and burnout in youth sport participants (Sapieja, Dunn, & Holt, 2011).

Strategies to Enhance Mastery Attempts

How can we help children and youth athletes move from home plate to first base in our baseball diamond model without their learning to be so fearful of failure or negatively perfectionistic? This base path involves helping kids develop and maintain a healthy attitude about sport and competition and providing them with skills to build their competence.

1. Commit to an athlete-centered philosophy and talk to the athletes about this repeatedly. Examples are provided in chapter 3, and a catchy phrase like "Athletes first, winning second" or "It's all about the kid" reminds adults and youth athletes of why we're here and what the focus should be. Make sure that kids see and hear about it at every practice and competitive event. Put it on their T-shirts and any written materials you hand out to athletes and parents.

2. Modify the practice and competitive situations to fit kids' needs. More specifics are provided in chapters 7 and 8, but we note here that you want to design activities that fit kids' physical sizes, maturational status, and learning abilities. You want more action and less standing around, variety in activities, strategies to get everyone involved in every practice, and plenty of opportunities to succeed.

3. Be (or find) a great teacher. Always remember that the recipe for long-term motivation and love of a sport requires the essential ingredient of skill. Maybe running around and having fun with friends is motivational for a while, but kids won't continue with an activity if they fail to develop skill in performing it. Developing fundamentals (e.g., prerequisite skills) is critical. Skill development can be emphasized in creative ways, without the joyless overemphasis on "kill and drill."

4. Validate the thoughts and feelings of athletes who express fear of failure, as opposed to telling them not to worry about it. For example, if a child says "I'm afraid I might lose," don't reply with "Oh, you won't lose" or "Don't worry about it." They *are* worried about it. Express your understanding of how they feel: "That must feel bad—tell me more about feeling afraid." Ask questions, validate their feelings, and lead into a discussion about how to think about and deal with failure. Learning is simply a string of failures and successes. Help them adopt a growth mindset, in which their mastery attempts are part of an ongoing effort to grow and expand their ability (Dweck, 2007).

5. Parents and youth sport coaches should give athletes permission to make mistakes. Let them know that mistakes show that they are trying hard and attempting new things, and are a necessary part of the learning process. Teach kids a mistake ritual (Thompson, 2010b), or a symbolic gesture to help them refocus after mistakes. Examples include brushing off your shoulder ("brush it off"), wiping fingers across

the brow ("no sweat"), taking off your hat and putting it back on, tapping your hockey stick on the ice, ripping the Velcro on your golf glove and then reattaching it, or swiping your foot across the rubber when pitching. You can even adopt a team mistake ritual, which helps kids realize that everyone makes mistakes and models productive responses to those mistakes.

Teach Athletes to Define Success in Personal and Controllable Ways (Base Path 2)

Our next goal in building competence motivation is helping youth athletes move from first to second base in our baseball diamond model (shown as base path 2 in figure 6.2). To do this, athletes need to learn to define success in personal and controllable ways. This is very difficult in a society where the media publicly trumpets athletes as losers and winners based on performance outcomes. But adults can help kids interpret their performance outcomes in ways that can enhance their motivation.

Goal Orientations

Success and failure are not concrete events and certainly should not be defined by newspaper headlines. They are psychological states based on whether individuals perceive they have achieved meaningful goals (achievement goal theory, Nicholls, 1989). Two motivational orientations based on goals have been shown to affect the perceived success, perceived competence, self-worth, and enjoyment of young athletes in sport: task and ego orientations. Kids are **task involved** when they focus on performing their best or mastering and improving their skills. Kids are **ego involved** when their focus is on beating others or demonstrating superior ability in relation to others.

Of course, kids can have both of these goals in sport, and often do. Striving to win is an inherent objective in any sport contest, yet developmentally appropriate youth sport emphasizes skill development and personal improvement as more important than the competitive outcome of winning. However, it's tough for kids to sort out these two competitive goals, and they need coaches and parents to help them focus on personally controllable goals in practice and competition.

It is crucial for kids to be highly task involved, which leads to greater effort, more persistence, and feelings of competence, self-worth, and enjoyment (Harwood, Spray, & Keegan, 2008). Ego involvement can also help focus resources on opponents to develop appropriate game plans and to maintain competitiveness in terms of playing with intensity in striving to win (Harwood & Biddle, 2002). However, ego involvement without any sense of task involvement leads young athletes to cheat, take shortcuts in training, and give less effort. And for kids who lack ability, ego involvement (without task involvement) is deadly because they are doomed to fail in relation to the superior ability of others, so they feel anxious, incompetent, and unworthy and often drop out of sport (Cervello et al., 2007).

Best Goal Orientations for Youth Sport Participants

We recommend two goal orientation strategies for youth sport participants (based on combinations of task and ego involvement). First, a motivational orientation of high task and low ego involvement allows young athletes to focus on their own performance and improvement, without concern for how they compare to others. This goal orientation is often adopted in sports like track and field, cross-country, and swimming, in which athletes receive clear individual information about their performance, irrespective of the position in which they finish in relation to other competitors (Harwood & Biddle, 2002).

Second, a motivational orientation of high task and high ego involvement allows athletes to pursue the goal of demonstrating ability and attempting to beat others in competition while simultaneously understanding that they can control only their own personal performance. The trick with this orientation is to concentrate during competition and performance on the process of playing and personal standards, which is the best mental strategy when one is competing against others (Burton & Weiss, 2008). Task involvement acts as an "insurance policy" for the times when youth athletes are unable to win or compete favorably with others. Young athletes can learn to identify successful aspects of their performance even in personal or team losses.

Strategies to Enhance Perceptions of Success

Base path 2 involves creating a motivational climate in which kids can experience success while being optimally challenged. This is important, because youth athletes' goal orientations have been shown to align with the motivational climate that directors, coaches, and parents provide for them (Boyce, Gano-Overway, & Campbell, 2009).

1. Help athletes identify specific task goals on which to judge themselves in sport. Examples include making contact with opponents to box out in rebound situations (basketball), using your backhand stroke more often (tennis), shaving time with more efficient flip turns (swimming), and starting on your pace, running strong on hills, and finishing with a power kick (cross-country running).

2. Ask youth athletes the right questions about competition. Questions like "Tell me about your game today," "Did you have quality at-bats today?" and "How was your front-row play (volleyball) today?" get the athlete focusing on task accomplishments. "Did you win?" and "How many points (or goals) did you score?" reinforce a purely ego-involved perspective.

3. Provide specific feedback loaded with information that is contingent on how the athlete performed. Positive feedback just to be positive isn't motivating; it's demeaning. It doesn't offer the challenge young athletes need to achieve success. Specific, informational feedback ("Jump high to front the cutter as she moves across the key") allows

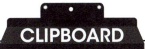

CLIPBOARD

What Is the Motivational Climate on Your Team?

Hey, coaches—want to find out how much you create a task-involved and an ego-involved climate on your team? Use the Motivational Climate Scale for Youth Sports (Smith, Cumming, & Smoll, 2008) in appendix F. Make copies of the MCSYS and provide it, along with pencils, to the athletes on your team. Explain to them that you're trying to be the best coach you can, and this will provide helpful feedback. Tell them not to write their name on their scale, and

ask them to be honest and thoughtful in their answers. Assure them that you will not be able to identify their responses, and thank them for providing you with helpful feedback. Follow the scoring instructions in appendix F to get your scores for Task-Involved and Ego-Involved Climate. Examine your total scores, but also look at your means (averages) for each item. Use the feedback to consider ways you can enhance the team motivational climate for your athletes.

the athlete to learn and improve, as opposed to general, evaluative feedback ("You're out of position on defense!"), which isn't helpful.

4. Reward effort (even unsuccessful effort), improvement, mental toughness, emotional control, and any other controllable successes you can observe in young athletes. When a basketball player uses her nondominant hand to correctly shoot a layup yet misses, verbally reward her decision and effort to use this developing skill in a game.

5. Explain to athletes that they should use competition as a way to test their personal skills and development (informative) as opposed to viewing it as an evaluative sorting out of who is better (normative) (Veroff, 1969). By test-driving their skills in competitive situations, athletes can assess how things are working and where they can improve and then revise their personal goals accordingly. Competition is useful for many things other than finding out who is number one.

Help Athletes Make Healthy Attributions (Base Path 3)

Still working our way around the baseball diamond model of competence motivation (figure 6.2), we're now on base path 3. This path involves helping youth athletes internalize their success to feel competent, worthy, and proud. The main way to do this is to help them make productive attributions for their successes and failures (attribution theory; Weiner, 1986).

What Are Attributions and How Do They Work?

Attributions are reasons that athletes accept to explain why they succeed and fail. Common attributions made by athletes include effort, luck, opponent's skill, officials, personal ability, injury, weather, and coaches. They're not excuses, but rather important self-reasoning explanations for personal outcomes.

Attributions are important because they influence the impact of success on perceived competence and self-worth more than the actual success does. Think about when you aced an academic exam in college. It's highly likely that you felt much more competent and proud if you believed that your success resulted from diligent study and mastery of the subject matter, as opposed to the exam's being easy and the professor's not challenging you. The reasons we believe we succeed are critical to building our perceived competence and expectations for future success.

All athletes, but particularly young ones, need help in figuring out the appropriate attributions to make when they succeed and fail. Our daughter's youth soccer team won all their regular-season games one year and made it to the state tournament, where they lost in the first round. As Brett, their coach, sat down with them after the game, all the players were crying and appeared upset over the loss. Coach Brett told them that it was okay to cry, because he understood the game meant so much to them and it was disappointing to lose. However, he told them how proud he was and how proud they should be of their accomplishments that season. He helped them understand that their opponent was skilled and deserved to win the game, but that as 9-year-olds in their first state tournament, they had learned a lot about how to get better at soccer and could continue to develop their skills. Coach Brett helped them attribute the loss to inexperience, the skill of the other team, and their need to continue to learn and develop their skills. This helped the players regain their sense of competence and made them excited to try again the next season.

So how are you going to help your youth athletes when talking to them after wins and losses? Here's a general recipe to follow for productive attributions. When kids fail, help them attribute this failure to things that they can control and change. Examples include better preparation, improvement of skills, continuing maturation and development, and better strategy and focus. An elite swimmer recalls how his father helped him make productive attributions when he failed as a youth swimmer, and credits his development of mental toughness to this: "My dad was usually there at the swim meets when I was younger, and anytime I lost, rather than having a defeatist attitude, he would tell me to work out what went wrong and then to work harder on these areas in training in order to be successful at future attempts" (Connaughton, Wadey, Hanton, & Jones, 2008, p. 89).

When kids succeed, help them attribute success to internal, controllable things, such as their ability, hard work, effort and hustle, preparation, and good decision making. An example might be "You should feel really proud of your IM [individual medley] race. That hard work on your butterfly is really paying off, and your backstroke technique looked really smooth and strong." Of course, there are often valid reasons why outcomes occur, but the motivational strategy is to internalize feelings of competence and pride and create an expectation for continued success in the future.

Learned Helplessness

Learned helplessness is a psychological state in which children feel powerless and unable to control the outcome of a situation (Abramson, Seligman, & Teasdale, 1978). It is characterized by maladaptive attributional patterns, with success attributed to external, uncontrollable things like luck or an easy task. And perhaps even worse, failure is attributed to a perceived unchangeable lack of ability. Because they don't believe they can get better or change their situation, athletes with learned helplessness "learn" to give up and not try very hard. This of course dooms their performance and validates their

beliefs that they lack ability and are powerless to improve.

When confronted with a learned-helpless athlete, coaches logically set up drills or situations in which the athlete can achieve small steps to success. But the problem of the maladaptive attribution pattern is still there. The athlete will say, "Oh, you just made it easy" or "It was just luck that I could do it this time," attributing their success to something beyond their control. So what should coaches do when confronted with learned-helpless athletes?

Setting up small steps to success is a good start. However, along with practicing skills in specially designed drills, coaches must also work with athletes to retrain their attributional thinking toward a renewed sense of personal controllability over their progress (Pelletier, Dion, Tuson, & Green-Demers, 1999; Rees, Ingledew, & Hardy, 2005). Four steps emphasizing the following aspects can help retrain attributions in young athletes:

1. The *commonality* of the problem ("Other kids your age in this sport found this skill difficult as well, and felt unsuccessful at first.")

2. The *developmental change* process ("Over time, the task became easier and they felt more successful. So let's give yourself time to learn it.")

3. *Strategy* ("You may not have found the best strategy yet for you to execute the skill, but we'll find it.")

4. *Effort and persistence* ("In time, practicing your new strategies will really help you improve.")

As the result of retraining attributions using steps similar to these, 11- to 12-year-old kids identified as learned helpless showed marked increases in perceived success, motivation, and controllable attributions on ball dribbling (Sinnott & Biddle, 1998). High school basketball players who underwent a four-week attributional training period developed more controllable attributions and greater improvement in their shooting as compared to other players who only received feedback (Miserandino, 1998). Motivating learned-helpless athletes requires a thoughtful game plan to get inside their thinking and enable them to perceive some control over their learning and performance. Working the process of small steps to success is useful, as long as it is accompanied by attributional retraining strategies.

Additional Strategies to Optimize Perceived Competence by Internalizing Success

We've provided several strategies for you to help athletes make the most productive attributions to internalize their success and build perceived competence and self-worth. Here are two final thoughts:

1. Praise young athletes for effort, not for performance outcomes. It's very easy to forget this, and to *ooh* and *ah* over great performances by young athletes when trying to be supportive and positive. While they should be recognized for their accomplishments, excessive praise of outcomes often leads to pressure. Try to focus your comments on the controllable efforts, practice, and persistence that allowed them to achieve the positive outcomes (e.g., "It's awesome that you worked so hard to bring your time down—congratulations!"). A study showed that children who were praised for their intelligence cared more about grades than about learning, and were less persistent when they failed as compared to kids who had been praised for their effort (Dweck, 2006).

2. Avoid attempting to boost children's self-esteem through praise and overattention. As shown in our baseball diamond model, self-worth (self-esteem) results from success at optimal challenges and earned perceived competence. The decades of the 1970s and 1980s overemphasized building kids' self-esteem

through praise and lack of challenge, which backfired and instead spawned narcissism and self-entitlement. Psychologist Roy Baumeister explains, "It was an honest mistake. The early findings showed that kids with high self-esteem did better. . . . It's just that we learned later that self-esteem is a result, not a cause" (Stein, 2013, p. 28). Self-esteem must be earned; it cannot be given.

Understand Developmental Changes in How Kids View Competence (Base Path 4)

Our final base path leads from perceived competence, self-worth, and enjoyment (third base) back to motivation (home plate). Volumes of research support this link (e.g., Weiss & Amorose, 2008), which has really been the point of the entire baseball game. When children perceive they are competent, they are motivated to participate in sport. And this sense of competence feeds feelings of self-worth and enjoyment, also stimulating motivation.

What might be helpful to wrap up our baseball diamond overview of competence is to explain how perceived competence is influenced by the psychosocial development of children. Perceived competence changes across developmental stages, and youth sport leaders should understand how this development unfolds.

How Competent Am I?

Children become more accurate in assessing their personal competence as they age (Horn, 2004). Young children (3-7 years) generally have inflated levels of perceived competence in relation to their actual competence. That's not necessarily a bad thing, and it might be valuable to drive their fundamental motor skill development, which is very important for this age. Kids this age are fun to coach in that they tend to work hard and persist, because to them effort and working hard means they're competent.

By middle childhood (8-11 years), children have developed cognitively to the point where they more realistically assess their own competence. This marks a period of vulnerability during which kids who are less competent in sport skills become aware of this and are candidates for dropping out of sport and becoming less physically active (Stodden et al., 2008). During adolescence (12-18 years), young athletes typically have developed a mature ability to accurately assess their competence, particularly across different social and achievement areas (e.g., sport, school, friends).

How Do I Know I'm Competent?

Children use different sources of information as they age to determine how competent they are in sport (Horn, 2004). When kids are very young (4-7 years), they base their perceptions of competence on three things: simple task accomplishment ("I did it!"), evaluative feedback from significant adults ("How was that, coach?"), and personal effort ("I worked hard, so I'm good"). In particular, teachers, coaches, and parents should be aware that their feedback and evaluation are extremely important in developing perceptions of competence in young children.

During middle to late childhood (7-12 years), children continue to use very concrete sources of information (such as winning and losing, personal statistics, praise), and peer comparison becomes a very important source during this time (Horn, 2004). In fact, peer evaluation becomes a more important source of competence information, while parent evaluation becomes relatively less important between the ages of 7 and 12. Coaches should focus on how best to socially engineer the youth sport environment during this time—for example, by constantly rotating warm-up partners and training groups to avoid ability groupings and cliques. Parents and coaches should also continuously emphasize the importance of focusing on personal performance goals, particularly to less competent kids, who often get teased or who feel inferior by comparison.

By adolescence (13-18 years), young athletes are able to weigh and use multiple sources of information to assess their competence, and they increase in their ability to use internalized or personal performance

Feedback and evaluation from significant adults is very important for very young children's developing perceptions of competence.

standards. This maturity to enable use of personal standards allows athletes to internalize a task-involved focus, which is important to support perceived competence and motivation.

Summary of the Baseball Diamond Model of Competence Motivation

So now you've been around the bases of our competence motivation baseball diamond. Youth athletes run the bases when they (1) make positive mastery attempts in sport based on their motivation to be competent, (2) define success in personally controllable ways, (3) internalize their success through productive attributions to feel competent and worthy, and (4) gain more motivation because they feel competent and enjoy their success. At this point, youth athletes are highly motivated to get back up to bat and start around the bases again. Remember that perceived competence is the foundation for kids' motivation in sport. Our job as adult leaders is to help them navigate these base paths to enhance their perceived competence and enjoyment, which makes them want to stay in the game.

AUTONOMY

In addition to competence, autonomy is a basic psychological need of children that greatly influences their motivation and behavior. **Autonomy** is the ability and opportunity to govern one's self. **Self-determination** is similar to autonomy in that humans are motivated when they perceive that they possess control over themselves and their actions—when they feel that they determine their own course of behavior (self-determination theory; Deci & Ryan, 1985). Self-determination leads to perceptions of autonomy. It's logical, then, that athletes' motivation is boosted when they are allowed to be self-determining.

But whoa, we're talking about sport here, where coaches are in charge of designing practices and controlling athletes' behaviors to induce them to learn skills and perform better. How in the world can we let athletes, particularly youth athletes, govern themselves, or be in control of their own training? It's a good question. The answer lies in understanding that many forms of motivation are available to coaches, and they all can be effective in building athletes' skills and sense of autonomy if used in the right way.

Intrinsic and Extrinsic Motivation

Most basically, motivation can be defined as either intrinsic or extrinsic. **Intrinsic motivation** involves doing an activity for the pleasure and satisfaction derived from engaging in that activity (Deci & Ryan, 1985). Kids play soccer and ice-skate and swim because they enjoy the feelings they experience when doing these activities. The reward is the activity itself. Obviously, intrinsic motivation is desirable, because it is self-determining and completely autonomous.

When kids fall in love with their sport via intrinsic motivation, you'll see them choose to train, persist to get better, and play with great intensity and engagement. The parents of basketball star Aaron Gordon (high school All-American and top-five college recruit in 2013) talk of how they were awakened in the middle of the night by the sounds of Gordon shoveling dirt in their backyard (Anderson, 2013). It seems he just couldn't wait to set up the new basketball pole and hoop he had received that day for his ninth birthday. In the morning he prodded his sleepy father, and by 8:30 the hoop was set and Gordon sat and watched, willing the concrete to dry so he could play. You probably know a story like this one, of a burning desire to play a sport that was evident at a very young age. Our objective as youth sport leaders is to create a motivational climate most fertile for the development of intrinsic motivation, or love of sport.

However, not all aspects of sport participation will be intrinsically interesting to kids. Sometimes extrinsic motivation is needed to fuel the repetitive practice required to build skill or the physical fitness training required for stamina and strength. **Extrinsic motivation** involves doing an activity to achieve outcomes or rewards beyond the activity itself. These outcomes are often tangible, material rewards like trophies, all-league recognition, and college scholarships. Extrinsic motivators can also be intangible, social rewards, such as approval from parents, popularity, and being thought of as cool and accepted by friends and teammates.

Autonomous and Controlled Forms of Motivation

Extrinsic motivation isn't always externally driven by the demands of coaches, pressure from parents, or acceptance sought from friends. Sometimes extrinsic motivation is autonomous, as when athletes choose to go on a training run or swim laps during vacation. They do these activities to gain some reward outside of the activity, but they make the personal choice to do it and "own" the behavior. Autonomous extrinsic motivation is important for young athletes to develop, because the fun-oriented intrinsic motivation of entry-level youth sport changes as they progress to higher levels of sport. Athletes need self-determined extrinsic motivation (along with intrinsic motivation) to commit to more intensive training and time spent in practice.

The Continuum of Self-Determination

A useful way to think about motivation is to situate its different forms across a continuum of self-determination[3] (see figure 6.3) (Lonsdale, Hodge, & Rose, 2008; Ryan & Deci, 2002). Intrinsic motivation anchors the high end of the self-determination continuum. Autonomous extrinsic motivation is also high in self-determination, because athletes have internalized the extrinsic reasons for playing as valuable and part of their identity. Controlled extrinsic motivation is the

[3] The continuum presented here is simplified and does not include the specific subtypes of controlled and autonomous extrinsic motivation as shown by Lonsdale and colleagues (2008).

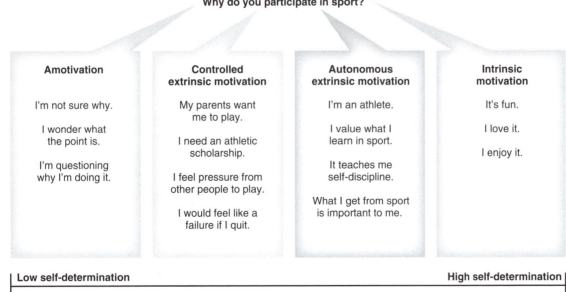

Why do you participate in sport?

Amotivation	Controlled extrinsic motivation	Autonomous extrinsic motivation	Intrinsic motivation
I'm not sure why.	My parents want me to play.	I'm an athlete.	It's fun.
I wonder what the point is.	I need an athletic scholarship.	I value what I learn in sport.	I love it.
I'm questioning why I'm doing it.	I feel pressure from other people to play.	It teaches me self-discipline.	I enjoy it.
	I would feel like a failure if I quit.	What I get from sport is important to me.	

| Low self-determination | High self-determination |

Figure 6.3 Continuum of self-determination and types of motivation.

least self-determined form of motivation and occurs when athletes participate to satisfy others, avoid shame and punishment, and obtain rewards. Even feelings of internal pressure, such as guilt or shame about skipping a workout, represent controlled motivation because the behavior is enforced, not freely chosen (Ryan & Deci, 2002). **Amotivation,** or the lack of any kind of motivation, anchors the low end of the continuum.

Different types of motivation often operate at the same time. It's quite typical for an athlete to play sport because he likes it (intrinsic), because he values the lessons and fitness it provides (autonomous extrinsic), and because everyone in his family is expected to play sports (controlled extrinsic). There are times when we need controlled motivation (e.g., I have to go to school today), but it works best when it is accompanied by autonomous extrinsic and intrinsic motivation.

Why Autonomous Forms of Motivation Work Best

Self-determined forms of motivation have been linked to greater attendance and participation in sport and physical activity, lower intentions to drop out of sport, greater effort, better concentration, goal attainment, enjoyment, and lower levels of burnout (Weiss & Amorose, 2008). Many coaches, even in youth sport, cling to the idea that autocratic coaching behaviors aimed at motivating through fear, intimidation, and punishment work best in training athletes. Controlling styles of coaching may work briefly to drive athletes using any means possible to win. However, to sustain an enduring program that meets the motivational needs of athletes and deepens their commitment to sport, autonomy-supportive youth programs and coaching styles are needed.

How to Be Autonomy Supportive in Youth Sport

Youth sport leaders who are **autonomy supportive** are those who listen to and attempt to understand their athletes, provide them with opportunities for input and choices, and minimize demanding or controlling behaviors. This doesn't mean that athletes are allowed to run amuck, but rather that choices are provided and athletes' voices are listened to within the specific structure, limits, and rules of a program (Mageau & Vallerand, 2003). Autonomy and independence are not the same. Athletes can feel self-determined even when following the training guidance and strategic decisions made by coaches. What is important is the way in which decisions are made, the way in which that information and feedback are provided, and the way in which coaches interact with athletes. Here are some of our suggestions, and we encourage you to develop your own creative ways to nurture feelings of autonomy in young athletes.

1. **Show authentic interest in and involvement with athletes.** Personally connect in a nonperformance conversation with each athlete regularly. Acknowledge athletes' feelings and inquire about how they're doing. Avoid patronizing comments like "Oh, you'll be fine" and demonstrate that you understand and accept what they're feeling.

2. **Provide a rationale for your decisions.** Explain *why* a lot, using words like "the reason for this is . . ." or "I think we should do this because. . . ." Point out how you think a certain activity or strategy will benefit athletes. Let athletes know your reasoning behind moving them to new positions, starting them, not starting them, asking them to try new roles, and not getting them into the game or having them playing a lesser role than they would like.

3. **Ask for athletes' input and give them choices within your team structure.** "How do you think practice went today?" "Is there something you think we should work on?" "What did we do well in the game last night, and what can we do better?" "What shooting drill should we end with today?" "Is our team warm-up getting

you ready to run? Any suggestions?" Athletes need to know you honestly listen and consider their feedback, but that doesn't mean you will always agree with them. They must understand that their ideas are important and heard, and sometimes implemented, but that the overall responsibility for the team still resides with the coach.

4. **Provide opportunities for athletes to take initiative and train independently.** Designate a player-coach occasionally, such that the designated player helps plan and organize the practice and actually runs drills and provides feedback in small groups. Divide athletes into small groups at various stations, where they are given a skill to work on and are asked to coach and provide

feedback to each other. Give athletes an extra day off, such as a Friday before the weekend break, and ask them to work out one day on their own. Provide some examples or ideas for what they could choose to do. Upon returning to team practice, ask them as a group how it went and what kinds of things they did to train.

5. **Minimize controlling feedback and behaviors.** Controlling statements to avoid might include ones like these: "It's about time you got a hit"; "Keep it up—we need that again next game"; "If you had listened to me, that wouldn't have happened"; "I'm counting on you today, so don't let me down." Conversely, these are examples of informational feedback: "Solid hit—you really rotated your

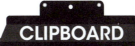

Autonomy and Discipline: Incompatible or Complementary?

A unique challenge for coaches at all levels is to discipline athletes to manage their behavior in accordance with established rules of conduct. Rules should reflect mutual respect and responsibility between the coach and athletes. Avoid the "I gotcha" game of looking to catch athletes doing something wrong. Instead, lead a discussion with them about rules for the team, and ask them for their suggestions about team rules. Keep it simple, without a long list of unenforceable, silly rules. Make this about them and how you wish to help guide their behavior, as opposed to being about you as the tough, controlling coach. Once the rules are established, ask if everyone can commit to them, which will help the team move toward important goals.

Avoid creating a "doghouse" where athletes remain in a prolonged state of punishment or banishment from the good graces of the coach for a previous misbehavior. Establish consequences that are viewed by most athletes as fair

and appropriate. Try to make the consequences logical, not punitive. If Natalie is late to practice, a logical consequence isn't to run laps. It would be more fitting, or logical, for her to be required to come 30 minutes early for the next practice or to stay 30 minutes after practice to help with equipment and secure the facility. It's important for the coach to link the logic of particular consequences to the athletes' behaviors when discussing issues with them.

Handing out random punishment to control athletes often backfires—for example, requiring all team members to run sprints because one athlete swore in practice. (This would probably create a lot more swearing!) Design and enforce a consequence that is logical, and make sure that when it's over, it's over. No doghouses! Overall, the purpose of discipline is to help athletes internalize an inner guidance system, which they value and make their own as an important part of being an athlete.

hips to get into the ball" and "Great attention to setting the block on defense today."

6. **Ask questions, as opposed to correcting athletes' mistakes.** Athletes improve the most when they develop their own intrinsic feedback system to evaluate their performance and correct mistakes. Help them do this by first asking their opinion about a performance outcome: "Why do you think you popped up on that pitch?" "If the setter's in the front row, where's the hole going to be for our attack?" Prod them to think and learn before you simply tell them what was wrong or what to do.

Autonomy-supportive teacher and coach behavior leads to positive outcomes in youth sport. A semester-long intervention to guide physical education teachers in being autonomy supportive resulted in higher levels of skill development, engagement, satisfaction, and autonomous motivation in youth as compared findings in a control group that did not use autonomy-supportive teaching methods (Cheon, Reeve, & Moon, 2012). Youth sport athletes who perceived that their coaches were autonomy supportive felt more competent and connected to teammates, and experienced less burnout and greater well-being (Adie, Duda, & Ntoumanis, 2012; Coatsworth & Conroy, 2009). We have noticed a strong trend in autonomy-supportive coaching in popular books written by nationally acclaimed coaches, from the youth to professional level. We urge youth sport directors to educate coaches and parents about specific ways they can adopt autonomy-supportive practices with youth athletes.

Caution! Extrinsic Rewards in Use

BOOK IT! motivates children to read by rewarding their reading accomplishments with praise, recognition, and pizza. So says the home page for the BOOK IT! reading program sponsored by Pizza Hut. Once kids achieve their reading goal, set with their teacher, they receive a free pizza. Millions of kids have participated since 1986, consuming many books and pizzas. So the program succeeds—or does it? The real question is, how much do former participants in this program read today? Did the program turn them on to reading, or did it induce them to read just enough to get a pizza?

A basic premise in psychology is that rewarding a behavior increases the probability of that behavior's being repeated. And this is often true, as we all have experienced. However, does an extrinsic reward (like a free pizza) serve to develop autonomous motivation (a lifelong reading habit)? The answer is that it has the potential to do this, depending on the reward, how it is given, and how the person perceives it. But it also has the potential to decrease kids' autonomous motivation and cause them to lose

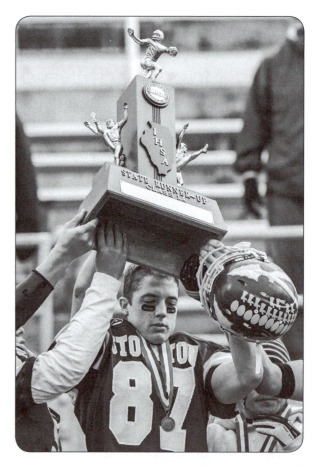

The overuse of or overemphasis on rewards can decrease kids' intrinsic motivation in sport.

interest in the activity. So we need to use caution in rewarding kids, particularly in rewarding them for doing things that they already love to do (e.g., sport).

Overjustification Effect

When you provide an extrinsic reward for something that is already intrinsically interesting, motivation can change from intrinsic to controlled extrinsic. This is known as the overjustification effect. You are overjustifying why people are doing the activity, so their perceptions about why they're doing it begin to change. Multiple research studies have shown that giving children an extrinsic reward (trophy or certificate) for doing an activity that was interesting to them ends up decreasing their intrinsic motivation for the activity (Deci, Koestner, & Ryan, 1999). Why might this occur? It sends the message that the task itself is not really interesting and focuses kids' attention on the reward, not on the engaging aspects of the activity.

Rewards as Controlling or Informational

Extrinsic rewards in youth sport affect motivation based on the meaning of these rewards to kids. An athlete may perceive an extrinsic reward (trophy) as a positive indicator of his sport competence (informational), whereas another athlete may perceive the same reward as coercion to keep him involved in sport (controlling) (Deci & Ryan, 1985).

How athletes' perceptions of rewards influence their motivation was examined in the "pay for play" studies of scholarship and nonscholarship collegiate athletes (Ryan, 1980). Football players on scholarship reported lower intrinsic motivation than did nonscholarship players. In contrast, wrestlers and female athletes on scholarship had higher levels of intrinsic motivation than nonscholarship athletes in these sports. The results were explained based on what the scholarships meant to the athletes. Because

football players knew that a large percentage of athletes in their sport were on scholarship, their scholarships were viewed as less special, less informational about their competence, and more controlling. For wrestlers and female athletes, particularly in the late 1970s, scholarships were not as prevalent, so they provided the athletes with special recognition for their competence.

Interestingly, more recent pay-for-play studies have found that coaching behavior was a stronger influence on the intrinsic motivation of collegiate athletes than scholarship status (Amorose & Horn, 2000; Matosic, Cox, & Amorose, 2014). Actually, it was coaches' use of autonomy-supportive behaviors that most strongly influenced the intrinsic motivation of athletes. So how coaches treat athletes and "use" scholarships is more important than the reward itself.

Overall, rewards have the potential to increase athletes' autonomous motivation if delivered in the right way. This "right way" means that rewards must support young athletes' competence and autonomy without attempting to coerce or control them. Here are some specific suggestions to consider in giving rewards in youth sport.

1. **The best types of extrinsic rewards are novel, creative, and underwhelming.** The reward should not be bigger than the activity itself (or bigger than the kid, as is the case with ridiculously large trophies). Our son's cross-country coach awarded lollipops in practice to those who bettered their times in the previous meet. My (first author) high school basketball team had the Purple Heart practice jersey, which was awarded to the player who demonstrated the most "game-changing hustle" in the previous competition. Start a tradition on your team by coming up with a creative reward that is highly valued by young athletes yet materially nonextravagant.

2. **Extrinsic rewards must be earned and given contingent on specific accomplishments.** Rewards quickly lose any

motivational effect when given indiscriminately. Avoid generalized participation trophies or certificates, which are earned only through being on the team roster and having a pulse. These rewards are meaningless to athletes unless they're attached to specific contingencies, like attending all practices. A good idea is to recognize all the team members but to provide them with a material reward or verbal recognition for their special and unique contributions to the team. Rewards must be earned, or they're viewed as meaningless and dishonest.

3. **Help young athletes process what extrinsic rewards should mean to them.** Congratulate young athletes on winning trophies or ribbons, and ask them to explain what the reward means to them. Help them understand that the material reward is just a symbol of the ultimate reward of feeling pride in your efforts and accomplishments.

4. **Downplay the controlling aspect of rewards, which creates a pressurized expectation for more achievement.** When athletes win honors or the attention of others, help them feel good about earning the honor based on how hard they worked, as opposed to feeling pressure to live up to the honor. Remember that praise is a powerful extrinsic reward that should be given honestly, not in a manipulative manner. Avoid the "Let's hope you keep it up" pressure.

RELATEDNESS

American swimmer Missy Franklin won five medals, four of which were gold, at the 2012 Olympic Games and was poised to cash in on numerous professional sponsorship opportunities. Instead, she returned to finish her senior year and swim on her high school swim team in Colorado. Franklin's motivation was simple—she savored her relationships with friends and teammates more than making millions as a professional athlete. In her last high school meet, she refused to wear a dome cap (often worn over one's normal swim cap) because "it was the last time I was going to swim with [my high school name] on my head, and I didn't want to cover that up" (Thomas, 2013).

The third basic need that drives motivation in youth athletes is **relatedness,** or our need to be connected to those around us and to experience a sense of belonging (Baumeister & Leary, 1995). Youth sport athletes' relationships with parents, coaches, and peers (teammates and friends) serve as important influences on their motivation (Keegan, Spray, Harwood, & Lavallee, 2010).

We've already discussed the strong influence of coaches on youth athletes' motivation in the way they structure practice and interact with athletes, and the role of coaches in youth sport is examined more in chapter 14. However, we can't emphasize enough the importance of emotional support from

---

Personal Plug-In

What Rewards Worked for You?

What rewards do you remember achieving in your youth sport experiences? Which ones meant the most to you or enhanced your motivation? Which ones backfired or decreased your motivation? Consider the reasons why these awards affected you both positively and negatively.

coaches as a key motivating factor for youth sport athletes. Young athletes desire an emotional connection with coaches, beyond the learning of skills and tactics (Williams, Whipp, Jackson, & Dimmock, 2013). Parental support, feedback, and modeling are also important influences on youth athletes' motivation and psychosocial development, as you might expect. The role of parents and families in youth sport is examined more fully in chapter 15.

As shown in the example of Missy Franklin, connections with peers are essential in meeting the need for relatedness in youth athletes. The need for this connection is especially heightened in late childhood and early adolescence. Overall, more positive connections with friends and teammates in youth sport relate to higher perceived competence and self-worth, greater enjoyment and less stress, more autonomous motivation, and a stronger commitment to continued sport involvement (Smith, Ullrich-French, Walker, & Hurley, 2006).

It is our observation that youth athletes' motivational need for relatedness is often overlooked in our zeal to build their skills and teach them competitive strategies. This is particularly true for those young athletes who have lower perceived or actual competence, as well as kids who are shy or new to the team or community. We have observed our own kids, particularly in early adolescence, experiencing sadness and lower self-worth and confidence when feeling that they didn't fit in with teammates or other peers. One could argue that our role as youth sport professionals is to build skills, not to facilitate children's social lives. But if the basic need for relatedness enhances young athletes' motivation and competence in sport, then we should act as social agents to connect kids in meaningful ways with each other.

Instead of just assuming that social connections are made in youth sport, we urge youth sport coaches and directors to thoughtfully and intentionally plan activities and strategies to ensure addressing the important need of relatedness for all participants. These could include meet-and-greet opening cookouts or pizza parties for athletes and their families, postcompetition stops for snacks, and parent–child competition days (which the kids love). Our son's summer swim program has a strong tradition of connecting kids at the city pool, where kids start at age 5 and swim through high school. They have team T-shirts, a special premeet psych-up circle with an elaborate chant and cheer led by the seniors, a preseason mock meet where they learn how to cheer for each other, and a swim buddy system in which premeet buddy packages are exchanged. Three nights of the summer are designated as Seahorse Swim Nights, with the pool open late only to team members for enjoyable games and relays. To be a Seahorse in our community means that you're connected.

Another way to meet kids' need for relatedness is to thoughtfully assign and rotate kids to different partners and groups in practices. Or coaches could simply direct athletes to partner up with someone new for different activities and ask them to learn one fun fact about their partner that they didn't know before. At the end of practice, athletes could share the fun fact about their partner with the entire team. Young athletes should be taught about the importance of supporting teammates—*all* teammates—and there are many easy-to-use team-building exercises that serve to deepen connections through these shared experiences. Put relatedness at the top of your clipboard as an important motivational need that should be addressed every day in youth sport.

WRAP-UP

To wrap up, we suggest that you remember the key aspects of motivation in youth sport by offering young athletes a motivational FEAST. Here's how to serve up the FEAST (figure 6.4).

F is for Feedback. Make your feedback specific, full of information so kids can learn, and contingent on their performance or behavior. Too much positive feedback hurts motivation because it isn't honest and makes kids feel less competent and coerced. Catch athletes doing something right, and tell them about it.

E is for Emotional Connection. Listen to and let your athletes know that you understand and care about them. Fill their "emotional tanks" (Thompson, 2010b) every day. Structure activities to build friendships and social connections among teammates, and teach and provide opportunities for team members to fill each other's emotional tanks. Don't expect this to happen—make it happen.

A is for Autonomy Support. Make sure your athletes feel they have a voice that is heard. Let them make choices within your structure and rules. Reward effort, not outcomes, so that they internalize feelings of control over their performance.

S is for Stimulation. Kids play sport because it is fun, and we believe it can and should be enjoyable at all levels. Be creative and use variety to help them fall in love with their sport, so they can internalize the autonomous extrinsic motivation needed to become a skilled athlete. Challenge them in training, because without optimal challenge, success doesn't mean anything.

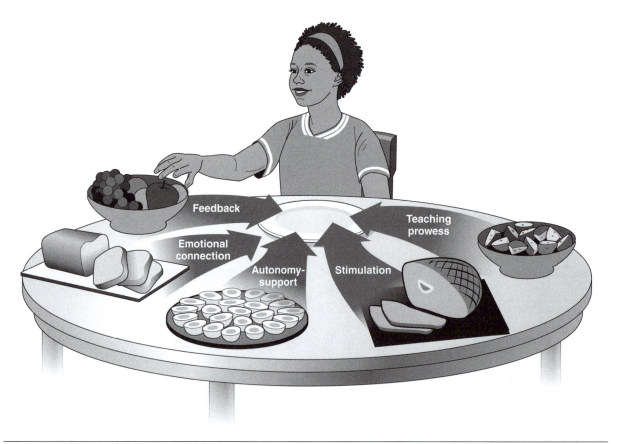

Figure 6.4 A motivational FEAST for youth sport athletes.

T is for Teaching Prowess. Be a great teacher. Study ways to more effectively help kids learn skills, because competence is at the heart of motivation.

Serving up a FEAST to youth athletes at every practice and competition provides them the motivational calories they need to succeed in sport.

LEARNING AIDS

Key Terms

amotivation—The lack of any kind of motivation.

attributions—Reasons that athletes accept to explain why they succeed and fail.

autonomy—The ability and opportunity to govern one's self.

autonomy supportive—Refers to behaviors that include listening to and understanding athletes, providing opportunities for input and choices, and minimizing demanding or controlling behaviors.

competence—Sufficient ability for some purpose.

ego involved—Focused on beating others or demonstrating superior ability in relation to others.

extrinsic motivation—Desire or intent to do an activity to achieve outcomes or rewards beyond the activity itself.

fear of failure—Fear of the consequences of failure, most typically a fear of shame and embarrassment, not being good enough, or letting down others (parents, coaches, teammates).

intrinsic motivation—Desire or intent to do an activity for the pleasure and satisfaction derived from engaging in that activity.

learned helplessness—A psychological state in which children feel powerless and unable to control the outcome of a situation.

motivation—Desire, intent, or drive to do something.

motivational climate—The ways in which various social aspects of a situation are conducted, which in turn influence motivation.

motivational orientations—Internal characteristics, such as beliefs, values, needs, attitudes, goals, and self-perceptions, that predispose people to think and act in certain ways in achievement- or goal-directed activities.

perceived competence—One's sense of personal ability or skill on a specific task.

perfectionism—Tendency to focus on and strive for flawless performance.

psychosocial development—The influence of social experiences, with parents, siblings, peers, teachers, coaches, and even popular media, on how individuals come to view themselves.

relatedness—Our need to be connected to those around us and to experience a sense of belonging.

self-determination—Athletes' perception that they possess control over themselves and their actions; when they feel that they determine their own course of behavior.

self-worth—One's sense of value or worth as a person.

task involved—Focused on performing one's best, or mastering and improving skills.

Summary Points

1. Motivated behavior is evident in choices, effort, persistence, and intensity.

2. Children say that having fun, learning skills, and being with friends are their main reasons for playing sport.

3. The three fundamental needs that drive children's motivation are competence, autonomy, and relatedness.

4. The baseball diamond model of competence motivation explains that kids' motivation leads to mastery attempts, which, if successful and optimally challenging, enhance their perceived competence, self-worth, enjoyment, and subsequent motivation.

5. Fear of failure and maladaptive perfectionism are motivational orientations that predispose youth athletes to focus on avoiding incompetence, as opposed to perceiving sport as challenging.

6. It is crucial for young athletes to be task involved, regardless of whether they are high or low in ego involvement.

7. Task involvement is emphasized when adults reward controllable successes such as effort and improvement, and when they help athletes identify specific task goals on which to judge themselves in sport.

8. Attributions influence the impact of success on perceived competence and self-worth more than the actual success does.

9. Coaches can help retrain attributions in learned-helpless athletes by emphasizing commonality, developmental change, strategy, and effort and persistence.

10. Motivation is enhanced when young athletes are praised for effort, not for performance outcomes.

11. Children younger than 7 years have inflated levels of perceived competence, but these become more accurate as they age.

12. As children age, they use different sources of information to determine how competent they are in sport.

13. Three forms of motivation are intrinsic motivation, autonomous extrinsic motivation, and controlled extrinsic motivation.

14. All forms of motivation are useful, although autonomous motivation is most directly linked to goal attainment, effort, and continuation in sport.

15. Extrinsic rewards have the potential to decrease intrinsic motivation if given in a controlling manner.

16. Positive connections with peers in youth sport relate to higher perceived competence, greater enjoyment and less stress, more autonomous motivation, and a stronger commitment to continued sport involvement.

Study Questions

1. What are the three reasons that kids give for participating in sport? How do these reasons relate to the three basic needs that drive motivation in children?

2. Why do fear of failure and perfectionism develop in young athletes, and what strategies can you use to help athletes overcome these orientations?

3. Why are attributions important, and what attributions should you help young athletes make for success and for failure?

4. What mix of task and ego involvement would you recommend for your sport? Explain why you think this orientation works best in your sport.

5. What is learned helplessness, and how can you work with youth athletes to overcome this negative motivational orientation?

6. Explain how extrinsic motivation can still be autonomous, and why this is an important type of motivation for young athletes as they develop.

7. Define autonomy supportive, and identify four examples of autonomy-supportive behaviors that youth coaches can use.

8. Explain the developmental changes in how children assess their competence and the sources they use to determine their competence.

9. Explain the overjustification effect in giving extrinsic rewards, and explain the distinction between controlling and informational aspects of rewards. Provide three guidelines for youth sport coaches for giving awards to athletes.

10. What is relatedness, and why is it a basic need that fuels motivation in youth athletes? Provide examples for how relatedness can be facilitated in youth sport practice.

Reflective Learning Activities

1. Choose a two-year age group (e.g., 9- and 10-year-olds) and a specific sport. Identify the rewards that you will use with this team, including the specific rewards that will be given and when and how they will be given. Provide a summary that explains how your reward ideas support the basic motivational needs of your athletes. Be creative.

2. Choose a two-year age group and a specific sport. Identify some specific areas in which athletes can be given choices or responsibility within the team. Explain the coach's and the athletes' roles in these choices and responsibilities.

3. Read the case studies provided in appendix G that represent different motivational issues. Explain what you think the motivational issue is in each case (using material from the chapter related to basic needs), and identify suggestions for how the case could be handled by coaches, directors, or parents.

Resource Guide

TEDxTalk by Ed Deci (YouTube) (www.youtube.com/watch?v=VGrcets0E6I). In this TED talk Dr. Ed Deci, one of the founders of self-determination theory (SDT), gives an overview of what SDT is, what it aims to explain, and how to use SDT to promote motivation in people. Throughout his discussion, Dr. Deci gives examples of what to do and not to do from a motivational perspective.

Supporting Athletes' Needs (YouTube) (www.youtube.com/watch?v=kxsJT6X-wNy0). This video covers motivational theories, particularly SDT and how it relates to athletes' needs. The video's target audience is coaches, and topics covered include internal and external motivators, sources of motivation, and suggestions for coaches to follow regarding motivation.

chapter 7

MODIFYING SPORT FOR YOUTH

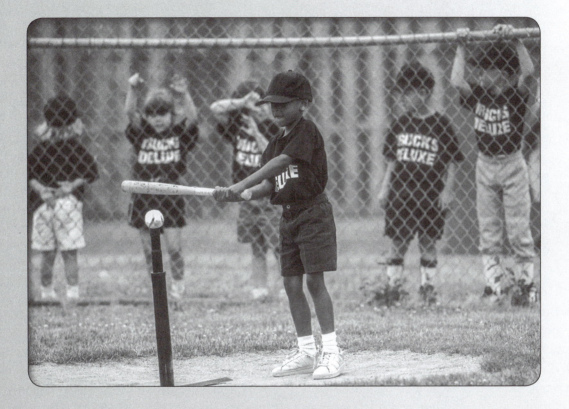

CHAPTER PREVIEW

In this chapter, you'll learn

» why modification is needed in youth sport,

» why modification is often resisted by adults,

» examples of how youth sport may be modified for kids, and

» the positive outcomes for kids when sport is modified.

Picture this. A 7-year-old is shooting at a 10-foot (3-meter) basket, and the ball never touches the rim. A team of 5-year-olds is playing football in full pads, 11 vs. 11, on a regulation-size field. A volleyball team made up of 13-year-olds practices five times a week, from May through October, because this gives the team the best chance to win. What's wrong with these examples? If your answer is kids playing adult games with adult-size equipment and rules, you're correct. In this chapter, you'll read about the importance of modification in youth sport, the benefits of modification for children's skill and psychosocial development, and how to implement developmentally appropriate modifications for kids.

Modification means adapting the sport experience to make it developmentally appropriate for children. Perhaps you can think back to your own sport experience and recall situations in which the rules, playing areas, or equipment for the sport were changed to meet your developmental needs. Here are a few common examples of youth sport modifications:

- Basketball size is smaller in circumference than a regulation men's basketball (27.25 vs. 29.5 inches [69 vs. 75 centimeters] in circumference).
- Striking object (e.g., bat, hockey stick, tennis racket) is shorter and lighter in weight.
- Target goal is lower (basketball hoop) or smaller (soccer goal).
- The field or court playing area is reduced in size.
- Fewer players are on the field of play during competition.
- Strategies are restricted (e.g., no pressing in basketball, no rushing the quarterback in football).
- Rules are changed to increase the amount of play for each child (e.g., every player bats in softball before sides change, every player plays all positions in soccer).

These are just a few of the many modifications that can significantly improve the youth sport experience for kids. As you read through this chapter, challenge yourself to be innovative in thinking about appropriate modifications that would help youth sport be a better experience for all children. A good rule of thumb is to match the activity to the kids, instead of trying to make kids fit into an adult activity.

WHY SHOULD SPORT BE MODIFIED FOR YOUTH?

Children do not automatically develop the physical skills and behaviors they need to safely and successfully participate in youth sport. It's up to the adults who structure youth sport to create an appropriate youth sport culture. This entails developing modified rules and guidelines for competition, practice, selecting teams, equipment, playing schedules, and tactics. When done correctly, modified youth sport increases the quality of play, maximizes the chance for success, and enhances enjoyment.

Developmental Differences in Children

Perhaps the most important reason to modify youth sport is that the participants are developmentally very different from adults. Children develop physiologically, mechanically, socially, and cognitively in different stages on their way to adulthood. These differences suggest that how adults play sport often does not fit or benefit kids. Children have smaller body size in height and weight, shorter levers (arms and legs), less strength and muscle endurance, and lower levels of coordination than adults. The differences in body proportions affect the mechanical parameters of skill performance, such as center of gravity, use of force, and angle of release. Yet, we often ask children to perform adult forms of sport with these physical disadvantages.

A study by the National Youth Sport Coaches Association (Engh, 2002) of 5- to 8-year-old athletes examined whether they had the skills necessary to participate successfully in their chosen sports. Fundamental motor skills such as throwing, catching, running, or kicking were tested. Of the over 1,000 children tested, 49% were found to be lacking skills they needed for minimum success. Without modification of sports for this age group, at least half of the children who played would not have been capable of performing even the basic skills found in traditional sports. Motor development experts have identified the need to acquire skill and technical abilities at a young age during sensitive learning periods for skill development (as discussed in chapter 5).

We know children have a better chance of learning biomechanically correct skills if tasks are adapted to their size, strength, and developmental level; otherwise, skill learning may be inhibited. For example, when Carly was age 6, her father wanted her to play tennis. He would take her to local tennis courts to practice. Carly's father had been a tennis player in high school, so he knew some drills and how to play the

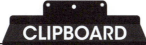

CLIPBOARD

How to Fit Sport to Kids

1. The rules of youth football are often the same as high school or college rules. However, many local organizations modify youth football rules to protect the players or allow for more competitive play. Here is a list of a few rule changes often used in youth football:

    - No defender may line up in a gap.

    - No blitzing is allowed.

    - There must be two backs in the offensive backfield.

    - No rushing punts or place kicks are allowed.

    - Only the 6-2 defense may be used.

    - The quarterback may not run with the ball.

    - All defenders must be stationary at the snap.

    - No more than five players can be on the defensive line, and at least two players should be 10 yards (9 meters) off the ball.

    - If your team is winning by more than 18 points, you have to take out your four best players (the other coaches pick the four players).

2. A youth basketball league in southern Ohio has modified the rules in the league so that every player has the opportunity to score a basket. Before the start of each quarter, the teams line up at the free-throw line of their basket and each girl or boy shoots one free throw. If the basket is made, 1 point is added to the game score. These scores are added to the overall team scoreboard as soon as they occur.

3. The Jack Nicklaus Learning Leagues introduces children to golf at parks and recreation facilities by providing user-friendly and safe equipment (www.snaggolf.com/jnll.html). Children, age 5 through 12, use plastic clubs, tennis-type balls, and Velcro targets. The goal of the program is to get children interested in golf at an earlier age and make the experience fun.

game. He gave her one of his old rackets and started hitting balls to her forehand and backhand. Of course, at age 6, she didn't have the hand–eye coordination or proper swing mechanics to hit the ball properly. To compensate, Carly found that if she blocked the ball with her heavy racket she would at least make contact and her dad would say "nice try." Over the many years of hitting tennis balls this way with her father, Carly's forehand and backhand strokes were learned incorrectly, which hampered her ability to play high school tennis.

Research confirms that children who are forced to learn tennis with an adult-sized racket tend to lean their trunk away from the ball when hitting (Ward & Groppel, 1980), which produces an inefficient and technically flawed movement pattern. Learning proper mechanics at an early age is like establishing a solid foundation for a building. Without the proper foundation, the structure is never really sound.

In some cases, adult forms of sport can be unhealthy for young athletes. An example is

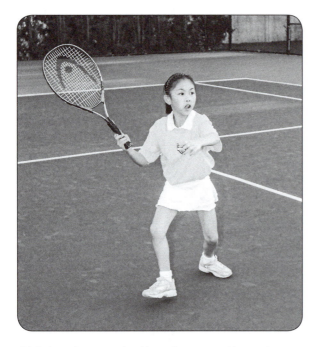

Children have a better chance of learning biomechanically correct skills if equipment and facilities are adapted to their size, strength, and developmental level.

young baseball pitchers throwing curveballs and too many pitches at a young age, which has the potential to damage their throwing arms (discussed in chapter 12). Overuse injuries have reached epidemic proportions in youth sport, chiefly due to designing youth sport training and competition such that they are similar in intensity to adult versions of the sport.

So what developmental factors should you consider when planning a modified youth sport experience? Here are some questions youth sport leaders and coaches should ask in designing youth sport practices and competitions to be developmentally appropriate:

1. What is the attentional focus of my players (e.g., how long can they sit and listen)?

2. Are their perceptual–motor skills (e.g., eye–hand and eye–foot coordination) ready for the demands of this practice drill or game situation?

3. What is a reasonable distance and speed at which they can perform the fundamental motor skills for this sport (e.g., throw, catch, skate, strike, run, swim)?

4. Do they have the cognitive ability to understand my strategy and tactics?

5. Can they physically execute the required skills of the game?

6. What are their neuromuscular and cardiovascular limits in this activity?

Children's Motives for Playing Sport

A second important reason to modify youth sports is that children play sports for different reasons than adults. As you learned in chapter 6, children play sport to have fun, learn and improve their skills, be with friends, and be part of a team (Sit & Lindner, 2006; Weiss & Williams, 2004). However, adults often focus on winning and championships. Unfortunately, we know that adult motives drive the culture of youth sport in many instances. When children are left on their own to organize their sport games, modified rules are often applied. Four basic principles apply to the ways children govern their own free play (Murphy, 1999):

Action. Games must be motivating and must be structured into competition. The competition is fun, and the rules make sense. Children decide how many players should be on each side to create the best action for competition, and they modify play for more action, fun, and competition with small-sided teams.

Personal involvement. Ask children this question: "Would you rather play on a team that may not win very often, or sit on the bench for a team that wins all the time?" The response is always the same. Children would rather play and lose than sit and win. For participants of every age, there is very little enjoyment in watching someone else play, and very little learning takes place without practice. Children often modify their rules to allow second chances at success. More importantly, they arrange the game so that everyone plays.

Excitement. Lopsided games are no fun for kids. If the teams turn out to be uneven, either the game is concluded and new sides are picked, or players trade places. With a new game comes a new chance for the losing side. Young athletes often modify their rules to create better, more exciting games.

Friendships. Youth sport participants enjoy being with their friends, competing against them, and competing with them. They also enjoy meeting new friends through sport. Friendships become a favorite outcome of participating in youth sport, so children structure their experience to build and maintain their relationships with other children.

Maximize Successful Experiences

The third reason modification is important has to do with the benefits of maximizing success for children. Research suggests that successful performances lead to feelings of higher self-confidence, whereas failure can lead to doubt about abilities and lower self-confidence (Chase, 2001). Self-confidence is important for children because it affects whether a child will choose to play, put forth enough effort to improve, and persist through occasional failures. Without the confidence to stick with a sport, children may drop out before they have the chance to learn skills.

If Alex joins the local swim team and starts competing in swim meets without the proper strokes or any modification to fit his experience level, he will continually fail. Alex begins to lose self-confidence in his ability to swim because he never experiences success. It's likely that Alex will decide that swimming is not fun, that he's not good enough, and he'll quit the team. If Alex decides that swimming is not for him and finds another sport activity, then there is little need for concern. But what if Alex never finds success in any sport because the sport culture does not provide successful experiences? Now we have a situation in which Alex drops out of sport completely, with low self-confidence and an opinion that sports are not fun.

So how can we maximize success for youth? While most coaches understand the importance of performance success to increase confidence, many adults define success using adult standards. Children, especially children under 10 years of age, see success differently than adults (Fry & Duda, 1997; Nicholls, 1989). Children under 10 years of age will most likely enjoy activities in which they can complete the skills or task (e.g., mere participation). A clear outcome of who wins and who loses is not as important as who finishes and who is praised for effort.

Once children are over 10 years of age and ability becomes more evident to them, coaches should structure the learning environment to provide opportunities for improvement. Children at these ages need to feel as though they can work hard to improve their skills and thus achieve successful performances. Therefore, when planning practice situations, coaches should make them age appropriate, avoid emphasis on the final outcome, and encourage progress toward improvement. Modification of rules, tactics, equipment, and playing areas increases the likelihood of successful experiences by matching sport demand and definition of success to the developmental level of children.

Research Support for Modification

Modification works! In this section we provide research support for this idea; we encourage youth sport leaders to use these

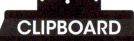

Other Modification Ideas

Modification for Youth Hockey: Doug Abrams (former college hockey player, coach, and law professor) suggests the following practice schedule for 8- to 9-year-olds in ice hockey (Bigelow, Moroney, & Hall, 2001). Practice is 1 hour long, broken down into 10 minutes of warm-up, 15 minutes of "skill drill" in stations, 15 minutes of "fun learning games," 15 minutes of scrimmaging, and, finally, 5 minutes for relay races. As the season progresses, more time can be spent on skill drills and scrimmaging and less on fun learning games. However, the practice must stay fun and active for all players. Specific modifications during practice to fit this age group include rotating stations every 5 to 8 minutes to match their attention span, scrimmage width-wise and not length-wise on the ice at the beginning of the season, playing two scrimmages side by side so everyone plays and no one watches, teaching the basic skills and basic position play, and then letting the kids play. Extended chalk talks are not necessary or productive for this age group. And finally, Abrams suggests rotating positions among all players, even the goalie position, so that all players learn to appreciate all positions and the skills necessary to play well.

Modification for Tee Ball: The best type of tee ball experience is one in which the main goal is for children to be active (e.g., bat more, field more, and throw more) during small-sided games. A modified tee ball game for 5- to 7-year-olds would keep children moving so they don't get bored. Here are several suggestions to accomplish that goal:

1. Create games with four or five players playing the field and four or five players at bat.
2. Sides change every time the batting team goes through one at-bat.
3. There are no outs and no score is kept.
4. Everyone bats off a tee—no coach pitch.
5. Players must throw the ball and not run with it.
6. The game should last four innings at the most or 1 hour for this age group.

When children drop out of baseball or softball at a young age, it's because there is very little action on the field while playing defense and they may get to bat only once every other inning. Structure tee ball so it's quick moving, with lots of running to field the ball and a chance to bat every inning.

findings to help convince others to set up youth sport in developmentally appropriate ways for kids.

The effect of basket height on shooting performance was examined from a biomechanical perspective by Satern, Messier, and Keller-NcNulty (1989). They found that changing the height of the basket affected the foul shooting performance of 7th-grade boys. Shooting performance was assessed on a 4-point scoring system that reflected whether the shot was successful or unsuccessful and whether the ball hit the rim, hit the backboard, or did not hit anything. With the use of two 16-mm high-speed cameras to evaluate shooting mechanics, the results revealed that the lower basket height was related to better shooting mechanics.

Chase, Ewing, Lirgg, and George (1994) conducted a study on the effects of equipment modification in youth sport basketball. They investigated the effects on success (number of baskets made) and player confidence of lowering the basket height from 10 feet to 8 feet (3 meters to 2.4 meters) and reducing the basketball size from a regulation men's ball to a youth size. Results of the study showed that children made more baskets and had more confidence when shooting at the 8-foot basket, regardless of the size of the basketball. Another study found that more dribbles, passes, and pass receptions were made in 9- to 11-year-old youth basketball when a smaller basketball was used (Arias, Argudo, & Alonso, 2012).

In a study by Kalyvas and Reid (2005), participation in and enjoyment of a Newcomb volleyball game were examined in youth ages 7 to 12 years. Of the 35 participants, 15 children had some type of physical disability and 20 had no physical disability. Modifications for the Newcomb volleyball game included (a) a lower net, (b) a balloon instead of a ball, (c) a rule that all members of a team had to touch the balloon before it was sent over the net, and (d) a serving line closer to the net. The results indicated that children both with and without disabilities

performed more successful passes, were more active, and spent less time inactive in the modified game as compared to the traditional game. The authors pointed to the importance of developing modifications that are challenging and interesting according to developmental age of the children.

A classic study investigated what differences would be found in batting, pitching, and fielding during baseball games played by 9- and 10-year-olds under either a traditional or a modified format (Martens, Rivkin, & Bump, 1984). In the modified format, coaches pitched to batters instead of kids pitching to batters as in the traditional league. The results clearly demonstrated that modifying baseball so that kids have pitches to hit substantially increased the amount of activity in the games.

In the traditional kid-pitch league, players were inactive at bat for 70% of the pitches. This means that nothing happened on offense or defense for 70% of the time! In the modified coach-pitch league, players were inactive only 29% of the time. One-third of all pitches were hit fairly in the modified league, whereas only 1/10 of pitches were hit fairly in the traditional league. Obviously, because of the increased offensive activity, defensive activity was increased in the modified league as compared to the traditional league.

Which game would you rather play in? If you're a baseball traditionalist and choose to play in the traditional format, we understand, because you're an adult. But this is youth sport, where kids want and need to develop their abilities—to throw, snag grounders, and catch pop-ups. Any way we can increase active time through modification in youth sport is preferred.

Research on sport modification in tennis, particularly racket size and ball compression, has demonstrated the effectiveness of modifying sport for skill development in kids. The International Tennis Federation modified tennis ball specifications in 2005 to create three types of balls that differ in softness, weight, and bounce, and the United States Tennis Association has done the same. Multiple studies have found that children experienced better technique development, longer rallies, greater enjoyment, and more net play when playing with lower-compression balls as compared to regular (adult) compression balls (Buszard, Farrow, Reid, & Masters, 2014; Farrow & Reid, 2010; Hammond & Smith, 2006; Kachel, Buszard, & Reid, 2015; Larson & Guggenheimer, 2013). Because the modified balls bounced lower, children swung low to high and struck the ball in front and to the side of the body more often than when the regular tennis ball was used. These techniques are critical for the development of topspin, an important component of the forehand shot (Buszard et al., 2014). Similarly, smaller court size and lighter rackets were related to better tennis performance in kids (Buszard et al., 2014; Farrow & Reid, 2010; Larson & Guggenheimer, 2013). A description of the modified tennis program sponsored by the United States Tennis Association is provided later in the chapter.

WHY DO ADULTS RESIST YOUTH SPORT MODIFICATION?

Parents are sometimes misguided in their perceptions of how children learn sport skills and become more proficient. They fear that their child will be left behind in the race to be a good athlete if she is not playing a regulation sport. Some parents want to get their son or daughter on the fast track to superstardom and the benefits that come with that stardom. Many parents are driven by the potential for college scholarships or professional contracts. They are trying to live out their own dreams of athletic stardom through their children (discussed in chapter 15). These irrational fears and thoughts may lead to serious, even fatal, consequences for youth sport participants.

According to a report released by the National Youth Sport Safety Foundation, more than 20 children were killed playing organized baseball games between 1973 and 1994. The cause of death was explained as children's being struck by a hard baseball. The report went on to say that because the children had not developed the motor skills of eye tracking, coordination, and timing to avoid being hit by a pitched or batted ball, they were struck in the chest or head, which caused extreme trauma and death. A simple solution would be to require the use of a soft, thus safe, baseball for any team with youth under the age of 12 years. The ball is the same size and is the approximate weight of a regular baseball, but it's softer, which means it's less likely to produce a deadly blow. Yet, the soft baseball is not mandatory, and children still die every baseball season because adults will not change the rules. Why wouldn't we make this equipment modification? Reports indicate that some coaches and parents fear that soft baseballs do not play the same as a traditional hardball, so players who use it will not develop the same level of skills as other players.

Some adults try to control youth sports and focus on adult goals instead of children's goals. One of the best examples of parents and coaches losing sight of the focus of youth sport is tee ball. All across the nation are tee ball leagues in which coaches refuse to use a batting tee, which is sort of the point of tee ball! Instead, the coach pitches to each batter a certain number of times (e.g., five pitches). Only after five missed pitches is the tee set up so the batter can hit off the tee.

The first problem with this situation is that coaches can't pitch to such short batters without getting close and lobbing the ball over the plate. The closeness of pitcher to batter reduces the reaction time for the batter, so if the ball does cross the strike zone, it happens too fast for the child to be able to swing. All the fundamental skills that

Personal Plug-In

How Modified Were Your Youth Sports?

Think about your personal experiences in youth sport. What types of modifications were made to the sports that you played as a child? What was the impact of these modifications? Was the game more fun or easier to play? Now consider any sports that you played as a child under the same conditions as in adult play. What were the outcomes of these types of games? Did any personal experiences you had with modification in sport influence your view of youth sport today?

could be gained through hitting off a tee is lost. And we won't even mention the time it takes and the boredom it creates to pitch five times to every batter and then bring in the tee. Any parent will tell you that tee ball can be excruciating to watch. But coaches and spectators struggle through tee ball games (that aren't really tee ball) because adults want players to bat a pitched ball.

WHAT CHANGES SHOULD BE MADE?

Youth sport modifications can be made for playing areas, equipment, rules, and tactics. Using these four categories, we challenge you to be creative, focus on the reasons children play sports, and consider how you could structure the sport culture so that all participants are active and improve their skills.

Playing Field

Because children are smaller and have less aerobic capacity than adults, a smaller area for play makes sense. It's also reasonable that in a smaller area that involves a ball or other object to control, children will spend less time chasing after the ball and more time throwing, catching, or kicking it to teammates (practicing the skills needed to play the game). The action of the game becomes available to all players and should provide more scoring opportunities.

Equipment

The equipment needs to match the size of the players so they can have some success during game play, can play without getting injured, and can develop sound fundamental skills. The wrong type of equipment (too heavy, too big) can cause children to improvise on their mechanics, which leads to poor fundamental skills and in some cases serious injury. Think about what the child needs to do with a particular piece of equipment and how you can make it easier to carry out that task. Is it better to catch a soft ball or a hard ball that hurts? Is it easier to control a short striking object or long one? In general, modification of equipment focuses on weight, height, circumference, color, texture (smooth or rough), or surface (soft or hard).

Rules

Modified rules in youth sport should align the game with the reasons why children want to participate in sport. Remember that children play sports to have fun, improve their skills, stay in shape, and be with their friends. Start by thinking about the sport season from the very first task (e.g., how do you select teams?) to the last task (e.g., do you have a league tournament?). How can you set up practice and game situations so that all children are highly active? The types of rules that are typically modified involve playing time, substitutions, position play, structure of game play (e.g., everyone bats before the inning is over), and number of players on a team.

Challenge yourself to think beyond the typical. For example, think of the tee ball game with only four players in the outfield. What would the game play actually look like? We would see children running to field the ball and throwing to a teammate who is moving to cover a base. Wow, that's a lot of activity for all the players! What a difference compared to the traditional game with eight children standing around out in the field. There will always be pushback from coaches and parents who want to challenge modified rules for all the reasons stated earlier. Hold your ground and adopt modified rules that make the game developmentally appropriate for children.

Tactics

Tactics are different from rules. However, the rationale for developing a tactic is the same as for developing rules: to align game play with the reasons children want to participate in sport. Tactics involve strategies (e.g., offensive and defensive) in game play and practice and should focus on keeping all players involved and learning skills. Be careful that your tactics don't backfire. Here's a tactic that we dislike because it rarely improves game play: Everyone must touch the ball before a teammate tries to score. Have you ever seen this tactic employed by children? The best players on the team hand the ball to the worst players and immediately grab it back. Then they continue on their way and try to score.

A better tactic is to play small-sided games, sometimes grouped by ability, so that all the "ball hogs" are on one field and other children get to play key roles in their games. Or, arrange the position play so that the dominant players can't dominate the game all the time. The key is to frequently mix up how you structure play so that the better players are challenged and the players who need to improve their skills have more opportunities.

USTA's QuickStart Tennis Example

The United States Tennis Association (USTA) launched the QuickStart Tennis program in 2008, which modified the court size, equipment, and rules of tennis for children 10 and under (www.usta.com). The program was designed to get kids playing the game immediately with a level of success that is enjoyable and motivational. As shown in figure 7.1, the balls, rackets, net heights, and court sizes are progressively modified to match the maturity and experience of learners.

For children 8 and under, the court is downsized and allows for four QuickStart courts to be set up crossways on a regulation tennis court (see figure 7.1). The net height is 2 feet, 9 inches (84 centimeters) (3 inches [7.6 centimeters] lower than regulation), making it easier for kids to rally over the net. Rackets are shorter, and the ball is a red low-compression ball made of lightweight foam or felt, which bounces more slowly and travels through the air more slowly. The modified scoring system is best of three games, with the first player to win 7 points winning the game.

For 9- and 10-year-olds, the court size is increased somewhat but is still not a regulation-size tennis court (see figure 7.1), although the net height is at the 3-foot (0.9-meter) tennis standard. Lower-compression orange balls are used; they are faster than the red foam balls but still have a lower bounce and speed compared to a standard yellow tennis ball. Rackets are still shorter (23-25 inches [58-64 centimeters]) than regulation (27-inch [69-centimeter]) tennis rackets but longer than the 8-and-under program rackets. Scoring for this level is best of three sets, with four games winning a set, and with the third set (if necessary) going to the first player to win 7 points.

Kids 11 years and older play on a regulation tennis court (see figure 7.1) and use green balls, which have a slightly reduced

USTA guidelines for 10 and under tennis

Stage	Red	Orange	Green
Age	8 and under	9-10	11 and up
Ball	Red felt or foam *Moves slower and bounces lower than orange ball*	Orange *Moves slower and bounces lower than green ball*	Green *Slightly reduced bounce from yellow ball*
Court size	36' x 18'	60' x 21' singles 60' x 27' doubles	78' x 27' singles 78' x 36' doubles
Net height	2'9"	3' center, 3'6" at net posts	3' center, 3'6" at net posts
Racquet	Up to 23"	23" - 25"	25" - 27"

Figure 7.1 QuickStart Tennis equipment and court modifications by age.

Reprinted from Sports Chalet.

bounce compared to the standard yellow tennis ball. The court is regulation size (78 feet [23.8 meters]), with rackets slightly smaller (25 inches [64 centimeters]) than regulation size (27 inches [69 centimeters]). Scoring at this stage follows the regular rules of tennis.

The USTA feels that the program will draw more kids into tennis and allow recreational and club programs to keep more kids active on the courts when using the 8-and-under format of four QuickStart courts across one regulation court. The QuickStart program has been adapted by junior clubs and programs, and equipment for the various levels is available online and in sporting goods stores.

The QuickStart Tennis program is an exemplary model for youth sport modification, with a slogan of "enabling children to 'play to learn' rather than 'learn to play.'" That sounds like a great idea!

WRAP-UP

Youth sport organizations are realizing that children require specific developmentally appropriate environments to cultivate their skills, enhance enjoyment, and maintain participation. Modifications in all types of sports are being more accepted as best practice for skill development. If you still aren't convinced that modifications in youth sport are a critical step for skill development, then think about your experience learning to ride a bicycle. Did your parents put you on an adult bike and send you down the nearest steep hill? Or, did you first learn to ride a small bike with training wheels? Once you mastered the pedaling and braking part, developed some confidence, and overcame your fear of moving fast, you probably removed the training wheels. And, as you grew each year, your bike would grow with you until the adult-size bike fit. This seems like a good model to follow for youth sports.

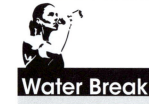

Water Break

Back to the Future for Skill Development

Don Lucia (2009), the highly successful men's hockey coach at the University of Minnesota, expresses his gratitude for the outstanding coaches he had as a player at the junior level. According to Coach Lucia, these coaches were all guided by a common theme—skill development. And he wishes that those coaches could go "back to the future" to model for today's coaches the ways they focused on building skills in kids.

Coach Lucia feels that adult coaches today tend to overstructure practice and competition for kids. He suggests finding ways for games that allow "the ice to be the teacher" as it was when he was a kid. He is a strong proponent of small-sided games, in which kids can improve both their skills in tight areas and their abilities to make quick decisions in pressure situations. He also advocates modifying the playing surface so that younger kids don't play or practice on a full sheet of ice. He suggests putting a couple of nets along the boards and playing cross-ice, which will allow players more puck touches and more shots.

Coach Lucia stresses that this freer type of skill development and modified ice hockey will build skills in kids that college and professional coaches deem important. He states, "They're looking for kids who can skate, stickhandle, pass, and shoot. They're not looking for how well they fore-check, backcheck, or where they are in the defensive zone" (p. 40)—these are things that can easily be taught later, according to Lucia. His take-home message for hockey modification is a great example of developmentally appropriate practice, in which skill development and the joy of playing are emphasized versus an overstructured emphasis on full-ice tactics and team play.

Keep this most important question in mind when considering whether and how to modify sport for children: Will this program, practice, or competition serve the needs of the children in this age group—all the children—or is it primarily serving the needs of the adults (Bigelow, Moroney, & Hall, 2001)? Clearly the needs of children should guide the choices we make in organizing and modifying youth sport.

LEARNING AIDS

Key Term

modification—Adapting the sport experience to make it developmentally appropriate for children.

Summary Points

1. Sport should be modified for kids because of children's smaller body sizes, shorter levers (arms and legs), lower muscular strength and endurance, and lower levels of coordination.

2. Children have a better chance of learning biomechanically correct skills if sports are adapted to their developmental levels; skill learning is inhibited without modification.

3. Children are motivated to play in situations that include action, personal involvement, excitement, and friendships.

4. Modified sport leads to greater success and the development of higher levels of self-confidence, which predict whether children stay in sport.

5. Research has shown that sport modifications increase skill efficiency, success, confidence, and activity in all participants.

6. Some adults fear that children will be disadvantaged in their skill development when participating in modified youth sport.

7. Youth sport modifications can be made in playing areas, equipment, rules, tactics, and objectives.

Study Questions

1. Identify several developmental differences in children that support the need for modification in youth sport.

2. Explain at least three possible negative outcomes for children when they play adult forms of sport.

3. Cite at least three arguments that you can use against parents who resist modification because they fear their children will be disadvantaged by the modification.

4. What do children seek from their sport participation, and how can we provide that in organized youth sport?

5. Describe how research has supported the positive effects of modification on children's sport experiences.

6. Identify and describe at least five modifications you would suggest for your sport.

Reflective Learning Activities

1. Identify at least three limitations or problems with current practices in your favorite youth sport. How could you modify this sport to be more developmentally appropriate for kids?

2. The QuickStart Tennis program is presented in the chapter as a national initiative to modify a specific sport for youth. Try to identify another program that has attempted to implement developmentally appropriate modifications. Explain these modifications and why you think they are useful (or not).

3. Choose one sport, and suggest several developmentally appropriate modifications to take participants through beginning, early, and intermediate levels of the sport.

Resource Guide

Educated Sports Parent (www.educatedsportsparent.com/developmentally-appropriate-program-modifications). This area of the Educated Sports Parent website discusses the importance of modification of youth sport programs. It not only addresses the importance of learning the basic skills necessary for sporting success, but it also discusses why not modifying sports for young athletes could lead to injury. At the bottom of this webpage is a list of sports and how they can be modified. These sports include basketball, baseball, football, hockey, and soccer; general modifications for any sport activity are also identified. These modifications are broken down into different age groups and encourage the development of the necessary skills in order for youth sport athletes to be successful now and in the future.

Start Smart Program, created by the **National Alliance for Youth Sports** (www.nays.org/sports_programs/start_smart/). The Start Smart program is a step-by-step approach to creating a youth sport program in which kids can learn the basic skills necessary for youth sport participation in a fun and safe environment. Baseball, soccer, basketball, golf, football, and tennis are sports included in the program.

chapter 8

TEACHING SKILLS TO YOUNG ATHLETES

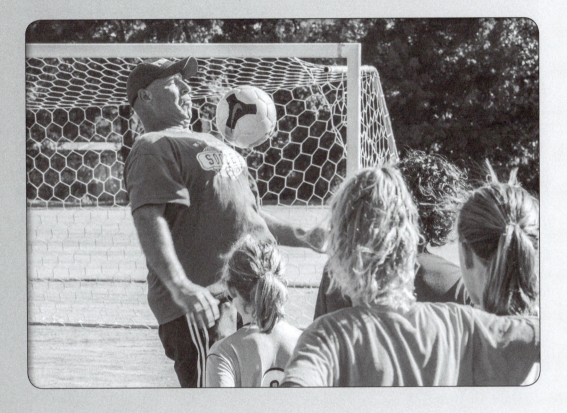

CHAPTER PREVIEW

In this chapter, you'll learn

» how children think and learn differently from adults,

» the five-step teaching cycle for youth sport,

» what makes a good instructor, and

» teaching tips to maximize learning in kids.

One of the most important objectives of youth sport is to help kids develop and improve their motor skills. Thus, youth sport leaders need to be effective teachers to help young athletes learn, improve, and perform. There are many different ways to teach skills to young athletes. Good teachers and coaches find a teaching style that fits their strengths yet also accommodates the readiness levels and different learning styles of young athletes.

Can you remember a teacher or coach who was especially effective in helping you learn a particular sport skill? Why was this person so effective in helping you learn? What made him or her a great teacher? We bet that you'll see this person as you read through the recommended practices of effective teaching in this chapter. We bet that your teacher or coach was able to understand you and your learning style, provide developmentally appropriate instruction and learning progressions, provide helpful personal feedback, motivate you, and make learning something that you wanted to do.

A book about legendary college basketball coach John Wooden's teaching principles and practices is titled *You Haven't Taught Until They Have Learned* (Nater, 2010). Explaining or demonstrating something to kids in practice doesn't mean they've learned it. **Learning** is the relatively permanent change in performance that occurs with practice (Wrisberg, 2007). Effective teaching that leads to learning in youth sport requires a systematic approach using demonstration, motivation, and practice in developmentally appropriate ways. We realize that many youth sport leaders are not professional teachers or coaches, yet we believe that they can improve their teaching skills by learning some basic principles and practices related to teaching effectiveness.

THE FIVE-STEP TEACHING CYCLE

Learning is a process that requires time, effort, and focus. It's also helpful to have a really good teacher. This chapter focuses on how to be that really good teacher. We begin by describing the five-step cycle of teaching: motivation, demonstration, practice, feedback, and practice (see figure 8.1).

Motivation

Today, kids ask, "What's in it for me?" and "Why should I learn this?" Thus, motivation to learn is the starting point for all instruction. Here are a few examples of motivational methods that may grab the attention of your athletes and prepare them for learning:

- Use a famous athlete (professional, collegiate, or high school) that they recognize as an example of someone who performs this skill. "When Rafael Nadal plays tennis, he talks about footwork being a key to his success. He works on his footwork every day to get better. Today we're going to start with a footwork drill for the forehand volley."

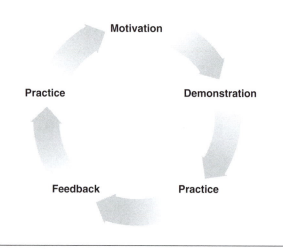

Figure 8.1 Five-step teaching cycle.

- Tell them that you are going to ask questions or quiz them later, so it's important that they understand what you are explaining. "We are going to start practice today with an explanation of a 1-3-1 zone defense. Pay close attention to the roles of each player in the zone. I'm going to quiz each of you before we move to the court."

- Explain the outcome or product that is likely to result if they learn this new skill. This is not a suggestion for an extrinsic reward that you will provide, but a consequence, such as improved play or scoring more points. "Today I want to stress the importance of team communication while we're playing. Members of good teams talk to each other during game play. As a result, they play better, they win more games, and they enjoy playing together much more than team members who don't communicate. Good teams communicate, so I want to hear you talking to each other during today's scrimmage."

Keep your motivational statements short. This is not a pregame pep talk. The goal is to get your athletes' attention, keep their attention focused on your demonstration, and provide motivation to work hard and learn what you are teaching.

Demonstration

The next time you're around a young child (4 to 5 years old), ask him or her to show you a skill that he or she has never seen before. For example, ask the child to show you a good athletic stance. Without a clear picture of what an athletic stance looks like, children will come up with all kinds of variations. Young athletes have to have a clear image or mental model of a skill before they actually try to perform the skill.

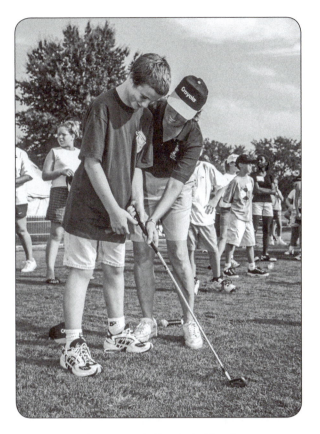

Adult coaches should be brief in demonstrating and explaining, taking anywhere from 30 seconds to a maximum of three minutes, before letting athletes themselves practice the movement.

There are several key principles to providing good demonstrations to learners (Rink & Hall, 2008). Teachers or coaches should demonstrate the whole skill several times at full speed, then break down the skill into parts (if appropriate), and then demonstrate the skill again at full speed several times. This principle provides the learner with an image of the skill, how it's performed as a whole and in parts, at the correct performance speed. Avoid demonstrating in slow motion or showing only parts of the skill because this does not provide the correct mental model the child needs in order to learn the skill. Also, provide the demonstration from several different viewpoints or angles so learners can view the skill from the front, back, and side.

After the whole–part–whole demonstration, provide learners with one to three instructional cues (labels) they can easily remember and say while practicing the skill. These cues are important in the learning process because they remind learners of the steps involved and the order of execution in performing the skill. For children, the instructional cues should represent mental images with which they are familiar (see table 8.1 for some examples). Be sure that the mental image is relevant and current for today's kids. Years ago, coaches used to teach players to shoot a basketball with the instructional cue, "Shoot like you are in a phone booth and the ball comes out the top." Today, young children would have a hard time imagining a phone booth since they don't exist anymore.

The last principle of the demonstration is to check for understanding before the athletes begin to practice. Ask your players questions related to the demonstration and performance of the skill to reinforce what they need to do. Ask them to recite the instructional cues, or labels, that they need to remember as they try the skill.

A common mistake made by coaches when teaching new skills is taking too long in their verbal instructions and demonstrations. They talk too much, with too many details, and demonstrate more than the players can remember. How long should the motivation, demonstration, and instructional cues take when you are presenting to youth athletes? Typically, less than 3 minutes is the recommended time. Depending on the complexity of the skill you are teaching, the motivation and demonstration may take 30 seconds. Let's time our example with the athletic stance. Start your watch and read through our example.

> *Today we are going to learn how to do a good athletic stance. Can someone name a famous athlete we all have seen play? (Sue Bird, point guard for the Seattle Storm.) When Sue plays basketball, she uses a good athletic stance when she guards another player. If you want to play good defense like Sue Bird, you'll need a good athletic stance. A good athletic stance means you are ready to move and play the game. Here's what an athletic stance looks like [drop into a stance three times, showing the stance from different viewpoints]. When I say 'go,' you are going to stand up and try an athletic stance. Remember these three cues when you practice your stance [demonstrate as you explain]: (1) Put your feet shoulder-width apart; (2) bend your knees and hips like you are almost sitting in a chair; (3) have your arms at your side for balance. Remember feet— sit—arms. Two questions: Who can tell me why you need to learn a good athletic stance? Name the three cues you'll say to yourself. I think you are ready to show me your athletic stance. On 'go,' spread out and begin. Go.*

Table 8.1   Instructional Cues (Labels) for Mental Images of Skills

Sport skill	Instructional cue for youth
Batting—back foot rotation	Squash the bug.
Follow-through in shooting a basketball	Arm looks like a goose neck—add a honk.
Start of a dash in track	Feels like you are shot out of a cannon.
Putting in golf	Arms swing like the pendulum of a clock.
Serving a volleyball	Pull your arm back like a bow and arrow.
Trapping the soccer ball	Pretend your foot is a pillow that absorbs the ball.
Serving a tennis ball	Bring the racket back like you are going to scratch your back.

This example should have taken you around 1 minute and 15 seconds. If you are sure your athletes have a clear understanding and clear mental image of the skill, they are ready to move on to the next step in the cycle of teaching skills: practice.

Practice

There is no substitute for repetition and practice when trying to learn a skill. Good coaches organize their practices to maximize success, **active learning time,** and fun. Active learning time is defined as the actual amount of instructional time spent learning and practicing a skill. Sitting and listening to directions about how the drill will be organized is not active learning time, because no one is engaged in a learning activity or active practice. Waiting in lines for a turn is not active learning time, because learning doesn't occur when kids stand and wait to participate. Research shows that effective teachers provide more active learning time for their students than do ineffective teachers (Kirk, Macdonald, & O'Sullivan, 2006).

Throughout the chapter, we'll discuss several ways to increase the amount of practice and active learning time by considering such things as use of space, equipment, or groups. For now, we want to highlight the importance of providing feedback. Other factors that influence practice are discussed in the next practice phase of the five-step teaching cycle.

Feedback

There are many different types of **feedback** to consider. These include internal feedback, external feedback, knowledge of performance, knowledge of results, nonverbal feedback, and verbal feedback. In addition, you should think about frequency (how often) and duration (how long) when providing feedback. As complicated as it sounds, there are some concrete principles that are easy to follow.

First, let's discuss what each of these types of feedback means. **Internal feedback** is the information your athletes gain from within their own body. It's the feedback from sensory receptors in muscles, tendons, and joints. For example, if you play golf and have ever hit a really good drive, you could probably "feel it" before you ever looked up to see where the ball went. Your swing felt good. When athletes are first learning a skill, it is sometimes hard for them to use internal feedback because of their young age and lack of experience. However, you should still ask them to try this type of feedback. Ask your athletes to *feel* the skill and remember the feeling. Tell them to use the information they receive from their bodies to provide helpful information. For example, if you are teaching a forward roll for gymnastics, ask athletes to remember where they feel the pressure on their back as they hit the mat properly.

External feedback is the information that athletes receive from outside their

---

My Best Teacher

Who was the best teacher you ever had in terms of teaching you physical or sport skills? Think back and try to identify the specific things this teacher did that made the difference in your learning and performance. What made her or him so good at teaching? What did you learn from this person, and how have you or can you incorporate these lessons into your work with young athletes?

bodies. This might be words, sounds, or visual images they receive from coaches, peers, parents, or their own performance. Using the same golf drive as an example, the athlete may receive external feedback from the sound of the club head hitting the ball in the sweet spot. The "pop" that you hear with the sweet spot of the club is different from the noise you hear when you top the ball. As with internal feedback, ask your athletes to remember this information to help them learn and perform the next time.

Knowledge of performance (KP) is information given verbally by a coach or others at the end of a performance or practice of a skill and contains information about the technique or form of the movement pattern. The feedback may include information about the parts of the skill that were performed correctly and the parts performed incorrectly. Knowledge of performance is critical for learners because the coach is providing subjective information that they cannot acquire themselves. The coach must be capable of observing, diagnosing, and communicating effectively to the learners information about their performance. Good coaches can watch a skill, or even an offensive-defensive series, and dissect what is right and what went wrong, and then provide the correct information to the athlete.

Knowledge of results (KR) is information given to an athlete at the end of the performance, usually by a coach or peers about the outcome of the performance. For example, the volleyball serve was in, or the hit baseball went to the outfield. Athletes also gain KR just by watching the outcome, which is typically objective. The object hit the target or did not hit the target. The ball scored or did not score. Coaches should avoid overemphasizing KR as opposed to KP. For young learners, the technique or correct form is far more important than the outcome. Typically, with good technique, athletes will eventually achieve a good outcome. The same can't be said for poor technique. Knowledge of results is useful for more experienced athletes who

already have an established technique and can make slight adjustments to alter the outcome without sacrificing form.

The impact of **nonverbal feedback** on athletes is often overlooked. Nonverbal feedback is information provided to athletes nonverbally, such as facial expressions, body language, and even actions such as the position a coach assigns a player. For example, a player assigned to right field or a less active position may think: "Coach doesn't think I'm very good." Athletes often interpret coaches' nonverbal behavior inappropriately. Coaches should focus on matching their nonverbal to their verbal feedback and should attempt to be as aware and consistent as possible in their nonverbal behavior.

The best type of verbal feedback contains information about how to improve, as well as a positive motivating phrase or nonverbal gesture. Young athletes prefer verbal feedback that contains helpful constructive information rather than only positive comments. Even young children understand that informational comments provide input that helps them improve and get better. And most importantly, children understand that a coach tends to provide informational feedback to athletes if the coach thinks the athletes are competent and can get better. (Some coaches avoid expending the time and effort needed to teach players with less athletic skill how to get better.) So avoid false "good jobs" and empty encouraging comments that contain no information. Children may perceive these comments as useless and an indication that they are not good enough to receive the coach's time and attention.

Feedback is so important to learning that you should make it your goal to provide a significant amount of informational feedback to every player, every day in practice. A positive motivating phrase or nonverbal gesture along with an informational comment reassures the athlete that you care about her, that you want her to succeed, and that you have confidence in her ability to learn. Examples of nonverbal gestures and positive phrases include a pat on

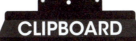

Four Tips for Teaching Youth Golfers

Here are some useful teaching tips from a top junior golf teacher (Patterson, 2013):

1. Kids learn more from not knowing. Let them make mistakes, and try *not* to tell them they're doing something wrong. Only offer ways to take what they're already doing and make it better.

2. If it's not fun, they won't keep doing it. They're typically not committed to the game until high school. Let them be themselves, without making things too intense.

3. If your kid tells you he or she wants to go hit balls, drop everything and go. But remember they're not asking you to teach them. You're only providing them the opportunity to play. Be ready to answer questions, but only when asked.

4. Golf works better when kids learn it with friends. There's protection in numbers, and the discussions will be on their level. This will help people stay engaged and might even get them hooked.

---

the back, high-five, thumbs-up, smile or wink, clapping hands, "I knew you could do it," and "You should be so proud of your effort."

Other Factors That Influence Practice

We've talked about the importance of active learning time for practice, but there are even more things you can do to make practice more effective for youth athletes.

Focus on Process, Not Product

Process involves the form or technique of performance and is more important to learning than the product or outcome, especially for young athletes. Therefore, during practice, athletes must focus on the process of performing a skill and not the product.

Sometimes parents are impressed by early results of their children's sport performance, only to find out years later that poor technique is limiting their true potential. For example, Scott is a high school senior on the baseball team. He has a very high batting average and has even hit a couple of cycles during the season (hitting a single, double, triple, and home run in one game). Everyone in his hometown thinks he will get drafted right out of high school into professional baseball because his batting results are so impressive. When the professional baseball scouts visit Scott and run him through some batting drills, it is apparent to them that Scott is not a good professional baseball prospect. Why do you think Scott will go undrafted? The baseball scouts have noticed that Scott has some serious flaws in his swing that will hinder performance at the professional level. His lack of attention to the process or correct hitting form as a younger player will prevent him from achieving long-term success.

Use Mental Imagery

Researchers have found that there is no substitute for actual physical practice. However, mental practice or imagery along with physical practice can improve performance (Vealey & Forlenza, 2015). Children are especially good at imagery because of their vivid imaginations. Take advantage of their imaginations and ask them to mentally practice or rehearse skills via imagery when they are at home (not during school!).

Just tell them to close their eyes and see and feel themselves doing the skill in their minds. They should attempt to see and feel themselves performing the skill successfully; tell them that by doing this they are strengthening their mental blueprint of the skill. They can mentally rehearse basic skills such as free throws and the footwork needed on layups from both sides of the lane in basketball. Young athletes may also mentally rehearse their specific positions within team formations or patterns of play. Encourage athletes to use the powerful tool of imagery when learning and practicing skills. Tell them that their minds don't know the difference between real and imagined events, which is true.

Use the Whole–Part Method

The motor learning literature offers two viable methods for demonstrating and practicing skills: the whole–part method and the part–whole method. Most people have a preference for one or the other. If kids prefer the whole–part method, they like to see the entire skill from start to finish first and then see parts of the skill (if the skill can be broken down into parts). Other kids might prefer the part–whole method, which means that they see all the parts first and then put them all together as a whole. When teaching young children, we believe it's better to use the whole–part method. We recommend showing the entire skill at full speed and then breaking the skill down into separate learnable parts, if appropriate. However, not all skills can be easily separated and practiced in parts.

Use Distributed Practice

Research examining distributed versus massed practice suggests that children learn best if practice is distributed. **Distributed practice** is defined as short amounts of practice time distributed over several days or weeks, as opposed to **massed practice,** which is defined as long amounts of practice time across one or two days. For example, when a softball coach wants to teach his players how to slide into second base, he will probably

choose distributed practice. The team would practice sliding into second base each day for 5 to 10 minutes every other practice day, for a couple of weeks until he feels they have learned how to slide. This approach makes more sense than spending an hour on sliding into second base for three straight days.

Also, **blocked skill practice,** in which people practice and learn one skill before moving on to the next skill, is not as effective as random skill practice. **Random skill practice** means learning and practicing to improve several skills at once.

In summary, practice situations work best when they focus on the process, use imagery to mentally rehearse skills, use a distributed and whole–part method, and include a lot of repetition.

INSTRUCTIONAL STRATEGIES TO MAXIMIZE LEARNING

You've now got the basics. Even without a lot of teaching experience, you can design practices and follow the five-step teaching cycle. But let's keep going! There are additional strategies you can use to enhance the learning of your athletes.

Progression, Extension, and Refinement

The main difference between good and poor coaches is in their abilities to design and use appropriate teaching progressions in their practices. A **teaching progression** involves designing the learning experience to proceed from a simple task to a more complex task. For example, a teaching progression in learning how to field a ground ball would be (1) going through the motions of fielding a grounder without a real ball; (2) fielding a slow-rolling grounder thrown by the coach; (3) fielding a faster-moving ground ball thrown by the coach; (4) fielding

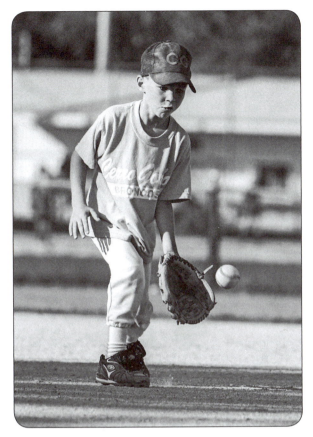

Good youth sport coaches teach skills using a progression of simple to complex, such as moving through the motions to field a ground ball without a real ball, moving to field a slow-moving ball, then fielding a faster-moving ground ball.

a slow-moving grounder hit off a bat; and (5) fielding a fast-moving grounder hit off a bat. Every skill and tactic in sport should be taught with an appropriate progression, one that doesn't skip a step, doesn't move too fast or too slow, and prepares athletes for all competitive situations.

An **extension** involves the sequence of difficulty, sometimes extending the task to become more difficult or extending it to become less difficult, depending on the learner. Here is an example of two extensions for kicking a soccer ball into the goal:

• To extend and make kicking the ball into a goal more difficult, a defensive player is added.

• To extend and make kicking the ball into a goal less difficult, there is no defense and the ball is moved closer to the goal.

A **refinement** is implemented to focus the learner on improving a specific aspect of the task. For example, a refinement for teaching a pick and roll in basketball might be more specific instructions for the person setting the pick, such as "Have a wider base with your legs, reverse pivot, and pin the defense with your backside as you roll." Refinements are taught when athletes are ready to refine or improve on the complexity of the skill or tactic.

When you teach young athletes new skills, you will need to be proficient at developing progressions, extensions, and refinements. For progressions, decide at what skill level most of your athletes (80%) are capable of starting. Begin with a simple task and move on to more complex practice as most of your athletes start to learn the skill. Be sure to use the teaching cycle of motivation, demonstration, practice, feedback, practice. As your athletes are practicing and you provide feedback, this is a perfect time to extend and refine practice. For athletes who quickly learn the skill, add a refinement or extend the task so that it is a little more difficult and challenge them to improve. For any athlete who is having difficulty, change the practice so that it is less difficult until the skill is learned. It's not uncommon for good coaches to have different athletes practicing different skills at different levels of difficulty. This individual approach meets the needs of all of your athletes and challenges each to improve at her own rate.

Developing teaching progressions, extensions, and refinements becomes easier with experience. As you learn age-appropriate abilities, you will know where to begin your teaching and can plan your progression from there. For most sports, moving from simple to more complex involves these types of refinements: type of equipment, playing surface, number of people involved, adding or deleting defense, speed, time allowed, number of skills combined, amount of space, and offensive or defensive tactics.

Game Tactics

A new and innovative way to teach skills is called the **tactical games approach** (Griffin, Mitchell, & Oslin, 1997). This approach focuses on teaching small-sided games to solve tactical problems that regularly occur in game situations. If you believe that kids can learn skills during game play, then this approach is worth considering. We like this approach because one of the issues in teaching skills to young athletes is the transfer of skills from practice to games. Sometimes the transfer is very poor, meaning that all that was learned in practice (correct form and rules) is forgotten once game play starts. In tactical games, children learn skills as they are playing in game-like activities so that skills and tactics and offensive and defensive strategy are interwoven.

For example, if a coach wanted his players to learn how to move and get open to receive a pass in basketball, he could teach backdoor, L-, and V-cuts. He could set up practice for players to learn these cuts and how to get open in practice drills (with or without defense) and then progress to game play. In a tactical games approach, the coach would explain the tactic: moving to get open without the ball. The coach would set up a small-sided game play for 2 vs. 2 or 3 vs. 3 to work specifically on moving to get open. He would supervise as his players tried various ways to get open so they could receive the pass, providing feedback and suggestions. As the players started to figure out how to get open, play would be extended to 4 vs. 4 and then 5 vs. 5. A tactical games approach takes more time to set up and organize, but the success for transfer of learning to game play is very high.

Arranging Players for Practice

One aspect of conducting youth sport practices that coaches don't typically think about is logistics. What's the best way to arrange or group athletes when teaching and practicing skills? The first issue to consider is grouping—what's the best way to group athletes during teaching? There are a variety of methods to use, such as grouping by gender, physical size, social compatibility, ability level, and random selection. We recommend that you use all of these methods, at different times during practice, as each has strengths and weaknesses.

If you always group by ability (highly skilled with highly skilled, lower skilled with lower skilled), the lower-skilled athletes do not get the advantage of practicing with players who are better. In tennis, if two lower-skilled players always practice together and neither one can return the ball very well, they have fewer opportunities to volley the ball. However, if ability level is mixed (high and low), then playing against someone better can improve the lower-ability player's skills. Of course, if the highly skilled tennis player is always grouped with a lower-skilled player, her skills might not improve because she isn't challenged.

Randomly dividing players into groups is fine as long as it doesn't take too long. Remember that players learn skills from lots of repetitions and practice, not from standing in lines and waiting to be divided into groups. Read the two following scenarios and decide which one is more time efficient.

1. Coach Mike decides to randomly group his team into four teams for practice. He lines up all his guys in a straight line. Then he moves down the line, asking the players to count off by 4's. As the players start counting, shifting of spots occurs down the line as some players are trying to make sure they are on a friend's team. When all the players finish counting, Coach Mike asks all 1's to go to the red cone, 2's to the blue cone, and so on. Jalen and Neal come up to coach because they forgot their numbers. When Coach Mike looks at the four teams, one team has 10 boys and another has three boys.

2. Coach Brett decides to randomly group his team into four teams for practice. He calls the boys in and counts quickly in his head how many are at practice today. He divides the total (22) by 4 and knows he will need two teams of 5 and two teams of 6. He tells the boys to pay attention and tells them that when he taps their shoulder they should go to their assigned team. He announces, "Team 1 go to the red cone," and then taps five boys on the shoulder. He says, "Team 2 go to the blue cone," and he taps six boys on the shoulder. He continues until all four teams are selected. Even though Coach Brett is randomly assigning boys today, he can still be sure that Charlie and Tim are on opposite teams, which is necessary because they tend to fight when they are on the same team.

Would you agree that Coach Brett's method is quicker and more efficient than Coach Mike's? When determining how you will group your players, keep the organizational instructions quick and efficient.

The second consideration when arranging your players for teaching a skill is group size. How many players should be in a group to practice? The guideline that we always use is to select the smallest number of players for a group that is needed to run the drill effectively. Our thinking is that this should provide the greatest number of repetitions or touches for each player. Sometimes situations demand larger groups, such as preventing fatigue or providing more game-like practice; but otherwise go with the smallest group size that works.

Small groups or station setups can work very well in providing a variety of opportunities to practice a skill or a combination of skills. Stations are an excellent way to hold young athletes' attention because they generally practice for 3 to 5 minutes at one station and then switch to a new station and new activity. Stations also promote a distributed type of practice that allows for the practice of several skills over several sessions.

Use of Space

Considering the use of space when you are teaching means you have designed a safe and effective learning environment. Ensure that there is enough space for athletes to practice skills safely. For example, softball players should not be practicing defensive cutoff plays in the field while teammates are taking batting practice. Throwing–catching warm-up in tee ball should be done using parallel lines, not perpendicular or random formations in which errant throws might injure a teammate. An effective learning environment means that you have considered the most effective way to organize your players for practice. Some of the most common formations are circles, two lines facing each other, squads of several lines, and scattered.

Organize your players so that you use all of the available space, with maximum participation by all players. For most single-skill practice, we favor a scattered formation with every player (or people in partners) having a piece of equipment (e.g., soccer ball). This formation can provide the greatest amount of active learning time. For small-sided game practice, like 2 vs. 2 or 3 vs. 3, set up multiple practice areas within the entire practice space. Instead of asking players to wait in lines and watch while only four or six players practice, let everyone practice as you move around the practice area providing feedback to all the small groups. It's important that as you organize players they are within hearing range of your direct supervision.

Use of Equipment

When teaching new skills to young athletes, you will need a lot of equipment. We suggest that you try to have at least one piece of equipment per player to avoid players standing and waiting. Skills are learned best through practice and repetition, so provide the equipment necessary to keep your players active. Another good idea when planning the use of equipment is to develop a routine for its distribution and collection. If athletes have to wait in line to pick up a soccer ball out of a bag to practice their dribbling, then you are wasting time during which they could be practicing.

Use of Time

Plan carefully how you structure practice, which skills you teach, and how long you spend on each skill. In your planning, consider your athletes' developmental abilities to maintain focus and engage in continuous physical exertion. Kids' physical and mental fatigue blocks the learning process. Build water breaks, changes of pace, and variety into activities.

Also, how long do you spend on athletes' learning any one skill? The answer is that it depends. It depends on the age of the athletes, their experience levels, and the length of the season. If the season is short (six weeks), you cannot spend four weeks on beginning fundamental skills. Use a distributed-practice model to introduce and practice all the skills players need to play the game and then keep refining as time allows. Compared to older athletes, younger athletes need shorter time on task before they take a break or switch to a new task. Use this guideline when determining how much time to spend on one skill before changing to another: The minimum number of minutes is equal to the athletes' age, and the maximum number of minutes is equal to their age times 2. So, an 8-year-old would practice a new skill between 8 to 16 minutes before changing to another skill. Of course, within this time frame there are extensions, refinements, and starts and stops for feedback.

Use of Reinforcement

Coaches and teachers often use **reinforcement** in the form of rewards or punishment

to change behavior. The idea is that children who receive a positive reward (pat on the back or candy treat) for a certain behavior will be more likely to repeat that behavior to receive more rewards. Children who receive **punishment** (frown, having to run laps, or sitting out) for a certain behavior will be more likely to avoid the negative consequence and change their behavior. In general, reinforcement works when one is teaching skills to children if it's used correctly. However, used improperly, too often, or with the wrong motives, reinforcement can create many unintended consequences. Read the Water Break section for an example of a coach's good intentions to reward her players gone wrong.

Why didn't Kelly's reinforcement idea work? Read the following guidelines for using reinforcement to see if you can determine what went wrong with Kelly's idea.

1. Different individuals can interpret the same reinforcement differently. Know your athletes well and match the reinforcement to their needs.

2. A positive reward works better than a negative punishment. Avoid punishing athletes as a way to change behavior when they are learning new skills.

3. The magnitude of the positive reward should match the magnitude of the behavior. Avoid overrewarding with big gifts that can't be given every time an athlete demonstrates the correct behavior.

4. Intermittent reinforcement is more effective than constant reinforcement when people are learning new skills.

5. A personal reinforcement (smile, positive comment) is more effective over time than material reinforcement (prize, medal, ribbon).

6. Reward effort and performance, not just outcome.

The use of punishment in youth sport, especially physical punishment, should not be the primary method used by coaches to

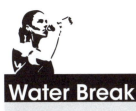

Water Break

Sticker Shock!

Kelly was coaching an 8-year-old girls' softball team. She decided that the girls needed to work harder in practice and set out to reinforce that behavior. Kelly told the girls she would reward one girl who had worked the hardest in practice that day with a softball sticker. This seemed like a good idea, and the girls were highly motivated to get a sticker. At the end of the practice, Kelly selected one girl, gave her the sticker, and noticed the joy in her eyes. The other girls seemed happy for their teammate, and practice ended as usual.

As the days went on, Kelly started to notice that the girls became nervous at the end of practice. Those who hadn't gotten a sticker but were working their hardest were terribly disappointed and almost embarrassed to be without a sticker yet. Those who had gotten a sticker seemed to slack off in practice because they soon realized that the coach was going to give one sticker to a different girl each day before anyone received a second sticker. By the time it came down to the last three girls on the team still without an effort sticker, Kelly felt terrible and could hardly face these girls. Realizing that her idea was a complete failure, she decided to give all three girls a sticker and end her sticker reinforcements.

change behavior (as discussed in chapter 6). When teaching skills, if you find you need to eliminate negative behaviors that are interfering with learning, then follow these suggestions:

1. Don't punish young athletes in anger by yelling or making physical contact.

2. Don't embarrass kids in front of their peers.

3. The type and intensity of punishment should fit the negative behavior (avoid overreacting and overusing punishment).

4. Remember that a simple verbal or nonverbal reward for good effort will set the expectations for the team.

5. Youth sport leaders should look for good behavior and catch their athletes doing something right, and then reward appropriately.

Maintaining Discipline

Your ability to teach skills to your athletes will suffer if you have to spend the majority of your time disciplining them or trying to gain control over their behavior. Be very clear from the start of the season what you view as acceptable and unacceptable behavior on the part of your athletes. Be clear with them about the consequences for unacceptable behavior, and follow through when they violate team rules. We suggest that you have a meeting with the parents before your first practice to make them aware of your expectations for behavior and consequences. Then conduct your practices and games in an organized, consistent, and disciplined manner. Young athletes appreciate both a well-organized routine with the flexibility to allow having fun as well as consistency in high expectations for their behavior.

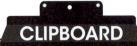

Ways to Maintain Discipline

1. Assess whether the behavior is aimed at getting your attention and so can be ignored or whether you need to take action. If it's the latter, run through the following steps until the behavior stops: Move closer to the athlete, make sure she knows you see her, make eye contact, and speak privately to her.

2. Put the athlete in time-out. Separate him from the activity for a time appropriate to his age and the misbehavior. Allow him to return to play after the time-out.

3. Speak with the athlete and her parents after practice. Be sure that they understand that the behavior is unacceptable and must stop. Inform them of the consequences should the misbehavior continue.

4. If steps 1 through 3 have not rectified the misbehavior, remove the athlete from participation. Be sure to inform your league director or athletic director of the severity of the discipline problem. Outline how the behavior needs to change in order for the athlete to return to the team.

One of the best ways to maintain discipline is to plan for and conduct a well-organized, active practice. Young athletes who have nothing to do, who are standing in long lines, and who are feeling bored will find something to entertain themselves, which usually leads to trouble. Establish a routine in practice to keep athletes moving. Develop a consistent start to practice each day. Athletes gather in the same place and begin with a warm-up. Activities can vary within the warm-up, but the athletes understand the organizational structure of practice. Establish a starting and stopping signal. Some coaches prefer a whistle that signals to athletes they should stop immediately and listen. If you prefer, athletes could drop to one knee or sit when you call them in for discussion or demonstration. Be clear about your signal to start activity, such as "when I say 'go'" or "on my whistle you may begin."

WRAP-UP

Sometimes volunteer youth coaches worry about their lack of technical knowledge in a sport. There are a lot of ways they can learn more about the sport and enhance their technical teaching and coaching abilities (using Internet resources, reading sport-specific teaching–coaching books, observing other coaches). However, the most important quality that youth sport teachers and coaches possess is their enthusiasm for teaching kids. Establishing personal relationships with young athletes and demonstrating sincere care about their learning and progress generally lead to quality youth sport experiences.

As we hope you've learned from this chapter, effective teaching and coaching require more than knowledge about a sport. Teaching skills is a science and an art, particularly with developing kids. Instructionally, our pet peeve is observing kids in practice who stand around a lot (e.g., one long layup line with three unused baskets, one athlete taking batting practice while everyone else watches, everyone listening to a coach talk for 10 minutes about how to do something). Take time in planning, and keep in the front of your mind the important instructional strategy of optimizing active learning time for every kid on your team. Not only will they learn more, they'll also enjoy it and want to come back for more.

LEARNING AIDS

Key Terms

active learning time—The amount of instructional time spent directly on learning and practicing a skill (not listening or waiting in line).

blocked skill practice—Format in which one skill is practiced and learned before moving on to the next skill.

distributed practice—Format in which short amounts of practice time are distributed over several days or weeks.

extension—The sequence of difficulty, sometimes extending the task to become more difficult or extending it to become less difficult, depending on the learner.

external feedback—Information that athletes receive from outside their body.

feedback—Information that athletes receive about their performance.

internal feedback—Information that athletes gain from within their own bodies.

knowledge of performance (KP)—Information given verbally by a coach or others at the end of a performance or practice of a skill; contains information about the technique or form of the movement pattern.

knowledge of results (KR)—Information given to an athlete at the end of the performance, usually by a coach or peers, about the outcome of the performance.

learning—The relatively permanent change in performance that occurs with practice.

massed practice—Long practice times distributed over a short period of time, such as one or two days.

nonverbal feedback—Information provided to athletes without words, such as facial expressions, body language, and even actions, such as the position a coach assigns a player.

punishment—A negative approach to control and change behavior.

random skill practice—Learning and practicing to improve several skills at once.

refinement—An attempt to improve a specific aspect of a previously learned skill.

reinforcement—Using rewards and punishment to modify behavior.

tactical games approach—Teaching small-sided games to solve tactical problems that regularly occur in game situations.

teaching progression—Designing the learning environment to proceed from a simple skill to a more complex skill.

Summary Points

1. The five-step teaching cycle is motivation, demonstration, practice, feedback, and practice.

2. Effective demonstrations use the whole–part–whole method, with performance of the movement at the correct speed.

3. Effective teachers provide more active learning time for athletes than ineffective teachers.

4. Feedback for learners can be given as internal feedback, external feedback, knowledge of performance, knowledge of results, nonverbal feedback, and verbal feedback.

5. Practice situations work best when practice focuses on the process, combined with imagery, in a distributed and whole–part method, with a lot of repetitions.

6. The difference between good coaches and poor coaches is in their ability to design effective practices with appropriate progressions, extensions, and refinements in their sport.

7. The tactical games approach involves using small-sided games to work on transferring skills from practice to competitive situations.

8. Reinforcement works, but if used improperly, too often, or with the wrong motives, it can have negative consequences.

Study Questions

1. What is the five-step teaching cycle?

2. Identify what makes demonstrations effective in teaching sport skills.

3. Explain the different types of feedback described in the chapter, and provide an effective example for each.

4. Provide three examples (beyond those in the book) of instructional cues that could be used in teaching a sport skill.

5. Provide an example for using progression, extension, and refinement in practice.

6. Identify some useful practice management strategies in relation to grouping athletes and using time and space effectively.

7. What are some do's and don'ts for using reinforcement and maintaining discipline when working with youth athletes?

Reflective Learning Activities

1. Select one sport skill and describe in detail a progression for practice, starting with the most simple and advancing to the most complex.

2. Plan one 60-minute practice that would involve teaching a new skill to your athletes. Be sure to explain how you would organize a teaching skills cycle, with specific details.

Resource Guide

Wrisberg, C.A. (2007). *Sport skill instruction for coaches*. Champaign, IL: Human Kinetics.

Baseball Throwing Fundamental Drills (YouTube) (www.youtube.com/watch?v=HYaOlDEamHY). Teaching video with multiple drills to teach throwing.

Intensity of Participation in Youth Sport

Welcome to part III of *Best Practice for Youth Sport,* which focuses on how much physical and psychological intensity is appropriate for youth sport participants. Here's a sampling of what you'll learn in the next four chapters:

- The amount and types of physical training appropriate for kids
- How kids develop talent and whether early sport specialization is good for them
- Why burnout occurs in young athletes and how to prevent it
- The main types of injuries in youth sport, including overuse, knee injuries, and concussions

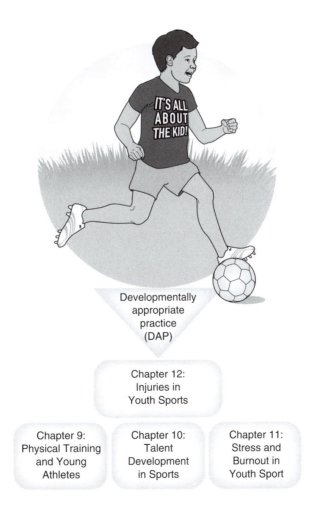

Developmentally appropriate practice (DAP)

Chapter 9: Physical Training and Young Athletes	Chapter 10: Talent Development in Sports	Chapter 11: Stress and Burnout in Youth Sport

Chapter 12: Injuries in Youth Sports

This part of the book focuses on the negative consequences of the "overs": *overtraining, overspecialization, overstress,* and *overuse.* The overs occur when adults find themselves on a slippery slope, forgetting that more isn't always better when it comes to training children in sport. Pushing for more often leads to physical training that goes beyond what kids' bodies can take and to early, exclusive specialization that can rob children of the joy of sport and a healthy multidimensional identity. So read on to become aware of the overs and how we can avoid these by following developmentally appropriate practice.

chapter 9

PHYSICAL TRAINING AND YOUNG ATHLETES

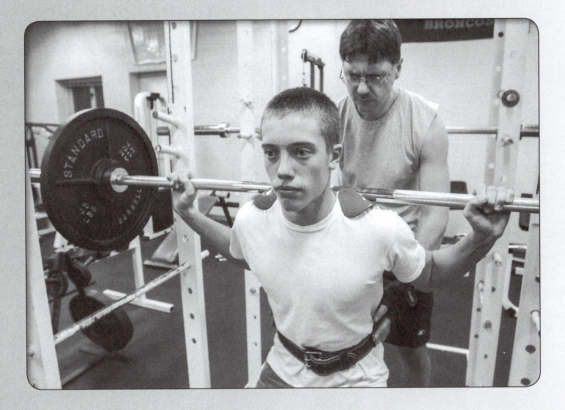

CHAPTER PREVIEW

In this chapter, you'll learn

- » the positive effects of physical training on kids,
- » how overintensity leads to disordered eating and drug use in youth athletes, and
- » physical training guidelines for young athletes.

"Child Bodybuilding: How Jacked Is Your Kid?" read the title of a popular magazine article (Spitznagel, 2011). The story features the strength training exploits of Giuliano Stroe, a 7-year-old muscle-ripped Romanian boy who held the world record for number of air push-ups. Air push-ups are like regular ones, except that one's feet aren't allowed to touch the ground—an amazing feat of strength and balance. Giuliano did 20 to set the world record, as captured on YouTube.

"Can Too Many Miles Ruin Young Runners?" led off another magazine article that questioned how far kids can safely run (Beverly, 2011). It featured a 14-year-old girl who ran 70 to 75 miles (113 to 121 kilometers) per week. Most medical experts state that it is safe for children to participate in long-distance running and training as long as they enjoy the activity and show no negative physical effects. However, not everyone shares this opinion. Participants must be 18 years old to run the Pittsburgh Marathon, while Houston requires that runners be at least 12 and Los Angeles has no age minimum.

Sport scientists have learned that children are capable of much more physical training than previously thought, although developmentally appropriate training guidelines should be followed. And although overtraining is a concern, the epidemic of childhood inactivity and obesity should impel us to design physical activities that are challenging and enjoyable for kids so that they learn to love physical activity. Childhood obesity has more than doubled in children and quadrupled in adolescents in the past 30 years (Centers for Disease Control and Prevention [CDC], 2015). In 2012, more than one-third of American children and adolescents were **overweight** (having excess body weight for a particular height) or **obese** (having excess body fat).

Obese youths are more likely than others to have risk factors for cardiovascular disease, cancer, prediabetes, bone and joint problems, sleep apnea, and poor self-esteem.

Thus, our focus in this chapter is on physical training in kids. What is good for their bodies and overall development, and what is or becomes harmful? How trainable are kids, and how can we get and keep them moving? What guidelines should we follow in different types of training?

POSITIVE EFFECTS OF PHYSICAL ACTIVITY AND TRAINING IN KIDS

Physical activity, including physical training in youth sport participation, provides many benefits for children. They are physically trainable (meaning that their bodies respond with higher levels of fitness), although their training responses are lower than those of adults.

Increased Lean Body Mass and Decreased Fat

Regular physical activity increases lean body mass and decreases fat in children. For example, a longitudinal research program[4] that provided four additional physical education lessons per week for two school years significantly improved the body composition (more lean and less fat) of 8- to 13-year-old children (Klakk, Chinapaw, Heidemann, Andersen, & Wedderkopp, 2013). The effect of the program was especially pronounced for overweight and obese children.

Similarly, participation in resistance (strength) training programs resulted in positive changes in body composition in children and adolescents who were obese or at risk for obesity (Faigenbaum et al., 2009). Children involved in organized sport and indoor physical activity programs during kindergarten and 1st grade showed a slower increase in body mass index (BMI, a measure of body fat based

---

[4] A longitudinal research study is one in which data are gathered for the same participants repeatedly over a period of time (months, years, or even decades), thus allowing researchers to examine change within the people being studied. This differs from cross-sectional research, in which data are gathered at one moment in time and different individuals are usually compared to one another.

CLIPBOARD

The "E" Word

When our daughter arrived home from 1st grade one day, we asked her what she did that day in physical education class. She replied with a downcast look, "Just boring exercise. Nothing fun." So here's a tip—don't use the word *exercise*. Kids often view it as boring drudgery. Similar to our suggestions in chapter 5 about ways to build fundamental motor skills in kids, our goal is to make physical activity fun for children so that they get hooked on it and want to continue. We love it when our son says, as he frequently does, "I want to do something *active* today."

Create a family atmosphere in which physical activity is the norm almost every day. But make it varied, creative, and something kids enjoy doing. Family walks, jogs, and hikes, or even fun runs sponsored by communities, are great activities. Check around for triathlons or marathons or half-marathons that allow team entries, and enter as a family or group. A great example is Bend, Oregon's Pole, Pedal, and Paddle Race in which contestants (often in teams, including families) race in a relay that includes alpine and cross-country skiing, cycling, running, and canoeing-kayaking. We're not all fortunate enough to live in Bend, but different types of races are available in many communities.

Buy kids different sets of "wheels"—including bikes, scooters, skateboards, in-line skates, and ice skates. Encourage kids to walk or bike to school, and advocate in your community for safe bike and walking trails that kids can use. Game your play. Buy backyard games and also improvise family outdoor games (even indoor games like balloon volleyball and basement soccer using a beach ball). Of course, children can begin organized youth sport programs around the age of 5, but we suggest that you continue family physical activities to internalize kids' commitment to moving their bodies. And start early. Fourteen percent of kids aged 2 to 5 are already overweight, so we want to model and provide an active lifestyle for them from the beginning. And remember: Be careful about using the "E" word!

---

on height and weight) from 6 to 10 years of age compared with children not involved in such programs (Dunton et al., 2012). And as you might expect, the amount of time spent watching television was significantly related to body fatness in kids (Marshall, Biddle, Gorely, Cameron, & Murdey, 2004).

Stronger Bones

One of the most important positive effects of physical activity is increased bone mineral density, or bone mass. Mechanical loading of the bones, as in physical activity, stimulates bone formation and thus enhances bone density, shape, and strength. Maximal bone mass is reached in our early 20s, and it gradually declines thereafter as we age.

This decrease is accelerated in women after menopause. Thus, weight-bearing physical activity during childhood and adolescence is extremely important, because that's when most of our bone mass is developed.

Active children and adolescents develop larger bone size and greater bone mass as compared to inactive youth (Faigenbaum et al., 2009; Nordstrom, Tervo, & Hogstrom, 2011). The best activities to stimulate bone health are weight bearing with high-intensity loading applied in varied directions, such as gymnastics, racket sports, volleyball, soccer, handball, and basketball. Good bone-strengthening fundamental motor activities are hopscotch, jump rope, skipping, tag, and dodgeball. Because bone mass during childhood and adolescence is a determinant of bone mass in adulthood, physical activity and sport participation in the youth years help to prevent against **osteoporosis** in later years (Baxter-Jones, Mirwald, Faulkner, Kowalski, & Bailey, 2009). (Osteoporosis is a disease that thins and weakens bones so they are fragile and break easily.)

Muscular Strength

Kids, even prepubescent children, show improvements in muscular strength through physical training. Strength is simply the ability to exert or resist force. We often notice how the performance of youth athletes is hampered when they lack the upper-body strength to shoot a basketball, throw a football, or execute the butterfly stroke in swimming. Or they might lack the core (torso) strength to physically hold off an opponent in soccer. Kids typically gain 13% to 30% in muscle strength through training, greater than the amount expected from normal growth and maturation (and significantly less of a gain compared to that in adult men).

Significant muscular hypertrophy (increase in size of the muscle) does not typically occur in prepubescent children. Rather, strength gains in young children result from neuromuscular adaptation as training increases the number of motor neurons that fire with each muscle contraction (Faigenbaum et al., 2009; Matos & Winsley, 2007). Of course, during and after puberty, hypertrophy of muscles becomes more apparent and accounts for increases in strength.

Aerobic and Anaerobic Fitness

Aerobic fitness is important for kids because it allows them to sustain physical activity for prolonged periods. Aerobic means "with oxygen," so it is a young athlete's ability to transport and use oxygen during endurance activities (like running or swimming, activities usually longer than 12 minutes in duration).

Kids do not respond to aerobic training as well as adults due to their smaller lung volumes and smaller hearts that pump less blood than in adults. In addition, children's endurance performance is limited by poor running economy. For a given pace, children require higher levels of oxygen consumption than adults. Their shorter limbs and smaller muscle mass result in lower mechanical power. Thus, children and adolescents can improve their aerobic fitness typically only around 5% to 10% (Matos & Winsley, 2007). In prepubertal children, gains from endurance training largely result from improvements in mechanical efficiency, not changes in physical aerobic power. After puberty, aerobic fitness is highly trainable, although there are genetic differences in aerobic trainability (Rowland, 2005).

Anaerobic fitness is a young athlete's ability to engage in all-out, short-term physical effort. Anaerobic means "without oxygen" and is an important type of fitness needed to perform high-intensity, short-duration activities (e.g., shifts in ice hockey, sprinting in swimming and track and field, running the bases, playing tennis). A higher anaerobic capacity also helps young athletes perform long-term endurance activities because they can function at the anaerobic level for a longer period of time. Children can improve their anaerobic fitness around 10% to 14% through sprint training (Matos & Winsley, 2007). As children move through adolescence and into young adulthood, their ability to generate anaerobic energy is greatly enhanced.

Psychological and Cognitive Benefits of Physical Activity and Training

Physical activity has been linked to improved self-esteem, lower depression, and higher perceived competence in children and adolescents (Sallis, Prochaska, & Taylor, 2000). And maybe most impressively, multiple studies have shown that physical activity leads to better cognitive performance (higher scores in math, language, general thinking, and memory tests) (Howie & Pate, 2012; Singh, Uijtdewilligen, Twisk, Van Meechelen, & Chinapaw, 2012), with aerobic training showing the biggest effect on cognitive outcomes (Fedewa & Ahn, 2011).

So physical activity and training make kids smarter! In the national bestseller *Spark: The Revolutionary New Science of Exercise and the Brain* (2008), John Ratey explains how physical exercise improves learning in kids:

1. It optimizes children's mindset to improve alertness, attention, and motivation.

2. It prepares and encourages nerve cells to bind together to receive new information.

3. It spurs the development of new nerve cells in the brain.

Summary of Benefits of Physical Activity and Training in Children

That's a pretty impressive list of benefits for kids, if we can get and keep them moving. Along with the benefits described, physical training conditions young athletes' muscles, tendons, ligaments, and bones to prevent injuries. In addition, it enhances performance, more so for adolescent athletes who have mastered basic skills and who can benefit from better fitness.

The benefits discussed in this section do require a certain level of training intensity. Parents need to understand that most entry-level youth sport programs do not involve physical training at high enough levels of intensity to build aerobic and anaerobic fitness. Most beginning youth sport programs are geared toward teaching basic skills and the psychosocial benefits of team membership. Physical activity (moving one's body and expending energy) entails a wide range and differing degrees of activity. **Physical training** specifically refers to a disciplined routine of specialized procedures performed by athletes to condition their bodies (Martens, 2012). At the higher competitive levels of youth sport, such as club, select, and middle and high school teams, more time and intensity go into physical training.

NEGATIVE EFFECTS OF OVERINTENSITY IN PHYSICAL TRAINING IN YOUTH

As youth sports became more professionalized and specialized, training and performance enhancement practices inevitably became more intense and extreme. When the intensity of training goes beyond what is physically and psychologically healthy for young athletes, several negative outcomes can occur. Some of these outcomes are discussed in the next chapters of this section of the book (overspecialization, burnout, and overuse injuries). Here we focus on the negative outcomes of the unhealthy female athlete triad, extreme weight gain and loss in male athletes, and the use of performance-enhancing drugs.

Female Athlete Triad

The female athlete triad refers to the interrelationships among energy availability, menstrual function, and bone mineral density (American College of Sports Medicine, 2007). As shown in figure 9.1, the healthy triad occurs when athletes have optimal energy availability through adequate nutrition, normal menstrual function, and optimal bone health. However, for many reasons, athletes may slide across the arrow shown in figure 9.1 to move toward or into the unhealthy, or pathological (involving disease) triad. This triad includes low energy availability (which may include eating disorders), **amenorrhea** (absence of menstrual periods), and osteoporosis.

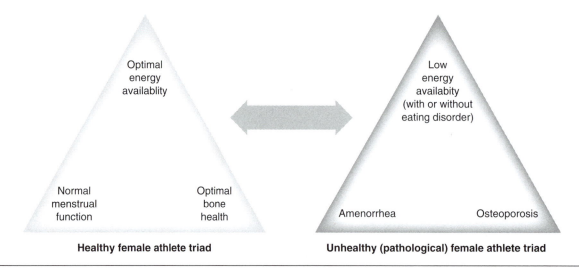

Figure 9.1　Female athlete triad.

The unhealthy triad can lead to irreversible consequences, including death. Christy Henrich, an elite gymnast who missed making the 1988 Olympic team by .0188 points, died of multiple organ failure at the age of 22 as a complication of an eating disorder. At the peak of her career, Henrich was 4 feet, 10 inches (147 centimeters) and 93 pounds (42 kilograms), but she became obsessed about her weight after a judge told her she was too fat. At the time of her death, she weighed 47 pounds (21 kilograms). The sobering health consequences of the unhealthy triad include cardiovascular complications (which can lead to sudden death by cardiac arrest), stress fractures from lack of bone density, gastrointestinal problems, electrolyte abnormalities, anemia, dental decay (from binging and purging food), fatigue, and temporary infertility.

What Is Disordered Eating?

Low energy availability is the keystone that leads to menstrual dysfunction and osteoporosis. Some athletes reduce energy by spending more time in physical training so that energy expenditure outweighs energy intake. Some practice abnormal eating behaviors like fasting, binge eating, purging, or using diet pills. These behaviors may lead to a full-blown clinical eating disorder

formally recognized by the American Psychiatric Association. **Anorexia nervosa** is an eating disorder characterized by restrictive eating in which the individual views herself as overweight even though she is at least 15% below the expected weight for her age and height. **Bulimia nervosa** is an eating disorder in which individuals, usually in the normal weight range, repeat a cycle of overeating and then purging, fasting, or exercising excessively.

Who Is Likely to Develop Disordered Eating?

Although both males and females can develop disordered-eating patterns, they occur in greater frequency with females. In adolescents, the incidence of clinical eating disorders has increased at an alarming rate over the past few decades. Anorexia nervosa represents the third most common chronic illness among adolescent girls (Bonci et al., 2008). Rates of eating disorders are higher for female athletes in appearance-oriented (gymnastics, figure skating) and lean (swimming, diving, track and field) sports as compared to other sports (Anderson & Petrie, 2012). Personality characteristics, including high-achievement orientation, self-motivation, rigid self-discipline, perfectionism, and concern with body image, have

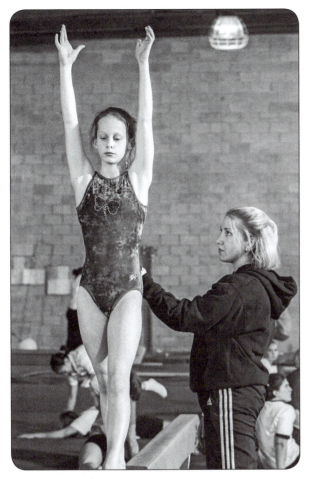

Anorexia nervosa is the third most common chronic illness in adolescent girls, and is more prevalent in appearance-oriented (gymnastics, figure skating) and lean (swimming, track, diving) sports as compared to other sports.

been linked to disordered eating. Tragically, Christy Henrich's nicknames were ET or Extra-Tough because of her commitment to training for her sport.

What Behaviors Might Indicate the Development of Disordered Eating?

You may notice a focus on or preoccupation with food that is different from what is seen in other athletes. You may observe eating extremes, from severe undereating to binging. Athletes may demonstrate changes in mood or personality or just start acting differently. For example, they might warm up alone, eat alone, or not socialize and joke around with teammates as much. One early indicator is a growing obsession with their bodies or weight, reflected, for example, in comments or questions about the topic or comparing themselves to others. They may be more self-critical, and tougher on and less accepting of themselves.

What Should I Do If I Suspect a Young Athlete May Be Experiencing Disordered Eating?

This is a very serious problem with dire consequences, so above all, you should act. Plan to approach athletes thoughtfully and with care. Ask to speak with them in private, and as much as possible, avoid using the term *eating disorder* (Selby & Reel, 2011). Describe their behavior, instead of evaluating or accusing them. You might say, for example, "I'm worried about you. I've noticed that you seem distracted and not as engaged with your teammates—like you're not having as much fun. I just want to make sure you're okay. Is there anything wrong, and anything I can do to help?" If you work at a school, talk to a counselor or school psychologist about your concerns. Parents should be involved and educated as well. As a teacher, coach, or youth sport administrator, you should have a list of potential referrals ready so that you can refer the athlete or parents (or both) to these professionals. For clinical eating disorders, a team of experts is needed, including a physician, mental health professional, nutritionist, and possibly athletic trainer and coach.

What Can We Do to Prevent Unhealthy Energy Expenditure, Including Disordered Eating, Among Athletes?

Mandatory educational programs for athletes, coaches, athletic trainers, and other athletics staff members should be implemented yearly. Female athletes should be educated about the health and performance consequences of menstrual irregularities and the importance of seeking medical guidance at the first sign of abnormalities. Coaches should avoid disparaging remarks about athletes' bodies or weights, as this behavior has contributed to disordered eating on the part of athletes (Arthur-Cameselle & Quatromoni, 2011).

Extreme Weight Gain and Loss in Male Athletes

Gymnasts are advantaged when they're smaller, and the opposite is true for football linemen. In 1970, there was only one 300-pound (136-kilogram) player in the National Football League (NFL). When

Water Break

Can Intense Training Stunt the Growth of Female Gymnasts?

Elite gymnasts are small. Gabby Douglas, who won the women's individual all-around gold medal at the 2012 Olympic Games, checked in at 4 feet, 11 inches (150 centimeters) and 90 pounds (41 kilograms). Since 1976, the average medal-winning female at the Olympics has been 5 feet, 1 inch (155 centimeters) and weighed 103 pounds (47 kilograms) (the 10th percentile for height and fifth percentile for weight [Mooney, 2012]). Is the intensive training they undergo responsible for their short stature? And is this training also responsible for their delayed maturation, which is later as compared to that of athletes in other sports and nonathletes?

There is no conclusive evidence that intensive training delays maturation and stunts growth in gymnasts. It is true that short stature and late maturity are characteristics of elite gymnasts. However, this is correlational,[5] and doesn't mean that gymnastics training *causes* growth to

be interrupted. Gymnastics "selects" girls who are shorter, and size and growth patterns determine who stays in the sport. Longitudinal research shows that girls who dropped out were taller, heavier, and earlier in maturation compared to those who persisted in gymnastics (Malina, Bouchard, & Bar-Or, 2004). Shorter and smaller body size fits the sport demands better, in terms of skill execution, but also the culturally prescribed expectancies of coaches and judges. In addition, the dietary practices of young gymnasts often lead to chronic undernourishment in their quest to maintain optimal body weight for performance. Although diet has not been causally linked to diminished growth in gymnasts, it is a concern and a possible factor. Overall, gymnasts are shorter than nonathletes and athletes in other sports, but no conclusive link has been established between gymnastics training and growth disturbances.

[5] Correlational studies examine the degree to which things are related to each other. Sometimes when people read the results of a correlational study, they mistakenly assume that one of the things being studied *causes* the related thing to happen. Correlational studies tell us only that things are related or that they are similar or correspond to each other; they don't tell us that one thing caused another to happen. Experimental research provides the best chance of determining causality, because experimental research attempts to control extraneous factors that could influence the outcome of the study.

the league kicked off for the 2013-2014 season, 358 players weighed 300 pounds or more. As college and professional players, particularly linemen, have gotten bigger, high school players now believe they have to pack on the pounds to perform effectively and get a chance to play at the next level. At the youth level, 45% and 43% of 9- to 14-year-old football players were overweight or obese, respectively (Malina et al., 2007). At least 127 high school offensive linemen in North Carolina weighed 300 pounds or more during the 2012 season.

So, along with the national trend of kids getting fatter, now we have kids who are intentionally getting fatter so they can impress coaches and earn playing time. However, the long-term health effects of such weight gain are problematic: diabetes, high blood pressure, heart disease, elevated cholesterol, breathing difficulties, and muscle and joint pain. The life expectancy for American males is 77.6 years. It's 55 years for NFL players overall, and 52 years for former NFL linemen (Hyman, 2009). The National Federation of State High School Associations challenges coaches to take responsibility for the issue, because they are in the best position to change cultural expectations about the need for extreme weight in the sport of football.

While football players focus on gaining weight, wrestlers, as they have for decades, focus on losing weight to qualify for lower competitive weight classes. Typical methods used are dieting, severe exercise, dehydration, and other even more extreme methods (wearing rubber suits, sitting in saunas, using laxatives and diuretics), sometimes by athletes as young as 8 years old. Despite repeated warnings from the medical community, weight cutting (rapid weight reduction) remains popular among youth wrestlers.

The American College of Sports Medicine encourages structural changes to prevent weight cutting, such as permitting more participants and more weight classes in meets, standardizing eligibility rules to discourage rapid weight loss at the end of the season (prohibiting dropping to a lower weight class), and providing educational programs for coaches, parents, and wrestlers ("Weight Loss in Wrestlers," 2013). The National Federation of High School Associations has implemented weight management rules for high school wrestling that include a hydration level not to exceed 1.025, body fat assessment no lower than 7% for boys and 12% for girls, and a monitored weekly weight loss plan limiting weekly weight loss to 1.5% of total body weight per week. This rule attempts to eliminate the drastic methods that result in dangerous weight loss attempts by youth wrestlers.

Performance-Enhancing Drugs

In their zeal to perform better, look fitter, and often in response to peer pressure and adult models, young athletes sometimes turn to performance-enhancing drugs (PEDs). About 1 in 20 teenagers report having used PEDs, including the following common types:

1. **Creatine,** an over-the-counter supplement used to improve performance in activities that require short bursts of high-intensity activity (wrestling, powerlifting, sprinting, football). High doses of creatine are associated with kidney, liver, and heart problems.

2. **Ephedrine** is a stimulant banned by the U.S. Food and Drug Administration. It is used to reduce fatigue, lose weight, and maintain mental alertness. Its use has been linked to strokes, seizures, and heart attacks.

3. **Anabolic steroids** are synthetic versions of testosterone that can be

taken orally, injected, or absorbed through the skin via creams and gels. Anabolic steroids build muscle and increase endurance but can cause many adverse physical and psychological health issues. Because anabolic steroids are legal only when prescribed by a physician, most are manufactured or traded illegally, which eliminates any quality control of the substances. Signs of steroid use include rapid weight gain and muscle growth; increased acne and facial bloating; mood swings; and aggressive, even violent, behavior. Anabolic steroids can have severe, long-lasting effects on health, including stunted height, cardiovascular problems, reproductive system problems, and damage to vital organs such as the liver and kidneys. Steroid-related deaths occur in the form of suicide or heart or liver disease.

4. **Steroid precursors** are substances the body converts into anabolic steroids, which are used to train harder, recover faster, and build muscle mass. Common ones are androstenedione ("andro") and DHEA (dehydroepiandrosterone).

The majority of steroid users are young male athletes. Many famous athletes have been identified as using PEDs (e.g., Lance Armstrong, Alex Rodriguez, Ryan Braun), and the U.S. Anti-Doping Agency has sanctioned cyclists, soccer players, weightlifters, water polo players, wrestlers, boxers, and track and field athletes. Although these athletes were sanctioned (meaning suspended for a period of time or fined), there seems to be a tacit acceptance of PEDs in our society that sends the message to kids that it's okay to use them as long as you don't get caught. We urge adult stakeholders in youth sports to take a strong stand against the use of PEDs.

Coaches and sport administrators should educate young athletes about the health risks associated with PEDs and create policies for dealing with PEDs in youth sport. Despite a 2002 Supreme Court ruling allowing states to randomly drug-test students, only Texas, New Jersey, and Illinois have implemented statewide procedures to do so. Coaches and youth sport programs can implement team policies for drug use that are available online. Of course, education that enables youth athletes to make autonomous and informed choices about their training and health is preferred to testing and enforcement policies. Dick Butkus' Play Clean program (www.iplayclean.org) educates and encourages high school students to make the right choice of "playing clean"—defined as training hard, eating well, and playing with attitude, instead of resorting to illegal and dangerous PEDs. Education has been effective in enabling young athletes to resist the social pressure to try PEDs.

Exertional Heat Illness

A final negative effect from overly intense physical training with youth athletes is exertional heat illness. This is a spectrum of conditions that range from muscle cramps to heat exhaustion to life-threatening heatstroke as the result of physical activity in the heat. Annually, there are many cases of exertional heat illness in youth football players, typically during heat in the late summer, which is the football preseason in the United States. Since 1995, 52 football players have died from heatstroke, 41 of whom were high school athletes (Kucera, Klossner, Colgate, & Cantu, 2014).

An important objective for our bodies is **thermoregulation**, or preventing our core temperature from rising or falling excessively. Contrary to previous thinking, kids

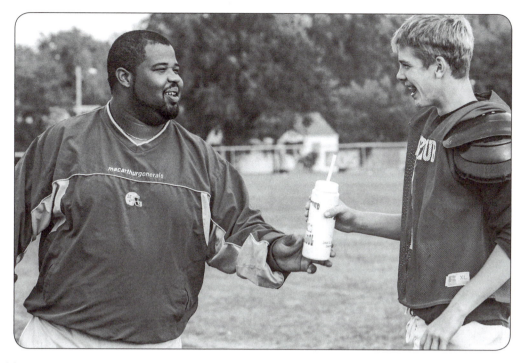

Since 1995, 52 football players have died from heat stroke, 41 of which were high school athletes.

do not have less effective thermoregulatory abilities compared to adults. Recent evidence indicates that children and adults have similar core temperature, skin temperature, and exercise tolerance time during exercise in the heat (American Academy of Pediatrics, 2011). Most healthy children and adolescents can safely participate in outdoor sports in hot and humid conditions. However, youth sport leaders should be aware of the risk factors for exertional heat illness and take appropriate actions to prevent and respond effectively to it.

Table 9.1 provides a list of such risk factors and recommended actions by youth sport leaders (American Academy of Pediatrics, 2011). Risk factors include climate, training intensity and frequency, clothing and equipment, and individual health factors. Recommendations include continuous hydration, progressive adaptation to climate and training, changes in intensity and frequency of training, knowing signs and symptoms of exertional heat illness, and having clear plans of action for when exertional heat illness occurs. Although these are general guidelines to consider, variations in youth athletes' health status and conditioning make some of them more susceptible than others to exertional heat illness. Consider this example (provided by the American Academy of Pediatrics, 2011, p. 3):

Even with a heat index of 95 degrees F (35 C), a very fit, rested, healthy 12-year-old who is acclimatized to the hot and humid conditions can likely safely compete in a soccer game without significant risk to his safety. However, with a heat index of 85 degrees F (29.4 C), an overweight high school football player who recently recovered from diarrhea and is running wind sprints at the end of a 3-hour workout on an unusually warm first day of training is much more likely to be at risk of overheating and exertional collapse.

Table 9.1   Exertional Heat Illness Risk Factors and Recommended Actions

RISK FACTORS
Hot or humid weather or both
Poor preparation (lack of heat acclimatization, inadequate prehydration, little sleep or rest, poor fitness)
Excessive physical exertion, particularly insufficient rest and recovery between repeated bouts of high-intensity exercise (e.g., sprints)
Insufficient access to fluids and opportunities to rehydrate
Multiple same-day sessions with insufficient rest and recovery time in between
Overweight or obesity and other clinical conditions or medications
Current or recent illness (particularly gastrointestinal distress)
Clothing, uniforms, or protective equipment that contributes to excessive heat retention

RECOMMENDED ACTIONS
Provide and promote, even mandate, consumption of readily available fluids at regular intervals before, during, and after activity.
Allow gradual adaptation to the climate, intensity, and duration of activities and uniforms and protective gear.
Modify physical activity by decreasing duration or intensity; increase frequency and duration of breaks (preferably in shade), and cancel or reschedule to a cooler time.
Provide longer rest and recovery time between same-day sessions.
Avoid or limit participation if the athlete is currently or was recently ill.
Closely monitor athletes for signs and symptoms of developing heat illness.
Have an emergency action plan with clearly defined roles and protocols.
Ensure that personnel and facilities for effectively treating heat illness are readily available on site.
In response to illness, promptly activate emergency medical plan and rapidly cool the victim.

Reproduced with permission from *Pediatrics*, Vol. 128, Page(s) 1-9, Copyright © 2011 by the AAP.

PHYSICAL TRAINING GUIDELINES FOR YOUNG ATHLETES

The purpose of physical training is to improve youth athletes' functional capacity to engage in physical activity, or to be able to play their sport better. So how can we help athletes learn to train hard, yet not suffer the ill effects of overtraining?

Basic Principles to Guide Training

All physical training programs should follow some basic principles that are easily applied in youth sport.

Overload and Progression

The basic physical training principle of **overload** means that athletes must do more than what their bodies are used to doing. Exceeding their current fitness capacity (causing fatigue and strain) induces their bodies to adapt to the increased demand. Applying overload (e.g., running a bit farther, requiring athletes to run the same distance more quickly, requiring more speed and movement in basketball practice) is fundamental in improving athletes' fitness.

The difficulty for coaches is determining the degree of overload appropriate for their athletes. If the overload is insufficient, the body doesn't have to adapt and there is no training effect. If the overload is too great, the body becomes overwhelmed, fatigued, and possibly injured. This is called **over-training,** the result of excessive training and inadequate recovery, which typically causes decreased performance and psychological distress (Richardson, Andersen, & Morris, 2008). A study of 13- to 18-year-old swimmers across several countries found that 35% had been overtrained at least once (Raglin, Sawamura, Alexiou, Hassmen, & Kentta, 2000). Signs of overtraining include decline in performance, increased muscle soreness, negative moods and irritability, decreased interest in training, and insomnia.

A general guideline is to avoid increasing the training load more than 10% from the previous training session. For example, a child running 20 minutes at a time four times a week could increase to running 22 minutes four times during the next week. In most team sports, the 10% guideline is estimated in terms of progressively increasing the amount and intensity of practice. This is based on the **progression** principle of physical training, in which the fitness levels of athletes are steadily improved by gradual increases in training intensity or duration. It's helpful for youth coaches to outline longer-term training progressions (e.g., weekly or monthly) so they can keep track of the degree to which they are increasing the training demands for their athletes.

Another important progression to consider in youth sport is how the time length of training sessions should be adapted as children age and mature. The length of training sessions should be developmentally appropriate not only to the physical capacities of kids but also to their abilities to pay attention and absorb information. Although it will vary based on types of sport and competitive level, here are our general guidelines for length of physical training sessions for kids:

- 45 minutes for 5- to 7-year-olds
- 60 minutes for 8- to 10-year-olds
- 90 minutes for 11- to 13-year-olds
- 120 minutes for 14- to 18-year-olds

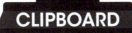

CLIPBOARD

Pain 101 for Kids

Adult athletes understand the difference between pain and injury, but children often don't. Explain to them that there is good pain and bad pain. Have them do a wall sit (back against wall with thighs parallel to floor) for 60 seconds or run up a flight of stairs, and then ask them if they feel the "burn" in their legs. It hurts, but it's good pain. Nothing is wrong or injured—the pain means you've overloaded your muscles in training them. Feeling the burn is good, as it means your muscles are working hard and you're getting more fit.

Then ask them if they've ever been sore the day after practice in their sport, particularly early in the season or after their first practice.

Ask them why this occurs and whether it's good or bad pain. Then explain that this is muscle soreness, which results from overloading the muscles more than they're used to being loaded. This is also good pain because it means you've worked hard enough to tax your muscles—to break them down so they'll grow stronger. This pain should go away in a day or two.

Then ask them, What is bad pain? Explain that this is typically a sharp, sudden pain that really hurts; it's an injury and is bad pain. When they feel this kind of pain, they should stop immediately and tell a coach or parent. Remind them that the adage "No pain no gain" is true for certain types of pain, but not for injuries.

Recovery

Recovery is the basic training principle that goes hand in hand with overload. To benefit optimally from training, young athletes must be given sufficient time between training sessions to rest and restore their bodies. Without recovery, the body doesn't have a chance to adapt to the training stimulus. Although recovery means rest and time away from the gym or pool, it actually starts at the moment the training session is completed. Coaches should build in active recovery time at the end of every training session. This entails 10 to 20 minutes of low-intensity exercise (e.g., jogging, walking, or easy sport drills) and 15 to 20 minutes of stretching all large muscle groups.

Variation

The principle of **variation** means that coaches should vary physical training over time to follow hard sessions with lighter ones and should use variation as well within single training sessions (easy to hard progression). With variation in types of activities in training, the muscles are "shocked" and must adapt as the different movement routines challenge the body in different ways. Variation also has to do with whether the training session is preseason, season, or off-season. Preseason training is usually much harder in order to get athletes into competitive shape, while in-season workouts are relatively lighter due to ongoing competitive events.

Coaches should provide a lot of variety in training sessions. It's okay to spend time on a specific skill or area of fitness, but the trick is to include many different activities (or types of drills) in the training. Always end a training drill or activity at the peak of intensity and enjoyment. Don't wait for energy to start to wane or for athletes to get bored or get tired of the drill. This timing and quick change of activities really picks up a training session.

Cross-training (doing another sport to build fitness) can be used for a psychological boost and change of pace, even during the competitive season. Our son's middle school cross-country coach always designated one day a week for the guys to play Ultimate Frisbee, a game that not only enhanced their fitness but also was a fun break from the distance running routine.

Specificity

The best way to develop physical fitness for a sport is to train the energy systems (aerobic and anaerobic) and muscles as closely as possible to the way they are used in competition. This is the principle of **specificity**. Soccer players have to be trained both aerobically, for endurance in running for 45-minute halves, and anaerobically, for the all-out sprints that they must make during competition. Baseball players or golfers don't need heavy aerobic training, although a basic level of aerobic fitness is helpful to all athletes.

For children under the age of 12, fitness training should be incorporated into the actual learning and practicing of skills. In soccer, dribbling games and relays can build fitness as easily as running, and they keep players from being bored. Using some of the ideas you learned in chapter 8, design imaginative games and drills in which kids play the game and build fitness at the same time. For athletes younger than 12, the emphasis should be on developing sport skills. Once good technique is mastered, physical training to build strength, endurance, power, and speed (or some combination of these) becomes more important. However, a guideline for ball sports is to spend at least 90% of training time with the ball (in skill or fitness activities specific to that sport) (Dicicco & Hacker, 2002), and perhaps even more time for very young athletes.

Strength Training

Strength training is the use of progressive resistance to increase one's ability to exert or resist force. Generally, the focus for children should be on strength training with an emphasis on progressive resistance, not weightlifting. The most practical way for kids to develop strength is to use their own body weight in climbing trees, swinging on ropes or trapezes, navigating monkey bars, and engaging in other active playground challenges. They can also engage in basic exercises such as sit-ups, crunches, or planks for abdominal or core strength; push-ups and pull-ups for chest and arm strength; and lunging and squatting while holding on to a partner for leg strength. Relatively inexpensive equipment that enables kids to use their own bodies in progressive resistance exercises includes elastic tubing and bands that can be purchased online or at most sporting goods stores, and the TRX, a body suspension training apparatus that can be used for full-body workouts.

Youth sport coaches can find many examples tailored to their sports on the Internet, and if interested, they can find books that focus on strength training for youth athletes (e.g., Faigenbaum & Westcott, 2009; LaCaze & Dalrymple, 2011; Martens, 2012). Here are some tips to follow in strength training with youth athletes (Faigenbaum & Westcott, 2009):

1. The most important aspect of progressive resistance exercises is technique. It is often a struggle to get kids to focus on correct technique because they're more interested in how many push-ups they can do or how much weight they can lift (if using free or machine weights). You must convince them that "cheating" detracts from the effects of strength training and that they're only cheating themselves.

2. Direct instruction and supervision should be provided by qualified adults who have an understanding of youth resistance training guidelines. Additional supervision may be needed during the first few weeks of a training program, when participants are learning proper technique.

3. Basic education on exercise room etiquette, proper exercise technique, the importance of individualized goals (not social comparison), and realistic outcomes should be provided by an adult who understands kids and youth sport.

4. Begin with very low resistance until proper technique is learned.

5. Complete 6 to 15 repetitions in good form before increasing weight or resistance.

6. Start each training session with a 5-to10-minute dynamic warm-up period (movement-based exercises for the upper and lower body).

7. Cool down with less intense calisthenics and static stretching.

8. Strength training should be at least 30 minutes in duration, two or three times per week on nonconsecutive days.

9. Keep the program fresh and challenging by systematically varying the training exercises.

Personal Plug-In

Getting Stronger?

What is your experience with strength training in youth sport? What did your youth coaches do, if anything, to build and maintain your strength? How might your performance and development have been different with better training?

Flexibility Training

Flexibility is defined as the quality of bending without breaking. That often applies literally to the human body. Physical **flexibility** is the ability of the body to move through its entire range of motion without injury. Flexibility of muscles and ligaments is important to kids' fitness in decreasing risk of injury and allowing for better performance. It's best to begin flexibility training when children are younger, because at adolescence kids begin to lose their natural flexibility (Lancaster & Teodorescu, 2008).

Stretching is the primary way to develop flexibility in young athletes. **Static stretching** (a stretch held at the maximum range of motion for up to 30 seconds) can be helpful in increasing flexibility. However, static stretching is not useful before physical training sessions as formerly believed by sport practitioners. Rather, the focus before training should be on **dynamic stretching**, which is movement through a challenging yet comfortable range of motion repeatedly, usually 10 to 12 times. Basketball or baseball players may slowly walk using lunging motions to dynamically stretch leg muscles. Volleyball players dynamically stretch their shoulders by slowly moving their arms through the complete range of motion, then making exaggerated overarm throws and bounce passes to each other in their warm-ups.

Dynamic stretching is not the same as **ballistic stretching,** which involves bouncing movements to force muscles beyond their typical range of motion. Avoid ballistic stretching with young athletes. Static stretching is useful after physical training sessions to stretch out the muscles after exertion. Youth sport coaches easily find appropriate flexibility exercises online (both dynamic and static) that are most appropriate for their specific sports.

ABC Training

An often overlooked area of physical training with kids is what we call ABC training (Balyi,

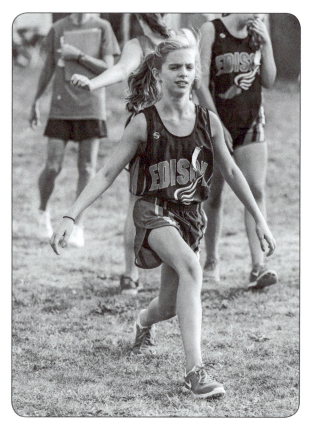

The focus prior to training should be on dynamic stretching, or repeated movements through a comfortable range of motion, such as walking lunges.

Way, & Higgs, 2013). ABC training is for agility, balance, and coordination. We emphasized the importance of these fundamental physical skills in chapter 5—they are critical for achieving physical literacy. **Agility** is the ability to change directions very quickly while maintaining balance, as when a football player cuts back and forth very fast. **Balance** is the ability to stay upright or in control of body movement, as required of a gymnast on a floor routine. **Coordination** is the ability to move body parts in a smooth and efficient pattern, as in executing a tennis serve. These abilities are closely connected, because you often enhance balance and coordination through agility training. Think of how a basketball player must be agile in moving forward, backward, and laterally while accelerating and decelerating, and also maintain body control and balance in coordinated movements with and without the ball in the air and on the floor. All sports have their unique ABC requirements.

For young children, the ABC can be trained in such activities as tumbling, obstacle courses (e.g., requiring forward rolls, jumping over hurdles, moving side to side), and creatively designed relay courses that require stops, starts, lateral movement, and forward and backward running. We remember long summer days hanging out at the pool and learning not only to move efficiently in the water but also to coordinate and balance our bodies going off the low and high diving boards. Games like follow the leader and jump dive are excellent for developing the ABC of sport. Riding bikes and skateboards, roller skating and ice-skating, and playing tag and dodgeball are all examples of children's activities that enhance their ABCs.

When kids enter organized youth sport programs, the ABC can be trained in very sport-specific ways, such as footwork drills and various eye–hand and eye–foot activities. For example, hockey goalies practice the Martin Brodeur drill (Brodeur was named top goaltender in the National Hockey League four times), which involves athletes holding a tennis ball in each hand and throwing the right-hand ball against a wall a few feet away. They catch that ball with their left hand after they have flipped what had been the left-hand ball over to their right hand. They continue this as fast as possible, switching the throwing hands. This drill builds eye–hand coordination and quickness in reacting. Small-sided games in training, such as futsal in soccer (discussed in chapter 10) or pepper in baseball and softball, enhance the ABCs of youth athletes. Examples of training activities for specific sports are plentiful on the Internet, and we urge coaches to incorporate basic ABC training activities in their workouts.

Aerobic and Anaerobic Training

Applying the principle of specificity, the amount and intensity of aerobic and anaerobic training should be based on the physical demands of specific sports. However, most team sports require basic levels of speed and power (anaerobic skills), as well as endurance (aerobic capacity). All athletes should first develop their aerobic foundation, preferably during the off-season. This puts them in the position to then either increase their aerobic capacity through more training or to move on to anaerobic training if their sport requires this quicker, more intense form of energy.

The most important factor in the training program is the intensity of exercise. There are instruments that can measure this, such as heart rate monitors. But in most youth sport situations, athletes and coaches have to estimate the intensity of the activity. Long, slow distance training (running, rowing, cycling, swimming, skating, skiing, or paddling) is what develops the aerobic foundation. The intensity for this type of exercise is 70% to 85% of a person's maximal heart rate. This is a pace at which athletes can talk to each other while exercising. To increase the aerobic capacity of children and adolescents, training should include a mixture of continuous and interval exercises for a minimum of three or four sessions of 40 to 60 minutes per week for a minimum of 12 weeks (Armstrong & Barker, 2011).

Aerobic training for kids should include variety and fun activities and should not be conducted in its entirety all at once during practice (Lancaster & Teodorescu, 2008). Coaches could incorporate different sports into their practices as conditioning activities; for example, they can have cross-country athletes occasionally play small-sided games like Ultimate Frisbee. Another idea is to set up obstacle courses across different terrains, which requires aerobic training yet offers some variety and some novel challenges. In general, endurance (aerobic) training on a track should be reserved for athletes 10 and older, as they are more focused and not as apt to become bored. Stick to activity-based aerobic training that is game oriented and gets their focus away from training and more toward playing (use your imagination or look for examples on the Internet or in books [e.g., Lancaster & Teodorescu, 2008]).

Training the anaerobic system requires intense, short bursts of exercise, usually 85% to 95% of maximum heart rate. The most common method used to train anaerobically is interval training. Thirty to ninety seconds of exercise working at 90% to 95% of maximal heart rate, followed by a recovery period four times longer than the exercise period, trains the anaerobic system. This could be sprints on the ice for hockey players followed by rest, full-court running and passing drills in basketball with intermittent rest, or four 400-meter runs with appropriate recovery between each. As much as possible, anaerobic training should involve sport-specific activities, such as short, intense basketball passing and shooting drills or short sprint soccer drills. With younger children, competitive relays are always popular and are an effective way to structure interval training.

Sprints are used for speed training and are done at 95% to 100% of maximum heart rate. Or, as we tell the young athletes, go all out. Individual speed ability is genetically determined, with the requirement of a high percentage of fast-twitch muscle fibers. Help young athletes understand this. Yet, speed is trainable. All athletes can improve their speed, but genetic factors limit their ability to match the speed of faster teammates or opponents. Speed is best trained at the end of warm-up or as a part of it, when there is no cognitive or physical fatigue (Balyi et al., 2013). Keep speed training exercises short, with full recovery between sets. Acceleration should be over a short distance, with proper posture and correct elbow, knee drive, and head positions. Remember, running is a fundamental motor skill that should be taught and practiced. Kids can improve their speed (and endurance) by learning the correct posture and mechanics of running.

Of course there are many physical training methods to build the aerobic and anaerobic fitness of young athletes. Our intent in this chapter is to help you understand the basic concepts and then enable you to seek out sport-specific guidance for the physical training strategies that best fit your needs. (A sample physical training session for 7th-grade [12- and 13-year-olds] basketball players is provided in figure 9.2.) At the very least, youth sport coaches should understand how to incorporate progressive fitness activities as part of their sport-specific drills in training sessions. Keep the activity fun and engaging, and kids will automatically extend themselves in their exertion to play the game.

WRAP-UP

Children are physically trainable, but they're not miniature adults and should not be trained like adults. They're growing and maturing and developing their relationship with physical activity. We want that relationship to be a loving one, so that young athletes are hooked on physical activity throughout their lives. But we don't want kids' relationships with physical activity to be obsessive. Physical training—and the outcomes it provides—sometimes becomes a seductive slippery slope for young athletes, particularly adolescents. Young athletes can slide from healthy training behaviors toward dysfunctional behavioral practices that threaten their well-being.

Physical training can also be a slippery slope for youth sport coaches, who zealously slide into thinking that more is better. We prefer the viewpoint that more and less are both better. More is better when it involves progressive overload and specificity in training. Yet, less is also a necessary part of the equation, where less involves adequate recovery, the clever use of variation to keep training fresh, and optimal (not excessive) amounts of physical training for different age groups. We hope you will develop your own ideas about how to follow the philosophy that more and less are better in using developmentally appropriate ways to get and keep kids moving.

A. Dynamic Warm-Up (10-15 minutes)

1. Without basketball (athletes engage in each movement from baseline to midcourt and back)

   a. Jog

   b. Backpedal jog

   c. Carioca (facing sideways, cross over leg in front and then in back to move down on the court)

   d. Skip with arm swing

   e. Defensive shuffle

   f. Walking lunge

   g. Jogging butt kicks

   h. Jogging high knees

   i. Straight-leg kicks

2. With basketball

   a. Figure 8 dribbling (between legs)

   b. Full-court half-speed dribbling

   c. Full-court dribbling (with crossover and spin at designated points) into layups

   d. Two-person full-court passing

   e. Two-person full-court passing with layup at end

   f. Three-person full-court passing weave with layup at end

B. Teaching Skills and Using Drills to Learn and Improve Individual Skills (30-40 minutes)

C. Drills and Games to Practice Offense and Defense (20 minutes)

D. Scrimmage (15 minutes)

E. Cool-Down and Light Static Stretching (5 minutes)

1. Calf stretch (gastrocnemius and soleus)

2. Quadriceps stretch

3. Hamstrings stretch

4. Hip flexors stretch

5. Trunk rotators stretch

Figure 9.2 Sample physical training session for 7th-grade (12-13 years) basketball.

LEARNING AIDS

Key Terms

aerobic fitness—The ability to transport and use oxygen during endurance activities.

agility—The ability to change directions very quickly while maintaining balance.

amenorrhea—Absence of menstrual periods.

anabolic steroids—Synthetic versions of testosterone used to build muscle and increase endurance.

anaerobic fitness—The ability to engage in all-out, short-term physical effort.

anorexia nervosa—An eating disorder characterized by restrictive eating in which the individual views herself as overweight even though she is at least 15% below the expected weight for her age and height.

balance—The ability to stay upright or in control of body movement.

ballistic stretching—Using bouncing movements to force muscles beyond their typical range of motion.

bulimia nervosa—An eating disorder in which individuals, usually in the normal weight range, repeat a cycle of overeating and then purging, fasting, or exercising excessively.

coordination—The ability to move body parts in a smooth and efficient pattern.

creatine—An over-the-counter supplement used to improve performance in activities that require short bursts of high-intensity activity.

cross-training—Participation in a second sport to build fitness.

dynamic stretching—Movement through a challenging yet comfortable range of motion repeatedly, usually 10 to 12 times.

ephedrine—A stimulant used to reduce fatigue, lose weight, and maintain mental alertness.

flexibility—The ability of the body to move through its entire range of motion without injury.

obese—Having excess body fat.

osteoporosis—A disease that thins and weakens bones so they are fragile and break easily.

overload—Training above one's current fitness capacity, causing fatigue and strain, to induce the body to adapt to the increased demand.

overtraining—Excessive training and inadequate recovery, which typically results in decreased performance and psychological distress.

overweight—Having excess body weight for a particular height.

physical training—A disciplined routine of specialized procedures performed by athletes to condition their bodies.

progression—Gradual increases in training intensity or duration in an effort to steadily improve athletes' fitness levels.

recovery—Sufficient time between training sessions to rest and restore the body.

specificity—Training the energy systems and muscles as closely as possible to the way they are used in competition.

static stretching—A stretch held at the maximum range of motion for up to 30 seconds.

steroid precursors—Substances that the body converts into anabolic steroids, which are used to train harder, recover faster, and build muscle mass.

strength training—The use of progressive resistance to increase one's ability to exert or resist force.

thermoregulation—Preventing core temperature from rising or falling excessively.

variation—Progressively mixing strenuous and easier training sessions, as well as easy and hard and different types of activities within sessions.

Summary Points

1. Physical activity and training can increase lean body and bone mass, muscular strength, aerobic and anaerobic fitness, mental health, and cognitive performance in children.

2. Prepubescent children's energy and muscular fitness systems are trainable, meaning that they can be enhanced, but not at the same level as in adults.

3. The female athlete triad refers to interrelationships between energy availability, menstrual function, and bone mineral density.

4. Certain personality characteristics as well as types of sport are related to the incidence of eating disorders in youth sport.

5. There is no conclusive evidence that participation in elite gymnastics stunts the growth and sexual maturation of young gymnasts.

6. Social pressures for excessive weight gain in football and weight loss in wrestling can have severe health consequences for athletes.

7. Anabolic steroids are illegal substances used to build muscle and increase endurance that can cause many adverse physical and psychological health issues.

8. Physical training in youth sport should be guided by the principles of overload, progression, recovery, variation, and specificity.

9. The most practical way for children to gain strength is through progressive resistance using their own body weight.

10. Dynamic stretching is recommended before physical training, and static stretching is useful after training sessions as part of the cool-down and recovery processes.

11. Aerobic training involves long, slow distance activities, while anaerobic training requires intense, short bursts of activity as in interval training.

Study Questions

1. Identify and explain as many positive effects of physical activity as you can.

2. Explain how physical activity and training as a child can prevent osteoporosis later in life.

3. Can prepubescent children gain strength through training? How so, if their muscles lack the appropriate hormones to undergo hypertrophy?

4. Explain how the healthy female athlete triad moves into the unhealthy or pathological female athlete triad.

5. What are the adverse health effects of the practice of gaining and carrying large amounts of body weight, a practice common for athletes in certain positions in American football?

6. Identify and explain the four types of performance-enhancing drugs commonly used by youth sport athletes, including their health risks.

7. Identify the five principles of training presented in the chapter, and for each, provide an example of how youth sport coaches can engage in appropriate physical training practices with athletes.

8. List five tips for using strength training with children.

9. What are the best types of stretching exercises to do before and after physical training? Provide examples of each type.

10. What are the key differences in training aerobically and anaerobically?

Reflective Learning Activities

1. Design a physical training workout for an athlete or group of athletes in your sport. Designate the sport, age of athletes, and time of season (e.g., preseason training or during competitive season). Incorporate specific warm-up and cool-down activities, including stretching exercises, in your workout. Explain how your workout enhances strength, flexibility, and the types of energy fitness needed (aerobic, anaerobic, speed, power) in this sport.

2. Design a brochure you could provide to parents to educate them about the use of performance-enhancing drugs in youth sport. Include the following information: types and use, availability, health risks, and warning signs.

3. Design a brochure to educate parents about eating disorders in youth sport.

Resource Guide

American College of Sports Medicine, or ACSM (acsm.org). ACSM is the governing body for sports medicine in the United States. On the ACSM website, guidelines are presented for strength training in children and adolescents. In fact, the ACSM has a position statement on youth strength training.

A Guide to Heat Acclimatization and Heat Illness Prevention, NFHS free online course (nfhslearn.com).

Strength and Conditioning, NFHS online course (www.nfhslearn.com).

chapter 10

TALENT DEVELOPMENT IN SPORT

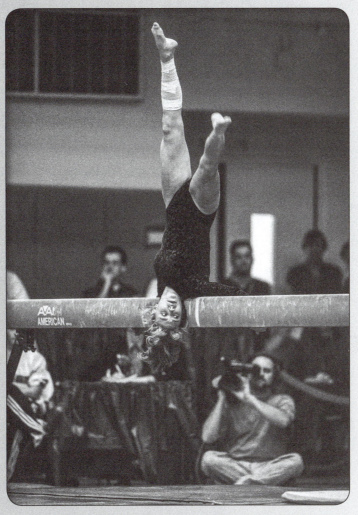

CHAPTER PREVIEW

In this chapter, you'll learn

» what talent is and how it is assessed in sport,
» the role of talent and practice in developing sport expertise,
» how overspecialization harms children, and
» strategies for developing talent in youth sport.

Elite athletes wow us with their expertise. Watching world-class gymnasts soar and flip and spin and balance is amazing enough, but observing them performing these complex, skilled movements on a beam 4 feet (122 centimeters) high and less than 4 inches (10 centimeters) wide is astonishing. There are numerous examples of astonishing expertise in sport, which includes not just physical execution of skills but also emotional control and focus under pressure, anticipation and decision making, and displays of mind-bending speed, strength, endurance, and body control.

We popularly refer to these abilities as talent, and we are consumed with the desire to know the best way to identify and develop such talent in children. How and when do we decide if kids are talented? Is it talent or practice that is more important in developing expertise? Should children specialize or diversify early in youth sport? Our objective for this chapter is to help you understand what we know about talent development in sport, with a particular focus on how youth sport is influenced by popular, and sometimes erroneous, ideas about developing talent in kids.

TALENT DEVELOPMENT BASICS

There are multiple terms that relate to talent development, which often mean different things to different people. So our first step is to clarify the meaning we give to these terms in this chapter.

What Is Talent?

Talent is usually defined as an innate (inborn) ability. Five elements characterize talent as a hardwired intrapersonal phenomenon (Howe, Davidson, & Sloboda, 1998):

1. It is based on genetic structures and thus is at least partly innate.
2. Its effects may not be fully evident at an early age, but there will be some

early indications, allowing trained people to identify the presence of talent before mature performance has been demonstrated.
3. These early indications of talent provide a preliminary basis for predicting who is likely to excel.
4. Only a minority of children are talented.
5. Talent is domain specific (that is, specific to certain sports or types of sports).

Talent refers to a quality (or qualities) identified at an earlier time that can lead to expertise at a future time, so the emphasis is on an individual's potential for success in a particular activity (Cobley, Schorer, & Baker, 2012). Here's how a freshman (high school) football coach described talent as potential in one of his players: "His ceiling is as high as any defensive player I've ever observed. He's a long, athletic young man, both quick and strong, and he's going to have a great future in this game." Researchers on the development of exceptional athletes found that parents, coaches, and the athletes themselves noted some evidence of talent or giftedness at a very early age (Bloom, 1985; Cote, 1999; Gulbin, Oldenziel, Weissensteiner, & Gagne, 2010).

Sometimes people use the word *talent* to refer to demonstrated ability on a sport task, but the execution of a sport skill or set of skills is more correctly termed **performance**. **Skill** typically refers to proficiency that is acquired through training and experience, while **expertise** is defined as consistent superior athletic performance over an extended period (Starkes, 1993).[6] We understand that this is confusing. "Talent shows" are really "expertise shows," according to our definitions. When people say that a team has a lot of talent, they often mean that the team is very skilled and demonstrates

[6] In research on giftedness in education (e.g., Gagne, 2009), *gifts* refers to natural abilities (what we call talent in this book), while *talent* typically refers to systematically developed competencies (what we call skill or expertise in this book).

expertise. However, some coaches state (correctly, according to our definitions) that their team has a lot of talent, meaning that this ability is unrefined and has the potential to be developed into higher levels of skill and expertise. So, in this chapter we are ultimately interested in how children's talents can be developed in the fullest ways to lead to sport expertise.

What Does Sport Expertise Look Like?

To know how to develop talent, we need to know what sport expertise it involves. To become an expert, athletes must possess or acquire expertise in four essential areas: technical, physical, cognitive (including tactical knowledge and perceptual skills), and psychological (see table 10.1, adapted from Janelle & Hillman, 2003). Weakness in any one area will impede an athlete's progress toward expert status. Elite athletes have repeatedly been shown to demonstrate higher levels of expertise in all of these areas

when compared to nonelite athletes (Epstein, 2013; Farrow, 2010; Helsen & Starkes, 1999; Krane & Williams, 2010). Athletes can achieve success without all the components of sport expertise, but they may reach their skill ceiling unless they are able to develop the component needed to move them to expert status.

What Is Talent Development?

Talent development refers to providing the most appropriate environment for athletes to stimulate their learning and performance. If talent is about potential, then talent development is about helping young athletes realize and achieve their potential. Through practice, experience, and coaching, athletes develop skills in specific sports—and with continued, dedicated practice, experience, and coaching, they may become experts in their sports (see figure 10.1). So talent is transformed into expertise only through skill development and refinement gained through extensive personal efforts.

Table 10.1 Essential Areas of Sport Expertise

Area of expertise	Description	Examples
1. Technical	Ability to perform sport skills in a coordinated, efficient, and refined movement pattern with a high level of automaticity	Executing a soccer corner kick on target Executing a triple Salchow jump in figure skating
2. Physical	Ability of the body's physical makeup and internal systems to enhance physical training and performance	Muscle fiber types, aerobic and anaerobic capacities, flexibility, size of body segments
3. Cognitive		
Tactical knowledge	Ability to determine what strategy will be most effective in different situations	Softball shortstop choosing the best defensive play based on base runners and number of outs
Perceptual skill	Ability to extract most relevant cues from the environment, quickly recognize patterns, and use advanced anticipatory cues and visual search strategies to produce best in-the-moment decisions or reactions	Soccer goalie stopping a shot by reading, anticipating, and reacting to opponents' positions and movements
4. Psychological	Ability to regulate behavior to enhance long-term goal striving, perseverance, self-belief, focus without distraction, and emotional control	Archer regulating arousal levels before shooting in competition Free throw shooter maintaining focus and routine under pressure of overtime and hostile crowd

Based on Janelle and Hillman 2003.

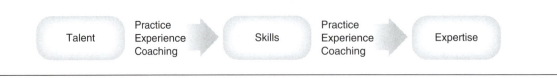

Figure 10.1   The talent development process in sport.

All youth sport should be about the development of talent in its more generic sense, or focusing on helping each child develop her talents as much as possible (an important objective for youth sport identified in chapter 3). However, another important objective of youth sport (also noted in chapter 3) is to develop athletic talent to create athletes with the expertise to compete at elite levels, such as the Olympic Games. Not all athletes have the talent or the commitment to move to the right side of figure 10.1 and become expert athletes as Rory McIlroy did. Most youth athletes practice, compete, and use coaching advice to develop basic sport skills (as represented by the left side of figure 10.1). Our 11-year-old son reminded us of this when we suggested to him that he attend a winter stroke clinic in preparation for his summer swim season, to which he replied, "Why would I take lessons? I already know how to swim." Right.

Although we embrace talent development for all youth sport participants, much of this chapter focuses on the entire sequence shown in figure 10.1. We think it's important for you to understand the process of talent development that leads to sport expertise, even though most youth sport participants will not become experts. The objective of developing expertise in sport is important, and it is a global phenomenon as national training programs around the world consider the best ways to develop athletic talent in their countries.

What Is Talent Identification?

Talent identification is the process of distinguishing (and usually selecting) children and youth who demonstrate potential for expertise in a particular sport. Other terms are sometimes used, such as *talent detection* and *talent selection,* but they all generally refer to the evaluation of young people to identify those with potential for success in a specific sport. Specialized talent development programs are then typically implemented for those identified.

Organized programs of talent identification and development began in the 1950s, led by the Eastern Bloc nations, including the Soviet Union and the German Democratic Republic, both of which achieved a great deal of international sport success in the 1970s and 1980s. As discussed in chapter 1, China employs a systematic, government-sponsored talent identification and development program that identifies and selects athletes for training in specialized sport schools.

After failing to win a single gold medal at the 1976 Montreal Olympic Games, Australia won 17 gold medals at the 2004 Athens Olympic Games and ranked fourth in number of medals won by a country. A major impetus for this surge in international sporting expertise was the decision in 1993 to award the 2000 Summer Olympic Games to Sydney, Australia. The Australian government committed $135 million to enhance athlete development in preparation for hosting the Games, including a national talent search program. It conducted nationwide searches and testing programs in the sports of athletics, cycling, canoeing, swimming, rowing, triathlon, water polo, and weightlifting. Australia won 58 medals in 2000, an increase of 114% in eight years (Baker & Schorer, 2010). The success of this program led to the establishment of the National Talent Identification and Development (NTID) program in 2006 (Gulbin, 2012).

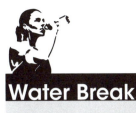

Water Break

A Talent for Golf

Rory McIlroy provides us with a great example of the talent development process shown in figure 10.1. McIlroy played in the British Open at age 15, became a professional golfer at age 18, and became the youngest player to rank among the world's top 50 golfers. By 2014, at the age of 25, McIlroy had won four major tournaments and was ranked as the number-one golfer in the world.

His talent for the game was apparent as an 18-month-old, when he would go to the range with his father to hit balls. Others noticed McIlroy's talent right away. Acclaimed golf teacher Jim McLean saw him at his first junior tournament at age 9 and told McIlroy's father, "This kid's good. I'm tellin' you, Mr. McIlroy, this kid has something" (Morfit, 2012, p. 64). He was featured on a television show pitching golf balls into a washing machine (because he practiced at home this way). Realizing his talent, McIlroy's parents worked multiple jobs and extra shifts to support his development.

Above all, however, McIlroy's talent was developed into expertise through his obsession with and commitment to the game of golf. McIlroy states that as a boy, he played golf from "half seven [morning] until 10 at night," typically 54 holes per day in the summer (Sampson, 2013, p. 53). His father called him a "strange wee boy" for wanting to practice all day. His teacher at the local club describes McIlroy's love of the process of learning, his ability to self-correct, and his autonomous striving to get better, without any push from adults. He begged to go to the range one cold snowy morning, and his parents tried to talk him out of it. But to no avail; the club cleaned a spot in the snow for him and gave him 200 balls to hit. His father describes another day of hitting at the range and then playing; on returning home, McIlroy asked if they could go back to the range. When his father suggested that they had played enough that day, McIlroy replied, "Dad, do you not want me to get any better?" (Morfit, 2012, p. 65). Unusual talent plus unusual commitment leads to outstanding expertise, as in the case of Rory McIlroy.

The United Kingdom implemented a similar talent identification and development program once it was awarded the London Olympic Games in 2012 (Vaeyens, Gullich, Warr, & Philippaerts, 2009). The UK Talent Team, as it was called, ran national recruitment campaigns and assessed over 7,000 athletes for recruitment into newly developed programs. One example was the Sporting Giants campaign, in which exceptionally tall athletic talent was sought through screening to fast-track into the sports of rowing, handball, or volleyball. The UK Talent Identification and Development program has continued to pursue international sporting success through talent profiling of youth.

The majority of athletes participating in youth sport will not be identified and included in national talent development programs. However, international talent development initiatives for elite performers influence youth practice even at the grassroots levels. So, in the following sections, we address some key issues about talent development that have implications not only for the few select athletes who go on to expert status but also for the vast majority of children who participate in youth sport.

HOW IS TALENT IDENTIFIED, AND WHEN DO WE DECIDE WHO IS TALENTED?

In the movie *Trouble With the Curve,* an elderly baseball scout (played by Clint Eastwood) showed that he could more accurately identify baseball talent from observation and experience than could other (younger) scouts who used computers and statistics. The National Football League's annual scouting combine, nicknamed the Underwear Olympics, is a massive talent identification affair in which college players are put through a dizzying array of drills, tests, and interviews to assess their abilities in relation to a prospective professional football career. Team executives differ in the value they place on the combine, with many using the event as a final evaluation of players' medical conditions and overall character. Draft day "busts" have served to embarrass several team front offices, which engaged in diligent talent assessment only to see their choices severely underperform. In 2009, 21 Major League Baseball teams passed on drafting 17-year-old Mike Trout, who within three years became the best player in baseball.

And this occurs when people are attempting to assess and predict the talent of adult athletes! Now consider the complexity in attempting to identify athletic talent in children, who are undergoing the greatest physical, psychological, and social maturational changes of their lives. How should we identify talent in kids? There are many different opinions about this in the sport science literature. Most people concur that talent is really hard to predict in sport, and we agree (the operative word being *predict,* which means to foretell the future). Others lament that there is no road map for definitive, scientifically based talent identification in sport. Of course there isn't—we don't have definitive scientific road maps for cancer treatment or language learning either. But the fields of medicine and education continue to work toward best practices to further understand these phenomena.

Methods of Talent Identification

Talent identification in youth sport has typically used anthropometric (size and proportions of the body) measures, maturational status estimates, tests of general physical abilities, and sport-specific skill evaluations (see table 10.2). To a lesser degree, talent evaluations have also been made using perceptual tests (reaction, anticipation, decision

Personal Plug-In

How Was Your Talent Developed?

Think about your early experiences in physical activity and in other areas. Did you recognize any special talents you seemed to have? Did others recognize these talents in you, or do you think that your talent was overlooked? Consider how your talent was developed, or not, and identify what you can learn from your own personal experience with talent identification and development.

Table 10.2 Methods Used in Sport Talent Identification

Method	Examples
Anthropometry	Sitting height, arm span, leg length
Maturational status estimates	Secondary sex characteristics
General physical abilities tests	30 m sprint, shuttle run, $\dot{V}O_2$max
Sport-specific skill evaluation	Dribbling, passing, and shooting skill in soccer
Perceptual tests	Force plates to assess reaction time, tracking of eye movements, anticipation tests
Tactical knowledge assessments	Interviews, Tactical Skills Inventory for Sport
Game or overall intelligence tests	Wonderlic cognitive ability test
Psychological assessments	Ottawa Mental Skills Assessment Tool (OMSAT-3)

making), tactical knowledge assessment, game and overall intelligence tests, and psychological inventories.

Anthropometric measures, coupled with maturational status, provide an estimation of a young athlete's adult physical features, with the objective of identifying body types that are most advantageous for performance in specific sports (Lidor & Ziv, 2013). For example, anthropometric features helpful for youth rowing performance include height, leg length, arm length, and body mass (Mikulic & Ruzic, 2008). General physical abilities typically assessed include strength, speed, aerobic and anaerobic capacities, and power. Although these abilities are trainable, there is a genetic predisposition that certainly influences athletes' fit for certain sports. For example, hand–eye coordination, upper-body strength, agility, and leg power are associated with performance in volleyball. Sport-specific skill evaluations are common in youth sport, such as ball control, dribbling, shooting, and passing accuracy in soccer.

Issues and Concerns With Talent Identification

Sport scientists have a great deal of concern about the ability of these evaluation methods to distinguish between more talented youth athletes (particularly prepubescent children) and those who have less talent (e.g., Abbott, Button, Pepping, & Collins, 2005; Lidor, Cote, & Hackfort, 2009). Performance and skill level at an early age are not always an accurate indicator of performance as an adult, as children grow, physically mature, psychologically and cognitively develop, and engage in opportunities that can radically influence their skill development (Abbott & Collins, 2002). Consider how late-maturing boys and children younger in relative age may be overlooked when talent is evaluated by size, general physical abilities, sport-specific skills, or some combination of these. The problem is that we may be overlooking young athletes with a great deal of talent because it is difficult to assess their potential when it is still dormant and not overtly apparent.

We understand the motivation of national sport organizations to engage in systematic talent identification initiatives to attempt to match young athletes with the sport activities in which they are most likely to succeed. This benefits the organizations and also may benefit the young athletes, who are fitted with a sport based on their physical characteristics and skills. We also understand that resources for developing talent are limited. National organizations, as well as school and club programs, have finite openings for membership on sport teams, so evaluation using the various talent identification methods must be conducted to decide who makes the teams. Although they miss out on selecting some individuals whose talent is still dormant, trying out in sport is an inevitability in select-type programs sponsored by national, club, professional, and school sport organizations. The trick is to do it better.

Suggestions to Emphasize Talent Development Over Talent Identification

It seems that talent development in the broadest sense should be emphasized over narrow, restrictive, premature talent identification. We strongly advocate finding ways to widen the narrow sluice that has restricted the number and type of children allowed to flow through into the stream of continued sport participation. Here are our suggestions:

1. **Focus on and create multiple pathways.** Our palm community model of sport participation was presented in chapter 3 to suggest structural and philosophical change in youth sport. The key is to think about multiple pathways that children can choose to follow in developing their personal talents.

Sport New Zealand has developed the Talent Development Framework, which attempts to provide alternative pathways for all children to reach their individual potential. The first objective is to develop fundamental motor skills and basic sport-specific skills to build competence and confidence in all children. Then children follow either the Participation or the High Performance pathway. The Participation pathway provides resources and opportunities for retaining kids in recreational sport experiences throughout their teen years. The High Performance pathway targets highly skilled and motivated children who wish to develop expertise and pursue elite performer status. The philosophical basis of Sport New Zealand's Talent Development Framework is the idea that talent is dynamic and not easily predicted and that gifted athletes can emerge at any stage of development. Similarly, the Australian Institute of Sport has instituted both a participation pathway and a talent pathway, a progressive program that focuses on building skills in all children, with some going on to elite sport careers while others remain active in recreational sport.

At the local level, school athletic directors, sport club directors, and community recreation directors could plan a comprehensive array of sport opportunities (using the palm community model from chapter 3) and then advertise, market, and educate community members about these opportunities. Because kids are conditioned to the pyramid model (up or out) of sport, once they are cut from a school or club team they often quit the sport altogether. We have to provide attractive alternative pathways for young people to continue to develop their talents. Several boys were cut from our local middle school team and had no place to play because our community recreational basketball league didn't have enough 12- and 13-year-old boys to offer a league for them. We worked with the recreation director to create an "in-house" league of just 14 boys who met twice a week with two adult coaches to continue their skill development in drills and games. We need more alternative opportunities beyond the "one school–one team" sluice that culls out kids before we, and they, have any idea of their talents.

2. **Emphasize psychobehavioral skills in sport talent identification and development.** Talent identification and development initiatives have been skewed toward physical skills and performance. Yet, research has shown that psychological skills (e.g., motivation, commitment, mental toughness) separate experts from nonexperts (Gulbin et al., 2010) and can be more predictive of elite status than physical skills (MacNamara, Button, & Collins, 2010a; Smith & Christensen, 1995; Smith, Schutz, Smoll, & Ptacek, 1995). Coaches at an elite Danish soccer academy known for producing expert players admit that they select athletes who have a little less talent and the mental ability to work very hard over hugely talented athletes who do not

work hard (Larsen, Alfermann, Henriksen, & Christensen, 2013). Similarly, the motivation, discipline, and autonomy that influence athletes' abilities to complete hard training sessions are emphasized over anthropometry and physical abilities at an elite Norwegian kayak school that has produced multiple Olympic athletes (Henriksen, Stambulova, & Roessler, 2011).

Young athletes will succeed (no matter the level of talent) only if they possess the attitude and mental skills required for the development of their talent. Of course, coaches subjectively assess mental skills

in selecting team members, but psychological assessments are underused in talent identification and development initiatives (MacNamara & Collins, 2012).

3. **Attempt to assess talent potential over static current skill level.** We understand that high school and middle school coaches must choose athletes for teams with limited positions, and typically those selections are made based on current skill level. However, to truly assess talent, coaches and teachers can try to estimate skill potential by evaluating maturational level in relation to body size and characteristics, coordination

Water Break

A Soccer Talent Development Machine

Germany had been a dominant player in men's world soccer for almost 50 years, but by the late 1990s this traditional brilliance was lacking and the international results had become mediocre. To remedy this, Germany created a new grassroots youth soccer talent development system that is the envy of most other nations. Across the country, 121 national talent centers were built for the training of 10- to 17-year-old soccer players, each with two full-time coaches. In addition, all 36 professional clubs in the Bundesliga, the professional soccer league in Germany, were required to build youth academies. In 2012, the 36 Bundesliga clubs spent a combined $100 million on youth development, more than any other professional sport league in the world.

Germany's national soccer association paid particular attention to identifying and developing talent in the very young

by setting up mobile coaching units, traveling across the country to visit schools and clubs, and advising local clubs on training methods for youth. The coaching philosophy is to develop technical ability, starting out by having athletes play four-a-side on small pitches to encourage individual skills. The national association director states, "We have a wide net in Germany. . . . It is virtually impossible for a talent to slip through the cracks" (Grohmann, 2013).

The result has been the youngest and most consistently successful national soccer team in the world, a team that won the World Cup in 2014. The national talent development program feeds the Bundesliga clubs with more than half of their squad members. Germany provides a prototypical model for how professional and national sport organizations can develop talent via a systematic grassroots approach.

in a wide range of fundamental motor skills, and specific fundamental motor and prerequisite skills for a particular sport. Young athletes may vary in their experience in the sport, but some may show raw signs of fundamental skills and abilities that may enable them to develop sport-specific skills more easily. Talent identification will never be an exact science, but the idea is to look for athletic qualities that could be shaped through training into specific skills. Interestingly, almost all coaches would tell you that they can identify these qualities, although it is difficult for them to explain exactly how they do it.

THE RELATIVE INFLUENCES OF PRACTICE AND INNATE QUALITIES ON SPORT EXPERTISE

What is your first thought when you observe the skilled performance of an accomplished athlete like Lionel Messi? Words like talent, genius, or prodigy often come to mind. Although we recognize that Messi engages in practice to hone his skills, it is common for us to explain his expertise as the result of innate, hardwired talent. What are the relative influences of innate talent and practice on kids who want to become elite athletes? The answer to this question is important because ideas about whether innate talent or practice is more important strongly influence what goes on in youth sport today.

Importance of Practice and Experience

David Beckham's father recalls how his son would kick a soccer ball from the same spot for hours as a young child. His father stated, "His dedication was breathtaking. It sometimes seemed that he lived on the local field" (Syed, 2010, pp. 61-62). The importance of practice and experience to the development

of expertise is widely chronicled, as in the Beckham example.

The 10,000 Hours and 10 Years Prescription

The theory of deliberate practice (Ericsson, Krampe, & Tesch-Romer, 1993) has strongly influenced ideas about sport training for expertise. In an initial study, Ericsson and colleagues examined the practice habits of three groups of violinists at an esteemed Berlin music school to find out why some were better than others. Group 1 included the stars of the school, on their way to world-class status as musicians. In group 2 were highly regarded violinists but still a step below those in group 1. In group 3 were violinists whose abilities were not at the performer level and who were slated to become music teachers. All the violinists started playing around age 8, and all decided to make music their careers around age 15. They all had the same teachers and the same schedule of instruction at the academy. So one could assume, as often is the case, that it was innate talent that created the differences in music ability between the groups.

However, upon examining training histories, Ericsson and colleagues found that group 1 violinists had spent an average of 10,000 hours practicing by the age of 20. In contrast, group 2 had averaged around 7,500 hours, and group 3 had averaged approximately 5,000 hours by that age. In a second study, Ericsson and colleagues (1993) found that expert pianists had similarly accumulated an average of over 10,000 hours of practice by age 20, compared to about 2,000 hours for amateur pianists. Thus, the 10,000 hours prescription for the development of expertise was born.

Along with the 10,000 hours prescription for expertise development, the 10-year guideline was proposed based on the finding that it takes chess players around 10 years to attain an international level of skill (Simon & Chase, 1973). Research has generally supported the 10-year guideline for expertise development in sport (Baker, Cote, & Abernathy, 2003; Bloom, 1985; Gulbin et al., 2010; Helsen, Hodges, Van Winckel, & Starkes, 2000). Although the two parts of the prescription don't have to go together (it could be 10 years or 10,000 hours), let's do the math for the hours within this time frame. To train for 10,000 hours in 10 years, you must train 1,000 hours per year, 84 hours per month, 21 hours per week, and ultimately 3 hours per day seven days a week—for 10 years. Wow. That's a lot of practice. But according to Ericsson, just any kind of practice won't do.

Significance of Deliberate Practice

According to Ericsson and colleagues (1993), the 10-year prescription for the development of expertise doesn't hold up unless it involves deliberate practice. **Deliberate practice** is a highly structured activity with the explicit goal to improve performance. It requires effort and is not inherently enjoyable. It involves not only repetition but also effortful, focused attention to enhancing skill beyond current levels. Thus, elite performance, or expertise, is the product of a decade or more of maximal efforts to improve performance through deliberate practice.

Although there are some qualifications to this prescription of deliberate practice for sport (discussed in a later section), the importance of deliberate practice in developing talent and expertise in sport has generally been supported (Baker & Young, 2014; Cote, Baker, & Abernathy, 2007). Not only do experts typically invest in greater amounts of deliberate practice overall, but they also devote more time to participating in the specific activities most relevant to improvement (such as advanced technical aspects of performance). Thus, these experts may not always do more of everything, but they tend to "do a lot more of the little things" (p. 86) that improve their performance in incremental steps not adhered to by less

expert performers (Young & Salmela, 2010). The deliberate practice prescription has spawned several popular books espousing the primacy of nurture over nature in developing sport expertise, including *The Gold Mine Effect* (Ankerson, 2012), *Bounce* (Syed, 2010), *The Talent Code* and the *Little Book of Talent* (Coyle, 2009, 2012), and *Talent Is Overrated* (Colvin, 2008).

Why Human "Software" Is Critical to Sport Expertise

At the 2004 Pepsi All-Star Game, Olympic champion softball pitcher Jennie Finch struck out Major League Baseball superstar Albert Pujols, who could not even foul off any of her pitches. At a later date, she did the same thing to Barry Bonds (Epstein, 2013). How could two of the greatest hitters in major league history, who regularly ripped 95-mile-per-hour (153 kilometers per hour) baseballs out of ballparks, fail to even make contact with the 68-mile-per-hour (109 kilometers per hour) softball pitches thrown by Finch?

Matthew Syed, an internationally recognized table tennis player and author of *Bounce* (2010), once asked Michael Stich, a former Wimbledon tennis champion, to serve him some tennis balls at his maximum pace. Stich had been clocked at 135 miles per hour (217 kilometers per hour) on his serve when regularly competing. It was a tall order to respond to such speed, but Syed had honed his table tennis skills at a young age and demonstrated exceptional reactions in returning table tennis serves and smashes against top international competitors. Surely, responding to a tennis ball would be similar to responding to a table tennis ball. Not even close. Syed admits that he could barely see the balls served to him by Stich and had no chance in returning them. How could this be?

The answer to both examples has to do with the ways in which athletes develop "software" in their brains that guide them in achieving expert performance (Epstein, 2013; Williams & Ward, 2003). The software that athletes develop through practice and experience is very skill specific. The typical time it takes a major league fastball to travel from the pitcher's hand to the plate is 400 milliseconds. Due to the time needed for initiating the swing, the batter decides whether and where to swing shortly after the ball leaves the pitcher's hand (Takeuchi & Inomata, 2009). This is a learned skill, not a reaction-time skill, which is why Pujols and Bonds could not hit Finch. Top tennis players look at the trunk and hips of the opponent serving the ball, picking up advance visual cues about where the ball will go. Syed had exceptional reaction speed in table tennis, but he did not possess the learned ability to use the visual cues and tracking specifically needed for tennis.

Human software, developed from extensive training, differentiates experts from nonexperts (Janelle & Hillman, 2003). This is different from the innate "hardware" component of general reaction time, which is typically no different between experts and nonexperts. A famous chess study conducted by a Nobel Prize winner demonstrated another type of software expertise (Chase & Simon, 1973). Grandmasters were able to reproduce the positioning of chess pieces, viewed as part of a typical competitive game arrangement, on a blank board after a few seconds of observation much more accurately than less skilled players. However, when the pieces were placed in a random arrangement that would never occur in a chess game, the recall advantage of the grandmasters completed disappeared. The expert grandmasters didn't have the hardware advantage of photographic memory. Rather, they were able to zero in on critical visual information and chunk it together for easier recall based on their vast experience in studying chessboards.

Expert athletes' software includes the ability to retain, recall, and recognize more information in structured game situations, better game knowledge of "how things work," and the use of advanced visual cues (knowing how and where to look) as compared to less experienced athletes (Helsen & Starkes, 1999). In our university classes, we like to show a YouTube segment that illustrates expert athletic software in action. In the segment, Portuguese professional soccer star Cristiano Ronaldo is shown repeatedly scoring from in front of the goal upon receiving a corner kick. The catch is that at the moment the ball is kicked from the corner, the experimenters turn out the lights, so that Ronaldo must play the ball without seeing it. Ronaldo's incredible ability to track, intercept, and score a ball in complete darkness is the result of his finely honed soccer software, acquired through years of training and experience.

Importance of Innate Characteristics

Do these fascinating athletic software examples mean that human hardware is not a factor at all in sport expertise? Of course not. Most prominent researchers agree that expertise is a function of both biologically endowed characteristics as well as environmental (e.g., training) influences (Davids & Baker, 2007; Gagne, 2009; Simonton, 1999).

Many examples of innate qualities that influence expertise in sport are provided in the book *The Sports Gene* (Epstein, 2013). One example is the enhanced visual acuity observed in expert baseball and softball players (on average 20/13 for all players, but 20/11 for major league position baseball players and 2008 Olympic softball players, as compared to normal vision of 20/20)[7] (Laby, Kirschen, & Pantall, 2011; Laby et al., 1996). Of course, this doesn't mean that all elite athletes, even all elite baseball and softball players, have exceptional vision. But it does indicate that

---

[7] Some research has shown that younger people, on average, have better than the standard 20/20 vision. Because elite baseball and softball players are typically young, that could affect the research findings. However, the visual acuity observed in athletes in these studies was beyond the typical vision advantage found in the studies of young people.

superior vision is helpful in picking up the anticipatory cues in these sports, making reaction speed less important.

Another example is the differences in physical trainability based on athletes' aerobic capacities and muscle fiber type composition. About half of individuals' abilities to improve their aerobic capacity with training is determined by their genetic makeup (Bouchard et al., 2010). So athletes can be categorized as low or high responders to aerobic training, and as one sport scientist puts it, "Unfortunately for the low responders in these studies, the predetermined (genetic) alphabet soup just may not spell 'runner'" (Bamman, 2010, p. 1452). And as discussed in chapter 9, the muscle fiber type distributions in athletes certainly influence their trainability. Distance athletes are advantaged when they possess a larger proportion of slow-twitch (type 1) fibers, which are facilitative to aerobic performance (Fink, Costill, & Pollack, 1977). Conversely, sprinters are advantaged when they possess a greater proportion of fast-twitch fibers. Training can enhance the capacity of both types of fibers (making fast-twitch more enduring and slow-twitch stronger), but it cannot make sprinters out of distance runners.

Consider the ways in which foot size (swimming), shoulder width (weightlifting), and length of legs (high jump) serve to influence the training and performance of athletes. All of the examples illustrate the key point about expertise made by Epstein (2013): "While physical hardware alone—like visual acuity—is as useless as a laptop with an operating system but no programs, innate traits have value in determining who will have a better computer once the sport-specific software is downloaded" (p. 44). Children born with some natural advantages in a specific sport type may be more committed to practice in that sport because it may be more enjoyable and internally reinforcing for them than it is for those children with less innate talent.

This effect, the **multiplier effect,** characterizes how a small initial biological advantage for a specific sport activity can interact with training to produce a larger effect for those athletes with this advantage (Ceci, Barnett, & Kanaya, 2003).[8] Young athletes who train extensively and have the biology suited for this training will certainly enjoy larger benefits from the training compared to athletes whose biology is less suited for a specific sport. To put this more simply, innate hardware $\times$ learned software = expertise. The more favorable the genetic predisposition to an activity, the more likely it is that dedicated practice will result in expertise (Singer & Janelle, 1999).

Some have begun to explore the idea of gene testing to predict a child's potential to become an elite athlete in a certain type of sport. Atlas Sport Genetics of Boulder, Colorado, offers genetic testing for young children for $169 to show "where their genetic advantage lies." The noninvasive technique requires only a cheek swab, no scary blood or muscle biopsy tests. The test assesses a gene called alpha-actinin-3 (ACTN3), which produces a skeletal muscle protein thought to influence two types of athletic ability: explosive power and endurance. From the test, the company tells parents if their child is more suited for endurance events, sprint–power events, or a combination of the two. However, using genetic tests to predict athletic potential is still very premature and does not reflect the complexity of genetic influences on athletic performance (Baker, 2012). Parents and coaches are advised to use typical physical assessments to ascertain if young athletes are more suited for speed versus endurance events, as this is easily inferred from observation. All the ACTN3 test can tell us at this point is who will not be competing in the next Olympic 100-meter final (Epstein, 2013), and that's almost all of us.

---

[8] The term *multiplier effect* is also used to more broadly describe any two factors that can work together to produce a larger advantage (e.g., deliberate practice and motivation).

WHAT IS THE BEST WAY TO DEVELOP SPORT TALENT?

Certainly, youth athletes' development of skills and expertise is influenced by their biological makeup. However, the influence of environment (amount and type of practice, coaches, parents, opportunity) is typically viewed as the most important factor in skill and expertise development. Therefore, it's important to turn our attention to what we know about the best ways to pursue sport expertise development in children.

How Deliberate Does Practice Need to Be?

Ideas about the length and type of training to build sport expertise should not be held to rigid standards such as 10 years or 10,000 hours of grueling and unenjoyable practice, and starting kids as early as possible. An inflexible deliberate practice and early technical training approach by practitioners is not appropriate for, and is even harmful to, young athletes.

Research with athletes has shown that expert (international) soccer and field hockey players accumulated hours of practice close to the 10,000 hours prescription (Helsen et al., 2000; Helsen, Starkes, & Hodges, 1998), which was higher than the accumulated hours of less accomplished (national and provincial) athletes. World-class triathletes and gymnasts accumulated over 10,000 hours to reach their elite levels, while less accomplished athletes in their sports trained less (Baker, Cote, & Deakin, 2005; Law, Cote, & Ericsson, 2007). However, other research showed that experts in several team sports (field hockey, ice hockey, netball, basketball) had accumulated between 3,000 and 6,000 hours of practice (Baker et al., 2003; Bruce, Farrow, & Raynor, 2013; Soberlak & Cote, 2003), well short of the 10,000 hours prescription. (These findings indicate only a relationship between practice hours and expertise; they do not lead to a definitive conclusion that practice causes expertise.)

Newer sports, or those with fewer competitors, may provide the opportunity for athletes to reach elite status with fewer hours of training. Australia created a specific talent identification program and immersed 10 athletes in intensive training for skeleton, a winter ice sliding sport that was reintroduced in the 2002 Olympic Games after a 54-year absence, as an attempt to fast-track them for international competition (Bullock et al., 2009). After 14 months of training and approximately 100 hours of sport-specific training, one of the athletes placed 13th in the 2006 Olympic Games. Of course, such a brief training period would not work for most sports, but the example shows that one size doesn't fit all when it comes to training for expertise. In this case, Australia used the concept of *talent transfer* to identify adult high-performance athletes with talent characteristics thought to transfer favorably to the skeleton event.

Conversely, the more complex the sport, the more crucial early practice is. Examples of sports involving greater complexity (e.g., highly developed muscle control and coordination, specific perceptual tracking) include gymnastics, baseball (hitting), ice hockey, and tennis. Sports that technically are not as complex, such as running, cycling, rowing, and kayaking, do not require earlier entry. For example, a sample of elite wrestlers began their sport at age 13, relatively later than for other youth sports but common for this sport (Hodges & Starkes, 1996). Track athletes admitted that they didn't engage in a lot of technical practice until later in their development, and instead relied on their "natural" talent and physical attributes to succeed in their early participation (Mac-Namara, Button, & Collins, 2010b).

Another aspect of deliberate practice in sport that varies from Ericsson and colleagues' (1993) original finding is that athletes generally report that they enjoy their training (Gulbin et al., 2010; Helsen et al., 1998, 2000). Indeed, enjoyment has been shown to be the strongest predictor of sport commitment among youth athletes (Scanlan, Carpenter, Schmidt, Simons, & Keeler, 1993). Here's how several former tennis champions remember their feelings about practice:

Monica Seles: "I just loved to practice and drill and all that stuff."

Serena Williams: "It felt like a blessing to practice because we had such fun."

Chris Evert: "When I woke in the morning, I couldn't wait to hit the courts to work on my game."

The goal of developing expertise is sorely misunderstood by many youth sport coaches, who equate joyless drilling and mind-numbing tactical training with effective coaching.

We're not saying that dedicated training, including effortful deliberate practice, isn't necessary to become a sport expert. It is. As my (first author) father liked to tell me, "There's no shortcut to anywhere worth going." We are saying that there is variability in approaches to developing expertise in sport, and there is not one formulaic prescription for everyone to follow. And significantly, sport research informs us that grueling, unenjoyable training is not what started elite athletes on their paths to expertise.

What Developmental Pathways Should Be Followed in Talent Development?

So what paths should young athletes follow in their quest to develop their athletic talent? Several development studies provide us with some insights as to how successful athletes developed their talent on the way to elite status. In addition, the long-term athlete development (LTAD) model (discussed in chapter 5) serves as a useful framework to guide the talent development of young athletes.

Bloom's Study of Expert Performers

Benjamin Bloom (1985) conducted a four-year longitudinal study on the development of expertise in 120 talented athletes, artists,

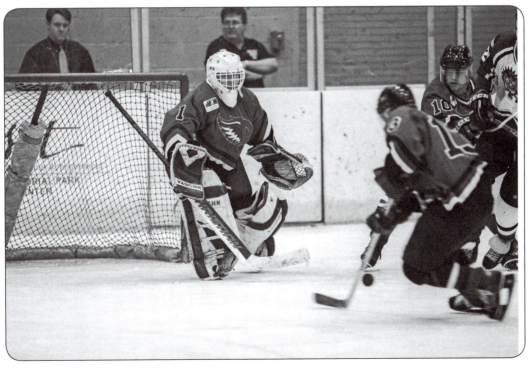

The more complex the sport, the more crucial is early practice.

musicians, and scientists. He found that talent development required years of commitment to learning, and that the amount and quality of support and instruction from teachers, coaches, and parents were critical to this process.

As shown in table 10.3, Bloom identified three stages of talent development and provided important insights into how the participants became experts. We like to think of the initiation stage as the "romance" phase, in which kids fall in love with the sport. The second development stage is when the kids become athletes; this technical training stage is characterized by a big increase in commitment and practice time. In the perfection, or expert, stage, the lives of Bloom's participants were dominated by their activities. Notice the changing role of parents and coaches across the stages, as well as the change in participant goals from fun to technique to high-level skill refinement. Another important finding was that coaches developed strong interpersonal connections with the performers during the first two stages of the process. And perhaps most importantly, the performers needed to fall in love with their activities (the romance stage) before committing to the technical training demands of the next stage.

Bloom's study emphasized that although the amount of time spent was crucial in developing expertise, it was not sufficient to ensure high levels of performance. Therefore, simply focusing on a number of hours or number of years of technical training does not automatically lead to expertise. As Bloom states, what learners do, how they do it, and how they feel about it are more important than absolute time spent on an activity.

Cote's Three Stages of Sport Participation

Jean Cote extended Bloom's original work to study expert athletes across a variety of sports (Cote, 1999; Cote, Baker, & Abernathy, 2003). Based on his research findings, Cote specified three stages of sport participation leading to expert status: sampling (6-12), specializing (13-15), and investment (15+) years. The characteristics associated with each stage are shown in table 10.4. Like Bloom (1985), Cote found that expert athletes didn't start off training intensely with high levels of deliberate practice. On the contrary, their entry or sampling years involved having fun in the sport, and this is critical in developing the love for one's sport, which enables athletes to later engage in dedicated deliberate practice. If that love isn't developed, athletes typically burn out or choose to drop out when the training intensity increases during the specializing years.

Also notice in table 10.4 that the sampling years involve what they sound like: sampling

Table 10.3 Conclusions From Bloom's (1985) Study on Talent Development in Experts

Initiation (romance) stage	Development stage	Perfection (expert) stage
Engaged in fun and playful activities	Became hooked on activity; identified selves as [gymnasts], not kids doing [gymnastics]	Became experts; emphasis now on development of extremely high-level skills
Focus on process-effort, not outcomes	Significant increase in practice time and increased focus on achievement and technique	Were radically obsessed by their sport, which dominated their lives at this point
Parents responsible for stimulating or nurturing interest in the activity or both	Coaches more technically skilled and took strong personal interest in children	Shift in responsibility for training and competition from coaches to athletes; athletes had to be autonomous and extremely knowledgeable
Coaches not technically advanced, but warmly supportive	Significant increase in practice time and required sacrifices by athletes and parents	Parents played lesser role at this stage

Table 10.4 Developmental Stages of Talent Development in Sport and Characteristics of Each Stage

	Sampling years (6-12)	Specializing years (13-15)	Investment years (15+)
Objectives	Fun and excitement; tried new things	Skill development but enjoyment and excitement still important	Skill development, elite performance, advanced strategy and tactics
Focus	Sampled a variety of activities, including sports	One or two sports (decreased involvement in others)	Achieving elite performance in a single activity
Parental involvement	Parents initially got children involved; provided opportunity for multiple activities; parents valued sport but focused on enjoyment for children	Parents emphasized school and sport achievement; strong financial and time commitment to their child; growing interest in child's sport	Parents as invested as athlete; athlete's sport involvement central to family activities; parents' emotional support critical due to difficulty of goals
Coach characteristics	Warm and supportive; good with young children; emphasized enjoyment and basic skill development	Coaches more technically advanced in sport knowledge and "serious" about practice and training	Sport specialist; advanced coaching and training at highest level of intensity

Based on Cote 1999; Cote, Baker, and Abernathy 2003.

a lot of activities. As stated earlier in the book, childhood should be a smorgasbord, not a feeding tube. Expert athletes are often involved in multiple activities from age 5 to 12, but then demonstrate a rapid decrease in number of activities from age 13 onward as they enter the specializing years and prioritize their time (Baker et al., 2003; MacNamara, Button, & Collins, 2010b; Soberlak & Cote, 2003).

Parents' roles changed across stages (discussed more in chapter 15), and particularly critical was the emotional and financial support for athletes as they pushed into the investment years. The roles of coaches also changed across stages. It was important for coaches to be warmly supportive and "good with children" during the sampling years. Later, in the specializing and investment years, coaches' technical knowledge became most important. These findings were supported by a large sample of Australian elite athletes who ranked "the ability to motivate and encourage" as the most important attribute of coaches during their basic junior years in sport, while "detailed knowledge of the sport" was noted as the most important coach characteristic at higher levels of competition (Gulbin et al., 2010).

The Long-Term Athlete Development Model

The LTAD is described in chapter 5 as a developmentally appropriate and systematic progression of activities for individuals to follow to optimize skill development and physical literacy (Balyi, Way, & Higgs, 2013). The first six stages of this model prescribe a pathway for young athletes to follow to develop their talent, culminating in the Train to Win stage, in which elite athletes with identified talent can pursue intense training suitable for international competition. However, as described in chapter 5, the early phases of this model emphasize developing a wide variety of motor skills, development over competition, and the discouragement of early specialization.

Summary of Developmental Pathways to Sport Expertise

The stage models of Bloom and Cote provide generalized age ranges that help us understand how kids progress from entry to expertise in sport. Similarly, the LTAD model provides a developmentally appropriate progression to help adults guide talented athletes to elite status. However, it would be an oversimplification to assume that all children follow exact, predetermined pathways in their development of expertise. There are many individual and cultural differences in the development of sport talent.

Alternatives to Deliberate Practice: Deliberate Play and Spontaneous Practice

As discussed previously, deliberate practice is important to develop sport talent. Yet, there is a lot of variation in exactly how much practice is required to achieve expertise for certain individuals in certain types of sport. But there's even more variation than that.

Deliberate Play

If practice can be deliberate, can't play be deliberate as well? The term **deliberate play** refers to informal sports or games that kids engage in for enjoyment but that contribute to skill development (Cote, Erickson, & Abernathy, 2013). These games are usually athlete directed, although adults may also be involved in the activity, and rules and guidelines are adapted for the specific situation or venue. Examples of deliberate play are the informal games of street hockey, backyard soccer, family softball, and pickup basketball, soccer, or football.

Many talented children who went on to become elite athletes spent more time in their sampling years engaged in deliberate play than deliberate practice (Berry, Abernathy, & Cote, 2008; Soberlak & Cote, 2003). In Brazilian football (soccer), *pelada* is the cultural term used to refer to soccer played with adapted norms and rules and played on streets, beaches, town squares, or dirt fields (Araujo et al., 2010). Here is how its role is described in the development of Brazilian soccer talent: "It is rare to see young players busy practicing isolated technical or tactical drills in an explicit way. [In pelada], learning occurs implicitly within the competitive

form of the street game, where children can learn from their mistakes, unaware of the technical, tactical, psychological, and physiological abilities they are developing through their less formalized scrimmages" (Araujo et al., 2010, p. 170). Brazilian soccer icon Socrates, recognized by the Fédération Internationale de Football Association (FIFA) as one of the top 125 soccer players in international soccer history, explains: "We started playing football on the streets with an avocado seed. . . . When you play in an orchard, with irregular surfaces and surrounded by trees, [you develop] a bunch of abilities to prevent injuries (Araujo et al., 2010, p. 170).

Freddie Adu, who was drafted into Major League Soccer at age 14, spent his early years engaged in deliberate play in Ghana before coming to the United States. He credits his expertise development to his skill development during play in Ghana, stating, "It's too structured in the U.S. You're telling kids to do one, two touches, and pass—when they get older, they can't learn the game. Plus, it's just boring" (Farrey, 2008, p. 103).

The game of futsal is a small-sided (five players a side) indoor version of soccer played on a hard surface, without the hockey rink-style walls used in U.S. indoor soccer facilities. The game of futsal has no goalkeepers, and uses a smaller and heavier ball with less bounce to allow for more control. Because of the frequency of touches and the close quarters inherent to the game, the popularity of futsal in Spain, Brazil, and Argentina has been identified as a reason for the technical superiority of soccer players from those countries. United States soccer officials have urged more of an emphasis on playing futsal for fun as part of youth development in hopes of improving the skills of American soccer players from a young age.

Spontaneous Practice

Most athletes, certainly most elite athletes, remember a childhood that included time spent practicing the sport they loved, for fun.

Children engage in **spontaneous practice** in their free time for skill development and enjoyment, with no adult-specified activities or supervision (Cote et al., 2013). This is in contrast to deliberate practice, but it is an important part of talent development. Sidney Crosby spent hours honing his skills by shooting pucks at the dryer in the family basement. Former Brazilian soccer star Zico, ranked 14th all-timer in the world by FIFA, describes his spontaneous practice: "I used to spend my whole day with the ball. Sometimes I made little sock-balls and sometimes I played with those rubber balls. I threw it at the wall and tried to master the ball alone in my room (Araujo et al., 2010, p. 170).

Deliberate practice, with focused attention on refining skills and technique under the guidance of coaches, is an important part of expertise development in sport. However, there are other methods that are just as important, particularly early in an athlete's career. Deliberate play and spontaneous practice are activities that kids should definitely engage in during the sampling years to enjoy the activity and experiment with their own personal skill development.

What Do Successful Talent Development Programs Look Like?

In chapter 1, you learned about the IMG Academy in Bradenton, Florida, as a sport academy site for youth sport talent development. Systematic research has begun to study such academies, called athletic talent development environments (ATDEs), to learn the most effective ways to develop talent in young athletes in these environments (e.g., Henriksen, Larsen, & Christensen, 2014; Henriksen et al., 2011; Li, Wang, & Pyun, 2014). The successful ATDEs, mostly studied in Scandinavian countries, had several common features.

First, they were structured as a strongly integrated and mutually supportive culture in which sport, school, family, and other demands were coordinated in an efficient way. This way, athletes didn't feel trapped and pressured between competing demands for their focus and time. Second, all athletes were included in one overall training program, with supportive relationships, despite differences in performance levels. The younger athletes learned how to train and compete from the modeling by the older athletes: "The relationship between the prospects and elite athletes is immensely important. The athletes learn training, culture, technique, everything. I call it osmosis because knowledge simply diffuses" (Henriksen et al., 2011, p. 349).

Third, there was a singular focus on long-term development rather than on short-term success. (Less successful programs constantly measured athletes' current performance levels and placed too much emphasis on short-term results.) Daily training was competitive, and winners were recognized in each day's session. However, the focus was on the process of winning as explained by a program director: "Our goal is to be world best, and it's true we applaud good results. But when a result comes, we help the athletes ask themselves why the result came at this moment. What were the steps that led up to the result? We try to teach a mastery focus; a focus on the skills and qualities needed to develop in daily training rather than a focus only on results. But we do this because we firmly believe this approach yields results" (Henriksen et al., 2011, p. 355).

Fourth, diversification was applauded and even recommended. This is surprising to those of us who envision athletes going off to a training academy to pursue excellence in one sport. But these successful programs reaped the benefits of athletes participating in sports other than their signature sport, and even integrated different sport training in their daily routines. The philosophy of these programs was that a diverse sport profile is beneficial to elite performance. Athletes tended to specialize late and to compete in other sports in the off-season.

So we're starting to learn some strategies that work best in developing athletic talent, particularly in ATDEs, or special talent development academies. Coaches and youth sport leaders may want to check out their own particular program culture to assess how effective it is in relation to preferred characteristics of talent development programs (see the Clipboard).

What It Takes to Get to the TOP in Sport

From what we've learned about how sport expertise is developed, let's boil it down to three essential elements necessary to become an elite athlete. We believe athletes need three things to get to the TOP in sport: talent, opportunity, and passion. As shown in figure 10.2, talent, opportunity, and passion all interact to create a fiery synergy whereby expertise development occurs.

Talent

Of course it begins with talent, meaning that the athlete has the necessary qualities to achieve success in a particular sport. However, this is still in the form of raw potential and isn't enough by itself to achieve sport expertise.

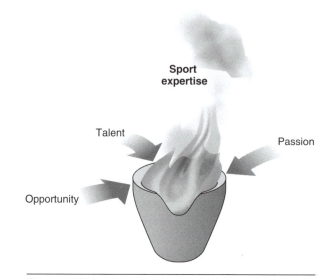

Figure 10.2 Three essential elements needed to achieve sport expertise (TOP).

Opportunity

Opportunity occurs when athletes spend their developmental years in a culture or environment where their skill is nurtured, often without their even realizing it. Opportunity doesn't mean that elaborate facilities are required. Some of the most enriching talent development environments in the world are the poorest in terms of equipment and facilities. Examples include the Spartak Tennis Club in Moscow, described in chapter 5 and the Brazilian soccer culture

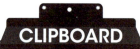

CLIPBOARD

How's Your Talent Development Culture?

An excerpt from the Talent Development Environment Questionnaire for Sport (Martindale et al., 2010), provided in appendix H, can be used to assess athletes' perceptions of the talent development environment in which they are participating. The questionnaire was developed for use with teenage athletes who are in programs designed to develop talent and pursue expertise. If you'd like to use the questionnaire with athletes, ask them to complete it anonymously, and then use their feedback to assess various aspects of the talent development environment in your program. For research or more formal evaluations, you should use the complete version of the TDEQ, available in the article by Martindale and colleagues (2010).

of *pelada* mentioned previously in this chapter. Serena and Venus Williams began their world-class tennis careers being taught by their father on the uneven, pitted courts of Compton, California.

In Kenya and Ethiopia, hotbeds for developing distance-running talent, children routinely run to school, and runners are revered in the same way that American basketball and football heroes are. Ethiopian distance runner Haile Gebrselassie, winner of eight world championships, two Olympic gold medals, and 25 world records, grew up in poverty but ran 10 kilometers to school every morning and 10 kilometers home every evening—at high altitude. The MVP Track Club of Jamaica, whose members have set world records and won Olympic medals in multiple sprint events, has a grass field for its training facility (Ankersen, 2012).

We do realize that many young athletes are denied opportunities to develop their sport talent. Their families may lack the financial resources, may be unable to commit to the time and travel required for many modern youth sports, or may live in areas without the facilities needed to train for a particular sport. Sports like golf and ice hockey require access to specific types of facilities and equipment, and some children live in blighted urban areas without access to safe areas to play and train.

Often, opportunity occurs by luck or just the right blend of circumstances. Matthew Syed (2010) attributes his international table tennis talent to the following: the table his parents bought when he was 8, a brother comparable in age whom he played with daily, and a teacher at his school who happened to be a national table tennis coach and who sponsored a table tennis club open 24 hours a day to kids who were members. There are many stories of expert athletes who grew up in a culture than enabled them to take full advantage of their potential. But . . . are talent and opportunity enough? We think not, because the potentially talented athlete has to seize the opportunity and apply his own efforts to maximize the opportunity. That requires passion.

Passion

Wayne Gretzky has said, "Maybe it wasn't talent the Lord gave me, maybe it was the passion." The fiery crucible of expertise development in sport (figure 10.2) requires the third essential element of passion to ignite talent and opportunity. **Passion** is the deep love of an activity that spurs athletes to invest time and energy in it and leads to the activity's becoming internalized into their identity (Vallerand et al., 2008). Passion provides the devoted, fervent energy to engage in deliberate practice and to persist when faced with daunting obstacles in the pursuit of sport expertise. Research supports passion as a precursor to deliberate practice and elite status in sport (Gulbin et al., 2010; Vallerand et al., 2008). A study of child prodigies found that they possessed a "rage to master," with their chosen activity becoming more important than anything else in their lives (Winner, 1996, as cited in Horton, 2012). Most people agree that such a deep-seated obsession with an activity comes from within, and is impossible to instill in an athlete.

SPECIALIZATION IN YOUTH SPORT

We've already learned that expert athletes tend to participate in many sports and activities, emphasizing deliberate play and enjoyment, until age 12. Generally, they begin to specialize, or narrow their focus, in one favored sport around age 13. So we know that early specialization is not required for expertise in most sports. However, many parents and coaches believe that there are still advantages to early sport specialization, so why not do it? And if athletes should specialize in their teen years, what does that mean? Should they drop out of all activities and do one sport to the exclusion of all other activities? How narrowly should they specialize? And, just because elite athletes have been shown to specialize in their teen years, does that mean that all youth athletes should follow that pathway?

Specialization, Diversification, and Overspecialization

Specialization involves an investment in a single sport through systematic training and competition, typically including year-round participation in that sport, to pursue proficiency and enjoyment in a signature activity. The opposite of specialization is **diversification,** which is an investment in a broad range of sports and activities. Although we tend to view specialization and diversification dualistically, as categorical opposites, in reality they are on a continuum representing the degree to which athletes specialize or diversify (see figure 10.3).

Degrees of Sport Specialization

Our daughter sampled soccer, tae kwon do, basketball, volleyball, and track (athletics) before age 14, at which time she chose to focus solely on volleyball. She participated in a fall school season, a spring club season, a summer camp season, and off-season conditioning in volleyball throughout high school. However, she also participated in the steel drum band, art club, and Academic Challenge team. So, you could say she

"specialized" in volleyball, but she chose to participate in other activities. Some youth athletes have a signature sport that is their favorite, which they engage in year-round (often achieving awards and opportunities for higher-level participation) while also engaging in other sports in the off-season for enjoyment and cross-training.

So our definition of specialization emphasizes a narrowing of focus and main emphasis on one sport as a signature activity, with the possible continuation of some complementary or secondary activities. Research has shown that elite athletes narrowed their number of activities to focus on their main sport in the specializing years but remained involved in a couple of other sporting activities for relaxation and cross-training during the off-season (Baker et al., 2003).

However, a growing trend in the United States has been to push for exclusive specialization, in which athletes discontinue all other sports and most other extracurricular activities, to train and compete year-round in one sport. This is often mandated by coaches who, for some unfathomable reason, have the power to cut athletes from their programs unless the athletes agree to quit all other sports and most activities. For example, a high school soccer coach in our area required attendance at a summer-long conditioning program and refused to allow athletes to miss a workout to go on summer vacations (even for a week) with their families.

Exclusive specialization has contributed to the epidemic of overuse injuries emerging in the past two decades by depriving young

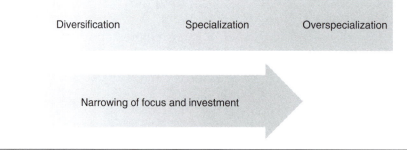

Diversification   Specialization   Overspecialization

Narrowing of focus and investment

Figure 10.3   Specialization continuum.

athletes of the benefits of cross-training and off-season rest. So although specialization is not inherently bad, the narrow ways in which it is interpreted by overzealous coaches have created negative outcomes for youth athletes.

The Problem of Overspecialization

When the exclusivity or intensity of specialization is so great that children suffer adverse mental and physical health effects, it becomes overspecialization. **Overspecialization** occurs when children, often controlled by parents or coaches, pursue expertise and extrinsic rewards in one sport through year-round systematic training and competition, and sacrifice their psychological development and well-being as well as participation in most all other activities typical of kids their age. Unfortunately, examples of overspecialization are common in sport.

The title of former elite gymnast Jennifer Sey's (2008) book says it all: *Chalked Up: Inside Elite Gymnastics' Merciless Coaching, Overzealous Parents, Eating Disorders, and Elusive Olympic Dreams.* Dominique Moceanu was the youngest (age 14) member of the American gymnastics team who won the gold medal in team competition in the 1996 Olympic Games. Her book, *Off Balance* (2012), describes a sickening overspecialization experience of emotional and physical abuse, including the ignoring and ridiculing of injuries. In his autobiography *Open,* Andre Agassi (2009) describes the abuse that he endured from his father as a child: "No one ever asked me if I wanted to play tennis, let alone make it my life. . . . I hate tennis, hate it with all my heart, and still I keep playing because I have no choice. . . . I beg him for a chance to play [soccer with friends]. He shouts at the top of his lungs: 'You're a tennis player! You're going to be number one in the world! You're going to make lots of money. That's the plan, and that's the end of it'" (pp. 27, 33, 57).

Emotional abuse has been documented across many youth sports (Gervis & Dunn, 2004; Kerr & Stirling, 2012; Stirling & Kerr, 2007). This form of abuse includes belittling, humiliation, threats, and denial of attention and support; and it goes beyond the strong communication and external regulation often used by coaches to push athletes in their training. Overspecialization involves adult behavior that crosses the line; the well-being of athletes is superseded by an obsession with attaining extrinsic rewards in sport (e.g., Olympic medals, college scholarships, or simply winning). This is called the **rationalization of sport,** whereby performance becomes more important than the human beings who are producing that performance (Donnelly, 1993). A swimming parent explains, "It was tough to see it [abuse] happening, but . . . once your kid starts winning championships it's easy to forget that she may be damaged along the way" (Kerr & Stirling, 2012, p. 201).

Summary of the Specialization Continuum

Overspecialization is specialization gone amuck, because it sacrifices the most important thing—the well-being of the athlete—for selfish adult motives. It should be avoided at all costs. Whether athletes choose to remain diversified or to specialize once they leave their early sampling years should be up to them.

There are athletes who choose to narrowly specialize in one sport because it is their passion, they enjoy it, and they choose to spend their time focusing on that sport. Professional Golfers' Association (PGA) star Rickie Fowler's mom recalls her son's devotion to golf: "When he was 7, he told me, 'Mom, I don't want to play baseball or do gymnastics anymore. Just golf. I want to be a pro.' And he worked on it every day. He sacrificed his social life. No parties. No vacations. Didn't go to football games. I was a little worried back then. He actually allows

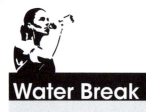

Water Break

The Marinovich Project

The Marinovich Project is a 2011 ESPN film about Todd Marinovich, raised by his father in a highly controlled environment with the goal of shaping Todd into the greatest football quarterback of all time. His father, Marv, stated, "The question I asked myself was, 'How well could a kid develop if you provided him with the perfect environment?'" (Sagar, 2009). Marv put Todd through special stretching and flexibility exercises while he was still in the cradle. Todd ate only fresh-cooked strained vegetables as a baby and continued a special diet throughout his development. On nonschool days, he regularly completed 4-hour workouts, including fitness training, stretching, weightlifting, plyometrics, and throwing drills. He had a stable of scientific specialists honing his physiological, biomechanical, and mental skills throughout his youth.

Marinovich's talent and training led him to huge success in high school, where in 1987 he amassed a national-record 9,194 passing yards and was the National High School Player of the Year. He chose to play college football at the University of Southern California, and although he was successful, he was suspended from the team multiple times for rules transgressions. He signed with the National Football League Los Angeles Raiders, but was released after two years of professional football. After that, he was arrested for numerous drug violations, and for years he was a full-blown drug addict. *Esquire* referred to him as "the man who never was," stating, "You could say that Todd missed his childhood. Sports took away his first twenty years. Then drugs took the second twenty" (Sagar, 2009).

In the film, Marinovich talks about his personal discomfort with his upbringing, admitting he felt like a "freak show." In reflecting back about when he won the starting quarterback job with the Raiders, he stated, "I'd done what I wanted to do, [which was] please the old man. I'd accomplished all I wanted, and I was done." He admits that his drug use was an escape from the intensity of his overspecialized world. It is not our intent to denigrate Todd Marinovich, but rather to use his story as an example of the perils of overspecialization.

himself a little bit more fun now. But either way, he loved it" (Diaz, 2014, p. 108). Earlier in the book, we offered similar stories about Rory McIlroy, Tiger Woods, Sidney Crosby, Serena Williams, and Chris Evert. Clearly, there are athletes who choose to specialize early because the sport is their passion. But the problem is that many adults see these examples and assume that early, exclusive specialization is the pathway for all kids to take. We forget that the passion and commitment must be inside of the young athletes, and the choice to specialize and train to the exclusion of most other pursuits is theirs.

Many teenagers choose to remain diverse and participate in many sports and activities. It's really an individual preference for the vast majority of youth sport participants who are not interested in pursuing expertise or elite status in sport. We have noticed that because the performance levels of youth sport continue to improve, it's getting more difficult to make high school sport teams. So some specialized commitment and focus on a sport may be necessary to continue participation at the high school or selective club levels. Athletes should decide for themselves whether and how much to specialize, with guidance and support (not mandates) from parents and coaches.

Merits of Early Diversification

The next issue to address is when, or how early, athletes should specialize in a sport. Most sport scientists and professional organizations advocate early (12 years and under) diversification as opposed to early specialization in sport (e.g., American Academy of Pediatrics, 2000; National Association for Sport and Physical Education, 2010). In this section, we've identified several reasons why early diversification is a good idea for most children.

• **Children can diversify early and still attain elite athlete status in most sports as an adult.** As discussed previously in the chapter, elite athletes in a variety of sports have achieved elite sport status after engaging in early diversification (or sampling) in their childhood years (typically until around age 12) (Baker et al., 2003; Gulbin et al., 2010; MacNamara et al., 2010b; Soberlak & Cote, 2003). A study of over 4,000 Olympic athletes found that the average starting age in their chosen sports was 11.5 years (Gullich, 2007, as cited in Vaeyens et al., 2009). Overall, specialized training at an early age was not a prerequisite for reaching elite levels across a range of Olympic sports. A study of 708 minor league professional baseball players showed that although their mean starting age was 6 years, the players' mean age of specializing in baseball was 15 years (Ginsburg et al., 2014). The majority of players (52%) did not specialize until at least 17 years of age. Most sports, like the ones in these studies, are considered late-specialization sports, in which exclusive specialization and extensive deliberate practice are not necessary before age 12.

On the other hand, gymnastics and figure skating have been designated early-specialization sports (Balyi et al., 2013; Vaeyens et al., 2009), in which elite levels of performance are achieved before puberty. Gymnastics and figure skating are subjectively judged, with performance expectations calling for smaller, lighter, more flexible bodies to execute the difficult skills required at the elite level. Thus, it is typical for gymnasts and skaters who aspire to attain elite status to begin extensive technical training very early, and there is evidence that expert athletes specialized earlier than nonexpert athletes in these sports (O'Connor, 2011). Former Olympian Dominique Moceanu began gymnastics at age 3, and by age 7 she was training six days a week for at least 25 hours per week.

Overall, research supports early diversification as facilitative to athletes' development in most sports. Kids can start their favorite sports early and also participate in other sports and activities. Early diversification doesn't mean that a young athlete can't spend a significant amount of time doing the sport he likes best. We would just recommend that early experiences in the late-specialization sports include a lot of deliberate play and spontaneous practice, as opposed to excessive levels of highly technical deliberate practice.

• **Early diversification develops a broad range of fundamental motor skills and different sport experiences that provide the athlete with more performance options and athleticism if they choose to specialize in one sport later.** A youth baseball academy coach discusses highly specialized athletes who can perform the mechanics of their sport but lack well-rounded motor skills: "My God, this kid is a horrible athlete. He can't run. He can't move. He's spent all his time in the batting cage. So many of these kids have played no other sport. They're one-trick ponies" (Sokolove, 2008, p. 204).

David Leadbetter, internationally recognized golf instructor, coaches Charles Howell III, a PGA tour player who has not yet realized the great promise he showed as a junior golfer. Leadbetter says of Howell (whom he has coached from the age of 12): "Charles has had a solid career, but he hasn't hit the heights some thought he might. I have always felt part of his problem is that he played only golf growing up. That hurts him. In other ball games you develop a feel for throwing and distance. But Charles never did that. He doesn't have the instinctive touch or hand–eye coordination you need to hit the ball close [inside 120 yards, or 110 meters]. If only he'd played baseball as a kid. That would have helped his awareness for distance (Huggan, 2013, p. 37).

- **Early specialization has been linked to dropping out of sport.** Ice hockey players who dropped out of their sport began off-ice training at a younger age and invested more hours per year in training at ages 12 and 13 as compared to active players (Wall & Cote, 2007). Both the dropout and active players enjoyed a diverse and playful introduction to sport, but the earlier specialized activities of the dropout players may have affected their motivation to continue in the sport.

A similar pattern was found in swimming (Fraser-Thomas, Cote, & Deakin, 2008a). Adolescent swimmers who dropped out were involved in fewer extracurricular activities and less unstructured swimming play during their early years, and also began more specialized training activities (training camps, dryland training) earlier than active swimmers. So although the starting ages of the dropout and active swimmers did not differ, the earlier specialized focus of the dropouts may have contributed to their discontinuation of swimming. Interestingly, dropout swimmers also reached "top in club" status earlier than active swimmers. The authors suggest that a comedown from child stardom to adolescent mediocrity, with resultant disappointment and decreased confidence, could occur for some kids who specialize and achieve early success.

Because dropping out is a motivational issue, it may be that early exclusive sport specialization does not allow youth athletes to experience the playful enjoyment found to be important to elite athlete development before age 12 (Bloom, 1985; Cote et al., 2003). A premature emphasis on technical training, deliberate practice, and competition may thwart the falling in love with a sport, which has repeatedly been shown to fuel the passion and commitment needed to continue to higher levels of sport.

- **Early specialization has been linked to burning out of sport.** Another negative consequence that has been associated with early sport specialization is burnout. Discussed more fully in chapter 11, burnout occurs when a previously enjoyable activity becomes drudgery, so that athletes feel physically and emotionally exhausted. Adolescent athletes specializing in swimming, diving, and gymnastics were higher in emotional exhaustion (burnout) when compared to more diversified adolescent athletes who participated in a variety of activities (Strachan, Cote, & Deakin, 2009). A sole focus on tennis at a young age has also been linked to burnout (and dropout) in elite tennis players (Gould, Tuffey, Udry, & Loehr, 1996).

- **Early diversification helps kids develop multidimensionality, or multiple pieces in their identity pie.** The development of a multidimensional identity, or self-concept, is important for the mental health and well-being of children. Exclusive specialization at a young age can restrict children to a unidimensional self-concept, which has been linked to burnout and psychological dysfunction (Coakley, 1992). Adolescent athletes who were engaged in other activities (e.g., performing arts, school, church) along with their sport participation have been shown to possess healthier psychological profiles than adolescents who participated only in sport (Zarrett et al., 2008).

A useful activity to do with young athletes is to ask them to draw their personal identity pie, labeling various pieces of the pie to represent who they are. The pie on the left side of figure 10.4 provides a multidimensional example: A young tennis player identifies other personally significant activities or personal strengths that define who she is. The pie on the right side of figure 10.4 might be drawn by another young tennis player; she is narrowly unidimensional and would be vulnerable to major blows to her self-worth and self-concept when encountering obstacles in her pursuit of expertise in tennis. A multidimensional identity is a good insurance policy for kids because it provides them with broad coverage of their sense of self. Help young athletes develop lots of pieces in their pies.

Structural Strategies to Avoid Overspecialization and Exclusive Specialization

To quell the rising tide of professionalization, overspecialization, and exclusive early specialization, policies and regulations should be instituted at the organizational level. "Developmentalizing" should always trump professionalizing when it comes to youth sport. Two examples are provided here, and we encourage you to consider additional ways to protect the interests of young athletes.

• **Continue and expand the practice of implementing minimal age restrictions for athletes to compete in professional or international sport.** The minimal age to compete internationally in gymnastics rose from 14 years before 1981, to 15 years in 1981, to 16 years in 1997 (one is eligible if one achieves the minimal age sometime in the Olympic or competition year). The age restriction is designed to protect child athletes from injury and exploitation, although it remains controversial, often with accusations of age falsification for international events. Professional tennis has a minimum age requirement of 14 years. The National Basketball Association requires draftees to be 19 years and one year removed from high school graduation, while prospects may be drafted right out of high school for Major League Baseball.

These restrictions are important because they have a trickle-down effect on youth sport. When Kevin Garnett signed as the

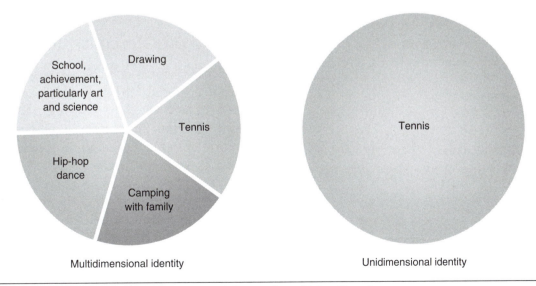

Multidimensional identity   Unidimensional identity

Figure 10.4 Multidimensional versus unidimensional identity pie.

fifth pick in the National Basketball Association draft in 1995 straight out of high school, the search for star players moved down from high school to elementary school (Dohrmann, 2010). It fueled the pressure on kids to play year-round and travel extensively at extremely young ages to compete in national tournaments. For example, the Amateur Athletic Union (AAU) has sponsored a 2nd-grade boys' national championship tournament since 2004. Sport organizations and youth sport leaders should continue to lobby for age restrictions to protect kids from pressure to specialize early and exclusively.

• **No athlete should be restricted from diversification through high school participation.** This recommendation is designed to preserve young athletes' rights to diversify their sport participation through their high school years. Others have recommended 15 years as the cutoff age for protected diversification (Wiersma, 2000), and we agree that this is a logical age cutoff. However, we see no reason that adults should mandate specialization before college when 98% of high school athletes are not going on to play at the collegiate level. Coaches and parents should guide young athletes in making important decisions about multiple sport participation versus more specialized approaches. But this should be discussed on an individual-case basis and should ultimately be the athlete's decision. We urge athletic directors and state and national high school sport associations to develop regulations that prevent coaches from having the power to restrict athletes' activities.

CATEGORIZING SPORTS BASED ON SPECIALIZATION DEMANDS

Previously in the chapter, you learned that the more complex the sport, the more crucial is early practice. More complex sports require highly developed muscle control and coordination, as well as refined visual tracking abilities. Sports that are not as technically complex do not require early entry. By assessing the complexity of various sports, we can categorize them as early- versus late-specialization sports. Different specialization categories have been proposed to help parents and youth sport leaders better understand the optimal or preferred times for young athletes to begin focused training in a particular sport (see figure 10.5, adapted from Balyi et al., 2013).

Early-Specialization Sports

As shown in figure 10.5, early-specialization sports include the acrobatic sports of figure skating, gymnastics, and diving. Early sport-specific training (ages 5 to 7) is needed for elite talent development. Specialization happens at approximately 9 to 13 years of age. Balyi and colleagues (2013) also recommend early specialization for sports that are highly kinesthetic and that require highly precise techniques, such as swimming (8-13 years) and equestrian events (early engagement in riding and then specialization around 14 years). Females typically specialize two years earlier than males in these activities, because of their earlier maturation.

Late-Specialization Sports

All other sports are late-specialization sports, although they can be categorized based on whether they require early engagement, which means that kids get involved in activities related to the given sport at early ages (e.g., younger than 8) (Balyi et al., 2013). Several sports require early engagement (not specialization, but early participation to gain the needed "feel," visual tracking, and decision making). These late specialization–early engagement sports are divided into kinesthetic, team, and visual sports (see figure 10.5).

Early specialization		Late specialization	

1. Acrobatic
   Figure skating
   Gymnastics
   Diving
 	
2. Highly kinesthetic
   Equestrian sports
   Swimming
	3. Early engagement
	  a. Kinesthetic
	     Skiing
	     Snowboarding
	     Luge
	
	  b. Team
	     Ice hockey
	     Basketball
	     Baseball
	     Softball
	     Netball
	     Soccer
	     Field hockey
	
	  c. Visual
	     Tennis
	     Badminton
	     Racquetball
	     Squash
		4. Common late
		   Football
		   Speedskating
		   Wrestling
		   Track and field
		   Canoeing
		   Volleyball
		   Bowling
		   Lacrosse
		   Rugby
		   Karate
		   Judo
		   Weightlifting
		   Boxing
		   Taekwondo
		   Curling
		   Golf
			5. Very late or transfer
			   Bobsled
			   Cycling
			   Rowing
			   Kayaking

Figure 10.5 Examples of early- and late-specialization sports.

Adapted from Balyi, Way, and Higgs 2013.

Kinesthetic sports categorized as late specialization–early engagement, such as skiing, require early engagement to develop feel and balance. Team sports in this category require kinesthetic feel (e.g., for the stick moving and receiving the puck in ice hockey), visual tracking (e.g., tracking the softball to strike and catch it), and complex decision making (as in soccer). Visual sports are those sports that require early engagement–late specialization, such as tennis, where the visual tracking of objects to a handheld implement is very important. Although early engagement (8 or younger) begins to code the brain for these activities, specialization is not necessary until age 14 to 16.

Late-specialization sports that are categorized as common include football, speed skating, track and field, volleyball, and golf (Balyi et al., 2013). "Common" here means that they require specialization at the typical time suggested by research, which is 13 to 16 years of age. Some of these sports do require earlier experiences in visual tracking activities (e.g., lacrosse) as well as eye–hand coordination and balance (e.g., golf). And certainly, there are specialized positions within these sports that may require earlier engagement, such as setting in volleyball.

Very late specialization sports include cycling and kayaking, where the requirements are high amounts of power and a high volume of training (Balyi et al., 2013). These are also known as transfer sports, because athletes can transfer from other sports and perhaps succeed in them.

The authors of this sport-specific categorization system have applied the LTAD model with a multitude of athletes and teams across several years (Balyi et al., 2013). This experience led them to propose these categories of early and late specialization, which is a useful model from which to begin studying the timing of training in relation to achieving elite status in various sports. Obviously, the exact categorization of specific sports is arguable, but the system is a valuable start to understanding specialization across sports.

However, we don't want parents and coaches to look at figure 10.5 and say, "Oh, swimming is an early-specialization sport, so let's get Aaron started at age 5, force him to swim and train year-round, and forbid any other activities." Remember that specialization is generally recommended at ages

13 to 16; and for swimmers, we're talking only about specializing a bit earlier than that age range. A useful feature of the model is the emphasis on early engagement for some sports, a concept that is developmentally appropriate when we think about the sampling of activities and multiple basic sport skills we want all kids to develop. It would be ideal for kids to experience early engagement in activities in all four different environments—that is, on snow or ice (skiing, skating), in the air (gymnastics, diving), in the water (swimming), and on the ground (most sports) (Balyi et al., 2013). If they want to be a baseball player, they should experience multiple activities in which they are visually tracking objects and developing eye–hand coordination, including learning to visually pick up and strike a ball pitched by another person.

The most important point to take away from figure 10.5 is that early specialization in late-specialization sports has a negative impact on the young athlete's development, as discussed previously in the chapter. When children try a number of sports, gain physical literacy, and choose to specialize later in their teens, they increase their chances of excelling (Balyi et al., 2013). Some sports require early involvement so that kids gain a feel for them and the brain-specific coding needed to succeed in these activities. But sampling and diversification early on is generally the best strategy for developing talent in young athletes.

TIPS FOR NURTURING TALENT AND WELL-BEING IN YOUTH ATHLETES

Here are some final tips for nurturing both youth athletes' talent and well-being. This is sometimes a difficult challenge because of the commitment and sacrifices needed to pursue expertise in sport, often by the entire family.

Separate Talent From Identity

A child who shows early talent and performance success in swimming may receive a lot of attention—"Oh, you're Zoe, the swimmer." Parents should help Zoe realize that she is a person who is an excellent swimmer, as well as an outstanding honors student, budding guitarist, and loving big sister and daughter. Swimming is what she does, and maybe what she does best, but it should not solely define who she is. Help talented young athletes add pieces to their identity pie. Swimming might be the biggest piece in Zoe's pie, which is fine, but it's important to include complementary pieces for a multidimensional self-concept. Parents should show interest in all of their children's activities, not just the ones in which they excel or the ones the parents like the best (Tofler & DiGeronimo, 2000).

Have a Plan B (and C and D If Necessary)

For athletes in the specializing and investment years, it's great to pursue a college or elite sport career . . . as long as they have a plan B, or alternative paths to pursue. "I'm going to do as much as I can to build my skills, to try to play in college" is a healthier approach than "Everyone expects me to get a scholarship to play Division I basketball, so I'm feeling a lot of pressure." As you learned in chapter 6, controlling extrinsic rewards, such as scholarships, can destroy the motivation of athletes. It's common for athletes to have important outcome goals (e.g., All-Conference recognition, playing in college), but help them also identify personal performance (e.g., assist-to-turnover ratio, free throw percentage) as well as process (e.g., patience and poise on the press breaker, push and penetrate with the ball in transition) goals on which they can focus. Too much emphasis and pressure on outcome goals and a rigid plan A with no alternatives is a risky, narrow approach to talent development, with possible negative outcomes for kids. Goals are wonderful motivators, but they must be flexible, with alternative paths if a particular goal is not achieved.

Focus on the Process

Sport is about winning, so it's easy to get caught up in early success measured by winning competitive events. But if we're truly interested in talent development, short-term results are not as important as developing the skills and qualities that will lead to success in the future. The director of an elite kayak talent development school explains: "Sport is about winning, but to win you need to be patient and smart. . . . We applaud good results, but we help athletes to ask themselves why the result came. What were the steps that led up to the result? We try to teach a mastery focus; a focus on the skills and qualities needed to develop in daily training rather than a focus only on results. We do this because we firmly believe this approach yields results" (Henriksen et al., 2011, p. 355).

Weigh the Cost of Sacrifice in Terms of Experiential Benefits for Children

Youth athletes sometimes leave home to train full-time at sport academies dedicated to develop talent in specific sports (e.g., Chris Evert Tennis Academy, Bollettieri Tennis Program at IMG Academy). We've read media accounts of the famous athletes who achieved professional sport stardom from these programs, such as Maria Sharapova, Serena and Venus Williams, and Monica Seles. But we don't hear about the many kids who attended full-time sport academies and did not make it to the elite level in their sports. Parents and young athletes who are considering the financial and emotional sacrifices necessary for academy training (or

any type of demanding deliberate practice training for a child) should weigh the costs of such a commitment against the benefits of the experience for the child if he does not advance to the elite level. Ask these questions (Tofler & DiGeronimo, 2000, p. 120):

- Will my child gain something valuable even if she doesn't rise above the rest?
- If my child's dream changes, will this still have been a valuable experience?
- Does the sacrifice bring my child something of value in the present?

Keep Things Family Centered as Opposed to Child Centered

In child-centered families, everyone's needs are subordinated to the star athlete's training and competition schedule. Besides being unfair, this creates pressure on the talented athlete to "pay back" the money, time, and attention in performance attainments. Talented youth athletes can be supported, even to the point of family sacrifices, but making them the center of the household is unhealthy for everyone.

We also observed that the race to engage our kids in multiple youth sport activities led to overscheduling and a frenzied household atmosphere. The sampling years involve trying out multiple activities, but parents should resist the tendency to compete with other parents for how engaged their children are in youth sport. By not overscheduling and by providing downtime at home, you send young athletes the message that it's okay to not be achieving all the time and that family time together is important.

WRAP-UP

We think it's great for kids to have dreams of fame and glory in the sport they love. It's part of childhood to dream big dreams, and these dreams are easily imagined in a world where the expertise of sport heroes is constantly displayed in the popular media. Dreams fuel the passion needed to develop one's talent. And if that talent, or the opportunity to develop it, is not enough to achieve sport expertise, kids typically move on to other dreams and goals. That's how we find the paths that are right for us in the world—most people become experts in something.

Yet, contemporary youth sport seems to have evolved into a frenzied push to develop children's athletic talents, with adults focusing on the prize (college scholarships, Olympic medals) instead of on the children to help them sample activities, learn what they're good at, and find the right paths for themselves. We hear it all the time at youth sport events. Parents of 10-year-olds talk about the athletic scholarship their children will receive or what sport to start their 4-year-old daughter in to give her the best chance of becoming a professional athlete. Of the 7 million high school athletes in the United States, 2% will play college sports. Only 1% of these will get full-ride scholarships to a National Collegiate Athletic Association Division I college athletic program. And a very small percentage of the 1% will become professional or Olympic athletes. These numbers show that the vast majority of youth sport participants who want to learn skills and enjoy sport shouldn't be forced to choose one sport and train for 20 hours a week.

It is we—the adults—who need to keep talent development in youth sport in perspective. Let the kids dream. Left alone, they figure things out pretty well. In a survey of junior (teenage) golfers, 92% believed they would reach the PGA or Ladies Professional Golf Association tours ("Junior Player Survey," 2010). However, 85% said that their talent development in golf was time well spent, even if they didn't make it as a professional. And 71% felt that a college degree was more important than earning their tour card. What a wonderful combination of belief, hope, and perspective! Let's learn from the kids, and let's keep our eyes on them as we help them develop their talent in developmentally appropriate ways.

LEARNING AIDS

Key Terms

deliberate play—Informal sports or games that kids engage in for fun.

deliberate practice—A highly structured activity with the explicit goal to improve performance.

diversification—An investment in a broad range of sports and activities.

expertise—Consistent superior athletic performance over an extended period.

multiplier effect—The ways in which an initial biological advantage for a specific sport activity interacts with training to produce a larger effect for those athletes with this initial advantage.

overspecialization—The process whereby children, often controlled by parents or coaches, pursue expertise and extrinsic rewards in one sport through year-round, systematic training and competition, sacrificing their psychological development and well-being as well as participation in almost all other activities typical of kids their age.

passion—The deep love of an activity that spurs athletes to invest time and energy in it and leads to internalization of the activity into their identity.

performance—The execution of a sport skill or set of skills.

rationalization of sport—A belief that performance is more important than the human beings who are producing that performance.

skill—Proficiency that is acquired through training and experience.

specialization—The investment in a single sport through systematic training and competition, typically including year-round participation in the sport, to pursue proficiency and enjoyment in a signature activity.

spontaneous practice—Athletes' practicing sport activities in their free time for skill development and enjoyment, with no adult-specified activities or supervision.

talent—An innate (inborn) ability or quality identified at an earlier time that can lead to expertise at a future time.

talent development—Providing the most appropriate environment for athletes to stimulate their learning and performance and help them achieve their potential.

talent identification—The process of distinguishing (and usually selecting) children and youth who demonstrate potential for expertise in a particular sport.

Summary Points

1. Talent refers to the qualities identified at an earlier time that can lead to expertise at a future time, so the emphasis is on an individual's potential for success in a particular activity.

2. To become an expert, athletes must possess or acquire expertise in four essential areas: technical, physical, cognitive (tactical knowledge as well as perceptual skills), and psychological.

3. National sport organizations have implemented talent identification and development programs to select and train athletes for international competition.

4. Talent development in sport has used anthropometric measures, maturational status estimates, tests of general physical abilities, sport-specific skill evaluations, perceptual tests, tactical knowledge assessment, game and overall intelligence tests, and psychological inventories.

5. Talent identification is difficult at an early age because of children's maturational differences.

6. Multiple pathways are needed so that all children can develop their individual talents, even those who do not pursue sport expertise.

7. Expert athletes' "software" includes the ability to retain, recall, and recognize more information in structured game situations; better game knowledge of "how things work"; and the use of advanced visual cues (knowing how and where to look) as compared to less experienced athletes.

8. The multiplier effect refers to how a small initial biological advantage for a specific activity can interact with training to produce a larger effect for those athletes with this advantage.

9. A prescription of 10 years or 10,000 hours has been recommended for expertise development, although research with athletes shows variation by sport type and individuals in terms of the amount of training necessary.

10. Bloom's study of experts emphasized that the developmental activities people engaged in at different stages were more important in leading to expertise than the number of hours in practice.

11. Cote specified three stages of expertise development in sport: sampling (6-12), specializing (13-15), and investment (15+) years.

12. To get to the TOP, sport expertise is achieved with talent, opportunity, and passion.

13. How specialized a youth athlete becomes lies on a continuum from diversification to overspecialization.

14. Early diversification is facilitative to athletes' talent and psychosocial development in late-specialization sports.

15. Sports can be designated as early and late specialization based on the need to develop feel, visual tracking skills, advanced technique, and decision-making skills.

Study Questions

1. How is talent different from skill? Why is this an important distinction when one is working with very young athletes?

2. Identify the essential areas that make up sport expertise, and provide examples of each area.

3. Name at least five ways in which talent has been identified in sport, and explain potential problems in identifying talent in youth sport. How can we ensure that all children have opportunities to develop their individual talents?

4. How was the 10,000 hours and 10 years prescription of deliberate practice developed? Explain how these guidelines have stood up in our studies of sport expertise.

5. Provide some examples of the human "software" that is acquired as part of expertise in specific sports. Provide some examples of some innate "hardware" differences in sport, and how this fits into the multiplier effect.

6. Explain the three stages identified by Bloom (1985) in his study of expertise development, and describe some important characteristics of each stage. Do the same for Cote and his specification of the stages of sport expertise.

7. Following the TOP prescription for sport expertise, explain why opportunity doesn't necessarily mean gleaming facilities.

8. Explain the concepts of specialization and diversification, and why they lie on a continuum. What happens to create exclusive specialization and overspecialization in youth sport?

9. Identify and explain five advantages of early diversification (over early specialization) in sport. When would there be an exception to early diversification?

10. Describe the continuum of early- to late-specialization sports, providing some examples and a rationale for early versus late. Explain the need to identify certain sports as late specialization–early engagement sports as compared to those where early engagement is not necessary.

Reflective Learning Activities

1. Choose a collegiate or professional athlete to interview. The purpose of the interview is to learn about the athlete's developmentally based sport experiences as he or she progressed through the various stages of sport participation (Horn & Butt, 2014). The main focus question is, "How did you develop your talent?" Specific information obtained should include (a) the ages at which the athlete began participation and began to specialize in his or her sport, (b) the factors that influenced the athlete's decision to select and continue participation in this sport, (c) the role of significant others (e.g., parents, coaches, siblings, teammates), and (d) positive and negative factors influencing transitions into higher levels of participation. Ask any other questions that you feel are important to understand this athlete's talent development. Write up your findings in a report that describes the athlete's talent development experience in relation to the material presented in this chapter.

2. Consider the accepted cultural practice of emotional, sometimes even physical, abuse by coaches in the talent development of athletes. Either write out or discuss your opinion on this topic with classmates. In particular, consider what would happen if teachers acted in abusive ways (similarly to coaches) toward students, and explain your position on why we allow this to occur with coaches and not teachers. Explain how the rationalization of sport (discussed in the chapter) influences these practices.

Resource Guide

The Marinovich Project, ESPN film.

UK Sport Talent Identification (www.uksport.gov.uk/pages/talent-id). This webpage gives you an example of the resources countries will put forward to identify and develop talented athletes around the world. The website provides multiple links to information about how the United Kingdom works to find talented athletes and about how it looks for keys to find other future talented athletes.

chapter 11

STRESS AND BURNOUT IN YOUTH SPORT

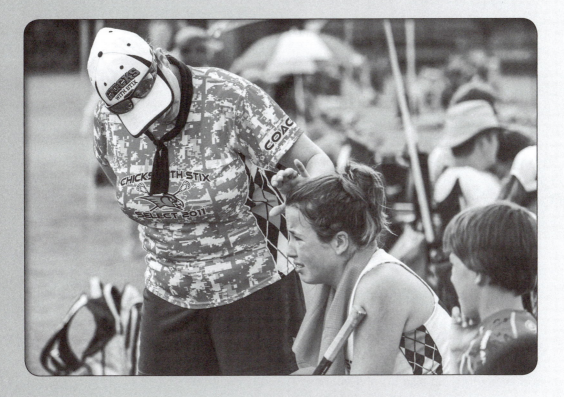

CHAPTER PREVIEW

In this chapter, you'll learn

» how stress can be good as well as bad for kids,

» strategies to prepare kids to manage stress,

» why flow is the ultimate goal of youth sport, and

» why burnout develops in some athletes.

Do you remember the top reasons kids give for playing sport? They play because it's fun and because competition is stimulating and challenging to them. However, the stimulation and challenge of competition often become stressful. In some cases, youth athletes experience burnout and even quit playing the sports that they previously enjoyed. That's a shame, and something that we want to help kids avoid. Our goal in this chapter is to educate you about the process of stress and to offer specific strategies to help kids effectively navigate this process.

Stress is a demand placed on a person, and is a necessary part of life. As you learned in chapter 9, overload (or demand) in physical training is needed to stress athletes' bodies to force them to adapt and grow stronger. But you also learned that progression, variation, and recovery are needed in physical training, and the same is true with stress. Stress without adequate recovery or stress in amounts that are too large is **overstress,** which creates adverse health consequences. However, we all need optimal amounts of stress in our lives to be challenged to develop fully. Although the worry and anxiety that accompany stress are uncomfortable, these feelings impel us to prepare for action. Worry is rehearsal, which focuses the mind on a problem so it can search efficiently for a solution (Goleman, 2005). So stress is useful when applied in the right amounts. But it doesn't always feel good, so an important developmental task is to get used to the feelings associated with stress and to garner the personal and social resources needed to manage stress effectively.

Young developing athletes need small doses of stress over time as "inoculation" that will stimulate the development of resources (antibodies) to deal with higher doses of stress when they're older (Martens, 1978). Living at home with their parents gives young children a chance to learn important life skills before moving out to independently take on life's demands. Youth sports should do the same, by gradually introducing kids to competition (as recommended in chapters 3 and 5), and allowing them to gain competitive experience in small doses that build up the coping skills needed to perform at higher levels of sport.

STRESS AS A PROCESS

Stress occurs as part of the process of competing (Martens, 1975). A youth swimmer goes through a lengthy process of deciding to join a swim team, meeting new teammates, training for competition, dealing with coach and parent expectations, thinking ahead about the upcoming meet, dealing with the jitters and excitement of swimming in the meet, and then experiencing joy and pride in swimming well or disappointment and embarrassment because she didn't swim well. It's a process that affects kids in many ways. Figure 11.1 illustrates the four-stage process of stress (adapted from McGrath, 1970):

1. A demand, or **stressor** (something that causes stress), is presented to the athlete. This could be the physical and psychological demands of competition or training, expectations from parents, or the social demand of having to fit in on a new team.

2. The athlete assesses the demand. Depending on her personality and available resources, she may assess it as an exciting challenge ("I'm fired up and can't wait to do this!") or a scary threat ("I'm stressed out and can't wait until it's over").

3. The athlete responds to the demand (physically, psychologically, and behaviorally). Does she perform well despite her nervousness? Does she accept the butterflies in her stomach as part of competition, or do they cause her to think negatively and choke?

4. What are the outcomes of the process for the athlete? Does she love playing the sport even more or dread having to compete again next time? Does she feel a sense of mastery and accomplishment, or does she think to herself "I'm not sure this is worth it"?

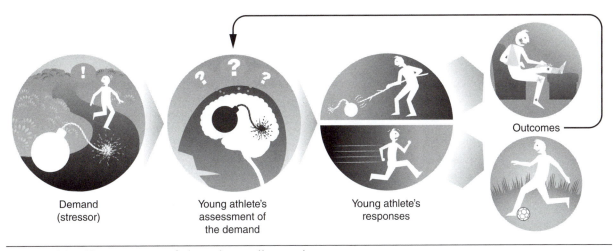

Figure 11.1   The process of stress in youth sport.

As shown in figure 11.1, the outcomes then feed back to influence the ways in which the young athlete assesses the next demand that she faces. So the process is cyclical and continuous. We want the process to be a positive one, or at least a growth experience, in which young athletes learn how to manage the stressors inherent in competition and life. In the following sections, the stages of the stress process are discussed to help you understand how stress occurs and how we can help youth athletes manage stress as they move through the process.

DEMANDS (STRESSORS) FACED BY YOUTH ATHLETES

Athletes face three underlying sources of stress that are inherent in competitive youth sport: social evaluation, importance, and uncertainty.

Social Evaluation

Being socially evaluated by others is what sport is all about, because sport involves public social comparison with opponents (you compete with others to assess your competence), often in front of spectators. Consider how this can be threatening for many kids who have played freely in their backyards without being publicly evaluated and who now must step up to the plate in a tee ball game in front of a crowd of family members, teammates, and opponents.

Social evaluation, or being publicly judged for the quality of one's performance, is a challenging stressor in youth sport. Many specific social evaluation stressors have been identified in youth sport, including fear of failure, being negatively evaluated by others, and being rejected by others (Reeves, Nicholls, & McKenna, 2009). Or as young athletes express it, "Knowing I've got to play well and win [makes me] think about failing" and "My dad is always on my case, so it's a worry, a pressure not to make mistakes" (Sagar, Busch, & Jowett, 2010, p. 222).

As the social evaluation increases in situations, kids perceive more threat. Individual youth sport athletes responded with higher **anxiety,** an unpleasant emotional state characterized by nervousness, worry, or both, as compared to team sport athletes (Martens, Vealey, & Burton, 1990). Athletes are more directly evaluated in individual sports as opposed to team sports, in which they may blend in with teammates. Youth wrestlers and gymnasts were found to experience more anxiety before competition than youth football, hockey, and baseball players (Simon & Martens, 1979). And interestingly, children performing band solos had greater anxiety than any of the sport participants,

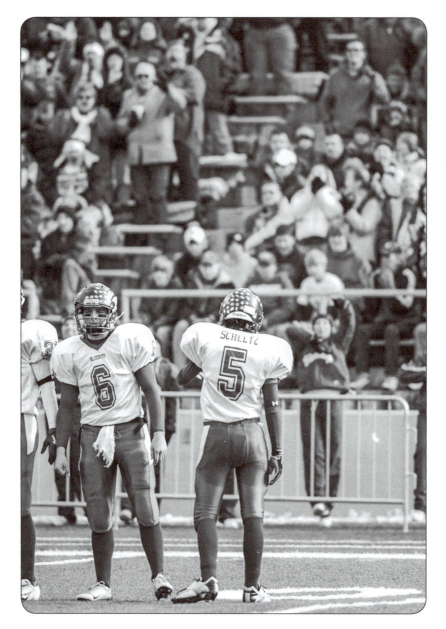

As the social evaluation increases in situations, kids perceive more threat and experience greater stress and anxiety.

which emphasizes that the social evaluation inherent in situations is what creates stress for kids (not just sport participation).

Importance

Events that are of greater personal significance, or more important, often create greater stress. The pressure of needing to perform well in situations with a high degree of importance has been linked to choking, in which athletes suffer significant and even unusual performance decrements in response to the pressurized importance of an event (Baumeister, 1984). There are many factors that increase the importance of a sport competition for youth athletes, such as family members in the crowd or playing against a particular opponent. Coaches and parents often create stress and anxiety for youth athletes by emphasizing the importance of winning the "big" game.

Uncertainty

Uncertainty creates stress for young athletes in two ways. First, they are often uncertain about their abilities to perform well, please their parents, or not let down their teammates. That is, they're uncertain they can meet the demands of the competitive situation (Martens, 2012). Second, they may feel nervous because they're unfamiliar with the nature of competition and don't have much experience with sport. Coaches often create uncertainty in athletes by not communicating with them about their role on the team or by expecting them to perform perfectly and not make any mistakes.

Understanding the Multiple Developmental Stressors for Youth Athletes

So, the demands placed on kids in youth sport can be summed up as social evaluation + importance + uncertainty. Now that's a recipe for stress! In addition, children and adolescents face multiple developmental demands. Their bodies are changing as they grow and mature, which creates not only physical but also psychosocial stressors for them (as discussed in chapter 4). They have the academic demands of school and various adolescent social stressors such as making friends, fitting in, developing their identity, and engaging in romantic relationships. A major stressor on young athletes who move into higher levels of sport is the time demand and the risk of being overscheduled. So the demands presented by the competitive sport environment are just one portion of the overall stressors typical in the lives of kids. Adult stakeholders in youth sport need to keep this in mind, because overstress may occur based not just on sport demands but also on the overwhelming crush of multiple stressors on kids, particularly during the challenging developmental phase of adolescence.

Strategies to Reduce or Optimize Stressors Faced by Youth Athletes

1. Youth coaches should reduce uncertainty in athletes by telling them before competition that they're prepared and to focus on doing what they've done in practice. Remind them that it's okay to make mistakes, which are part of learning and part of sport. They should play hard and focus on and enjoy the game.

2. Coaches should personally connect with each athlete on the team so that all of them are clear on their role and what's expected of them. Our daughter became very anxious during her freshman volleyball season when she was called up to the varsity squad to replace a senior who was injured. The coaches reassured her by explaining that she was ready, that she had trained for this, and that she was expected to play "her game" (not someone else's) in the front row. They encouraged her to not worry if she made mistakes, just to play hard and focus on her job. Such coaching communication is helpful in decreasing the uncertainty that comes from sudden challenges faced by young athletes.

3. On our son's community swim team, all kids are welcome to be a part of the team and train but are not required to swim in competitive meets. Some young children prefer to use the time during their first year in the program to learn the strokes and to swim in the intrateam mock meets to get used to competing. This is an excellent way to ease children into competition and help them get used to social evaluation.

4. For entry-level team sports, we suggest considering ways to decrease the evaluation potential of competition. This is typically done in tee ball, in which an inning involves every player on the team batting, no matter the number of outs. Also, no score is kept (except by certain kids and parents!). Many of the suggestions in chapter 7 about how to

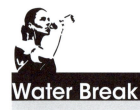

Water Break

Eyes on Michelle Wie

It's hard to identify a sport superstar who has endured more social evaluation scrutiny than Michelle Wie. A talented junior golfer, Wie appeared in the 2003 Kraft Nabisco Ladies' Professional Golf Association (LPGA) tourney (a major event) and made the cut as a 13-year-old. She then went on to achieve seven top-10 finishes in majors, nearly winning three at age 16. Arnold Palmer said, "She's going to influence the golfing scene as much as Tiger [Woods], or more" (ESPN, 2012). She signed lucrative endorsement contracts with several companies, including Nike.

Riding the public's fascination with the power of her game, Wie (managed by her parents) began to play in (men's) Professional Golfers' Association (PGA) events without ever having won on the LPGA tour. This was unprecedented, and it invited even more publicity and social evaluation. Her scores ballooned and she didn't make cuts, much less win. Most articles written about Wie have used phrases like "disappointing career," "confounding journey," and "stop waiting for Wie to be a superstar." After joining the LPGA, Wie had only two wins from 2009 to 2014. People attributed her problems to a host of factors, including overbearing parents, bad career management decisions, and the crushing pressure on her to live up to expectations. Wie did break through to win the prestigious women's U.S. Open in 2014 and spoke about how much the win meant to her because of her career-long struggle in the social evaluation spotlight.

A trend for younger athletes to compete in elite golf is evident. Lexi Thompson became the youngest LPGA winner in history by winning at age 16, after she had participated in the U.S. Open at age 12. Fourteen-year-old Guan Tianlang made the cut at the Masters tournament in 2013, astounding the golf world with his mature performance. However, these golfers did not receive as much public scrutiny as Michelle Wie. Lessons learned from her saga can hopefully influence parents and the media to avoid exploiting precocious youth athletes before they are ready.

modify sport can be implemented to engineer a progressive degree of social evaluation in youth sport.

5. Coaches and parents should de-emphasize the importance of outcomes, such as winning competitive events. Helping young athletes develop healthy perspectives on winning and losing actually enables them to perform better in pressure situations. Dan Jansen, 1994 Olympic gold medalist in speed skating, credits his father with helping him develop the perspective he needed to pursue Olympic and world championships. When Jansen failed to win in his first national championship event as a 12-year-old and cried all the way home in the car, his father sat him down and explained, "Dan, you know there's more to life than skating around in a circle" (Jansen, 1999, p. 6). Jansen admitted that he still loved to

compete and win, but his father had helped him to look at success and failure with a healthier perspective. This perspective enabled him to concentrate on the process of racing without allowing the expectations of others to add pressure that would have hurt his performance at important competitions like the Olympic Games.

6. Emphasize over and over the pursuit of individualized mastery goals in competition, which reduces the worry and anxiety of competition for kids (Morris & Kavussanu, 2009). In swimming, track, and cross-country, kids should focus on the goal of beating their previous best time. In team sports, coaches and parents should talk with kids about specific things they can concentrate on, like rebounding in basketball, passing well in volleyball, or making good decisions as a soccer goalie.

An interesting study showed that parental pressure created anxiety in youth swimmers only when the parents focused on outcomes, such as winning or beating opponents (O'Rourke, Smith, Smoll, & Cumming, 2011). Parents who engaged intensely with their children to encourage effort, learning from mistakes, and focusing on self-improvement were viewed as pressuring their children in an adaptive manner; this actually reduced evaluative pressure because the kids could concentrate on controllable goals. This study is valuable in emphasizing that stress in the form of parental demands can be helpful to kids as long as the focus is on individual mastery. Life is about demands, and who better to teach this to kids than their parents?

YOUNG ATHLETES' ASSESSMENT OF DEMANDS

Stage 2 in the stress process (figure 11.1) is about young athletes' assessment of the demands presented to them. Most basically, this comes down to whether kids view the demand as a challenge or a threat.

Coping in Youth Athletes

Young athletes perceive sport demands as a challenge when they savor the opportunity to perform the skills they've practiced and are in pursuit of mastery and personal growth. The key to the demand's being viewed as a challenge is athletes' beliefs that they possess the resources to cope and manage the situation. **Coping** refers to conscious attempts individuals make to manage situations that they perceive as stressful and as a danger to their well-being (Compas, Connor-Smith, Saltzman, Harding Thomsen, & Wadsworth, 2001). Threat occurs when athletes perceive that they lack sufficient resources to cope with the demands, and what is typically threatened in sport is one's sense of self-worth and competence. Thus, young athletes' assessment of demand is based on how well they believe their coping resources can handle the situation.

The ways in which children cope matter because certain types of coping are better than others in terms of psychological adjustment and personal growth (Compas et al., 2001). Generally, **active coping**, in which youth athletes learn and use strategies that help them solve problems or reduce and manage stressors, is associated with better adjustment as compared to avoidance, withdrawal, or just the soothing of negative emotions (Nicholls, Perry, Jones, Morley, & Carson, 2013). An example of an active coping strategy for youth athletes is for them to set specific performance goals for the competition and then mentally rehearse performing with a focus on these goals. It is also helpful for athletes to identify one or two things that happen in competition that cause them to lose confidence and feel pressure (e.g., a bad performance moment, getting criticized by coaches), and then to mentally rehearse a productive response they could make when this occurs.

Parents and coaches are important at this stage of the process in helping young athletes maintain perspective about the upcoming competition and helping them prepare to accept their performance mistakes as well as triumphs. As you might expect, kids become more effective in coping with the demands of sport as they age. Through experience, they develop a wider repertoire of coping resources (Tamminen & Holt, 2010). Actually, athletes apply coping skills throughout the stages of the stress model (figure 11.1) as they physically and mentally prepare themselves for competition (stage 2), attempt to manage stressors during competition (stage 3), and then manage their thoughts and feelings about the outcomes of the event (stage 4).

What Types of Kids Tend to Perceive Threat Over Challenge?

Certain individual characteristics of children and adolescents influence how they assess the demands of competitive youth sport. As discussed in chapter 6, some kids develop *incompetence-avoidance* motivational orientations (Kaye, Conroy, & Fifer, 2008) that increase their tendency to perceive threat in sport situations. Failure-oriented young athletes focus more on dreaded negative consequences of failure as opposed to the challenge and prospect of success. Kids who are negatively or excessively perfectionistic strive unrealistically for flawless performance and are overconcerned with mistakes. **Trait anxiety** is a personality characteristic that predisposes people to view competition and social evaluation as threatening (Martens et al., 1990). A questionnaire that assesses youth athletes' levels of trait anxiety is provided in appendix I.

What accounts for the formation of these personality characteristics that heighten children's susceptibility to stress? Although a definitive answer to this question is lacking, early childhood social interactions and experiences with success and failure appear to contribute to these characteristics. For example, trait anxiety has been linked to such parental child-rearing behaviors as excessive regulation of activities and routines, encouraging dependence on parents, less acceptance, and inconsistency in feedback (McLeod, Wood, & Weisz, 2007).

Another individual characteristic that influences young athletes' assessment of demand as threat, as opposed to challenge, is the way in which they've learned to view competitive anxiety. Through active coping, mental skills development, and competitive experience, athletes can learn that anxiety is their bodies' normal response to competition and that it can even help their performance by making them focused and activated (Jones & Hanton, 1996). It is critical that young athletes develop the ability to assess demands as challenging and anxiety provoking but within their abilities to manage, so that they can still perform effectively. Elite athletes admit that as they gained more experience in competition, they became more familiar with anxiety symptoms induced by competition and were able to rationalize their thoughts and feelings to effectively cope with the anxiety (Hanton, Cropley, Neil, Mellalieu, & Miles, 2007). They even learned that the anxiety symptoms they had interpreted as threatening when they were younger were actually necessary for good performance.

Strategies to Optimize How Youth Athletes Assess Sport Demands

1. Explain to athletes that they need to be willing to be anxious and to accept the jittery feelings that are a normal part of competition. Know that the nervousness will appear, and plan to be okay with that.

2. Expose athletes to many different types of pressure in training. Examples include performing in front of others who are judging you, performing while being videotaped, and performing through many types of distractions. The idea is to get athletes used to performing despite facing what they fear the most by exposing them repeatedly to a

wide range of very challenging stressors and pressure conditions. An outstanding example of this was carried out with elite late-adolescent cricketers, who were systematically exposed to pressure training and "punishment-conditioned consequences" designed to build mental toughness (Bell, Hardy, & Beattie, 2013). The experimental program led to enhanced performance under pressure.

3. Athletes should identify and plan responses to competitive demands that typically trigger anxiety. They can mentally recreate the typical thoughts and feelings that come with these stressors and then mentally rehearse their productive responses to them. This might include deep breaths, a productive go-to statement that keeps them focused on the task at hand, and the development of a routine that enables them to feel comfortable and ready before the performance.

4. Explicitly give young athletes permission to make mistakes. Tell them this shows they're playing hard and attempting new things, and that it's part of the learning process.

5. Help young athletes gain perspective by learning to zero in on aspects of their performance that they can control. An exercise to help them do this is provided in appendix J. In the exercise, athletes are asked to identify their "controllables" and "uncontrollables" for an upcoming competition. The exercise is an example of active coping, in which athletes identify strategies that help them manage competitive demands.

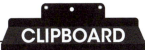

CLIPBOARD

A Training Example to Prepare for Pressure

Christy was a 14-year-old tennis player, ranked in the top 25 of her national age group, who needed to improve on two key aspects of her game. First, she had a poor net game because she was fearful of coming to the net for volleys. Second, she tended to choke on her second serve, worrying about double faulting, even though she had the technical talent to execute the serve.

Christy began working on her net game by physically practicing net volleys on shots that began very easy and progressed to harder. She verbalized the trigger word *seams* out loud; this made her focus her attention on the seams of the ball coming toward her and also occupied her mind to prevent negative thinking or worry. She mentally practiced net volleys in various situations, using her trigger word to create the correct visual picture, as well as net tactics for different competitive situations. She set a performance goal to hit at least one winner per game from the net. In training, she did not win the game or end the drill until she had accomplished this goal. Her net performance improved over the course of the 25-week intervention so that she won, on average, 4 points per match from the net.

To deal with her double-fault problem, Christy developed a preservice routine to relax, focus, and prime the automatic execution of her serve. The routine started with bouncing the ball four times and catching it. Then she took a relaxation breath, during which she imagined exhaling tension, and then visualized the ball kicking successfully in her opponent's service box. She used the word *stop* to put any irrelevant and worrisome thoughts out of her mind. Her routine was developed and practiced in parts and was refined over three months of practice. Christy was able to gain fluidity and smoothness in her second serve and significantly decreased her double-fault percentage as the result of her training.

Adapted from Mamassis and Doganis 2004.

YOUNG ATHLETES' RESPONSES TO STRESS

We've now arrived at the third stage of the stress process (see figure 11.1), and this is where the rubber hits the road, so to speak. The athlete has processed the demands and now must respond to them in terms of physical performance as well as psychological responses. Hopefully, his development of active coping strategies, such as mental training, physical training under pressure, and individualized performance goal setting, will help him in responding to the competitive demands of the situation.

Arousal

One's task at the response stage is to manage and attempt to optimize one's level of arousal. **Arousal** is a state of physical and mental readiness, or how revved up a person feels at a particular moment in time. Generally, athletes perform best at moderate levels of arousal. So, as shown in figure 11.2, most athletes perform best in the 4 to 6 range, with the numbers crudely approximating levels of arousal.

However, individuals may differ on what levels of arousal work best for them in helping them perform better. And different types of sports require lower (golf, archery)

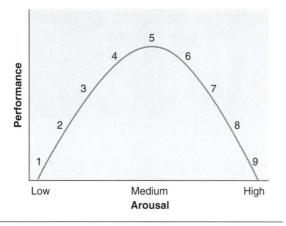

Figure 11.2 Inverted-U relationship between arousal and performance.

or higher (football, rugby) levels of arousal for optimal performance. Optimal arousal levels differ even within the same sport. Basketball players perform at high arousal levels when engaged in full-court defensive pressure, but then need to lower their arousal levels abruptly to shoot a free throw. That's why most basketball players have learned to take a deep breath and follow a focused preshot routine to optimize their physical and mental arousal before shooting.

Youth athletes need guidance in understanding how arousal affects their performance. Help them understand when they might need to psych up versus calm down. Ask them to identify the best number for them—that is, what level of arousal enables them to perform the best in their particular sport. They can then plan some strategies to manage their number to keep it in optimal range.

Attentional Focus

Along with managing arousal levels during competition, young athletes have to manage their attention. Of course, the best focus to maintain is on the present moment and the task in front of you. But as we all know, achieving that isn't that easy in the heat of competition.

Distraction

Stressors in competition often distract athletes from honing in on the relevant aspects of the task. Youth athletes are especially susceptible to distraction due to their lack of competitive experience and relative immaturity with respect to prioritizing thoughts and keeping emotions in check. As discussed in chapter 4, children and teenagers are not as biologically equipped to respond rationally and nonemotionally as adults (based on timing of brain development). So it's harder for kids to manage irrelevant thoughts, such as concerns about negative evaluation from others, letting the team down, or worrying about the outcome of the performance.

Self-Focus

Although anxiety can prevent athletes from focusing optimally on the execution of a skill, it can also cause them to focus too much on it. When a skill is well learned, an athlete executes it automatically. For example, a skilled golfer can focus on his target and execute his swing without having to think about each part of it. However, when he feels pressure to perform well in an important situation, he may turn his attention inward and think about each part of the swing in his extra effort to perform well. Self-focus during performance in those who are skilled is a main reason for choking, defined as performing poorly in response to wanting to do well in an important situation.

Strategies to Optimize Athletes' Responses

1. Teach athletes simple physical arousal regulatory strategies, such as taking a deep breath. An easy cadence to remember is count 5 (inhalation) and 5 (exhalation). They can think of, and even hum, a song that matches their number, or preferred level of arousal. For example, a young golfer's worries about her bunker game often make her rush her swing. She can hum a slow waltz in her head when preparing to hit a bunker shot. The waltz cadence cues her in to slowing down and swinging with the right rhythm. Another physical arousal strategy is for athletes to maintain physical poise and a confident posture even if they're not feeling it. Remind them to "fake it 'til they make it" in terms of acting confident and poised.

2. Athletes should keep their focus of attention simple and directed outward, concentrating on their job right now or on the next play. They can use a go-to word or phrase to direct their attention externally. More advanced or skilled athletes should use a holistic word or phrase to prime their performance, such as "strong and soft" (basketball free throw), "target" (softball pitching),

or "aggressive" (hockey). Holistic here refers to a focus on the whole, as opposed to parts of something. The literature shows that skilled athletes perform better using holistic process cues (words that suggest a feeling or rhythm or overall picture), while beginning athletes need more part-oriented cues to focus on the "how to" to prime correct performance. Beginning athletes still learning skills may want to use a key phrase or word that helps them execute the skill, such as "throw your hands" (baseball hitting) or "pendulum" (putting stroke).

3. At tough moments when athletes are not feeling confident, they can still focus and perform well. An important strategy for them is not to fixate or panic over not feeling confident. They should accept that these are typical thoughts that come up in competition, and that they're prepared to focus and execute even without feeling confident.

OUTCOMES FROM THE STRESS PROCESS

The final stage of the stress process involves the outcomes that result from the athletes' responses (typically how they responded in training or competition). This stage is important because it feeds back (see figure 11.1) to influence how athletes will tend to assess competitive stressors in the future. Obviously, we would like the outcomes to be positive, or at least personal growth experiences.

Strategies to Optimize Outcomes for Youth Athletes

1. Adults should encourage a "growth mindset" (Dweck, 2007), whereby kids view their competitive performances as continuous mastery attempts that are part of an ongoing effort to expand their abilities. Learning is simply a string of failures and successes. Remind them that it's called trial and error, not trial and success.

2. As discussed in chapter 6, adults need to help young athletes make attributions (identify reasons to explain why events occur) that allow them to feel proud that they earned their success by being prepared and working hard. Productive attributions also give athletes feelings of controllability, the sense that they can improve their skills and get better after experiencing failures. Attributions help to psychologically cement feelings of competence (for success) yet also help to provide hope and renewed commitment to improve in the future (after failures).

3. Parents should be thoughtful and patient in helping youth athletes work through the outcome stage. The dreaded parental PGA (postgame analysis) in the car ride going home is the last thing many kids want, particularly when the outcome was negative for them. Allow kids some time and space, or ask open-ended questions to invite them to debrief with you, such as "How did you feel about your match today?" When the emotion of the event has subsided, it is always helpful for athletes to systematically go through their performance mentally to rationally assess how things went and understand how and why things happened as they did.

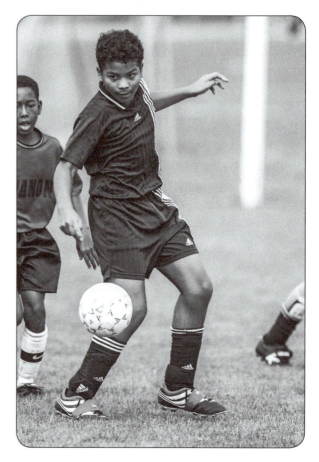

Youth coaches should avoid constant feedback, instruction, and evaluation to allow athletes time and space to experience flow, or total absorption in the sport experience.

FLOW: THE ULTIMATE GOAL FOR YOUTH SPORT PARTICIPANTS

One of the most important outcomes from the process of competing is developing a love for sport. It's an outcome we wish we could prescribe for every youth sport participant. One sure way to achieve this outcome is to create opportunities for kids to experience flow. **Flow** is an optimal mental state characterized by total absorption in the task (Csikszentmihalyi, 1990). Remember that magical state of immersion you experienced as a child when you were outside playing with friends and lost track of time? That's flow, a deeply rewarding experience of focused, pleasant energy.

Flow as the Ultimate Balance Between Challenge (Demand) and Skill

Flow fits into our discussion of stress because it occurs when athletes experience a balance between their skills and the challenges that they perceive in the situation. As shown in figure 11.3, the skill–challenge balance must be at a high enough level to be interesting, or the result is apathy. Low levels of skill and challenge are not enough to stimulate flow, even if they are in balance (dotted line area in figure 11.3). When the competitive challenge far outweighs athletes' skills, they become anxious. Conversely, when athletes' skills far outweigh the challenges they face, they are bored.

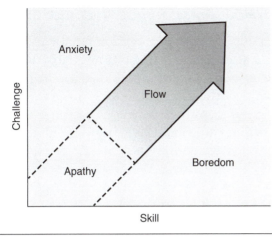

Figure 11.3 Flow as the balance between perceived challenge and skills.

Along with being enjoyable, flow leads to better performance, and it's easy to see why. In flow states, athletes lose their self-consciousness and thus forget to worry about how others are evaluating them. Their concentration is locked on the task of playing with complete focus, without distraction. Although they may be expending a lot of energy, it feels effortless because they are "inside the activity" as opposed to looking at it as something they have to do. Flow experts call this a merging of action and awareness, and athletes experience it as "going on autopilot." Flow is intrinsically motivating, and athletes engage in flow-like activities for no other reason than just to play (as with the free play of childhood).

Providing Opportunities for Youth Athletes to Experience Flow

Wow, can we bottle flow and let athletes drink it before competition? Unfortunately, flow can't be force-fed or even directly manipulated. Instead, we want to help athletes get in a position for flow to occur. Elite athletes use mental preparation strategies to help them attain the focus and positive feeling states associated with flow. Even then, it doesn't always occur, and of course athletes need

to prepare themselves to perform whether they're in the flow zone or not.

At the youth sport level, we can attempt to create conditions that are challenging and stimulating (not boring), yet not threatening or too difficult. Read the following checklist for youth sport coaches, which assesses their abilities to provide experiences that promote flow for their athletes:

- Do you use a variety of drills and activities in practice, and change pace often (instead of spending too long on one drill)?

- Do you plan and then ensure that all kids are as active as possible during practice (instead of having kids wait in lines or sit out waiting their turn)?

- Do you carefully consider and choose activities and drills that challenge the athletes but aren't too difficult based on their levels of ability?

- Do you build in occasional drills or activities that you know the athletes enjoy or that are fun for them?

- Do you create periods of time in practices and games in which you let the kids play, without providing constant instruction?

- Do you provide evaluation for your athletes at appropriate times, without overdoing it and constantly evaluating everything they do (overcoaching)?

- If an athlete is performing great, do you take it in stride without making a big deal about it (instead of saying "You're playing great—what's gotten into you?")?

What did you learn from the checklist? Young athletes need to be challenged, to be stimulated by variety and change, and to be able to engage in periods of playing their sport without constant instruction or evaluation. Coaches, sit down sometimes and just let athletes play. Constant feedback from coaches distracts players from what they're doing. In addition, take time to carefully plan training sessions. A real flow killer is to do the same activities and drills day after day, which is boring for the athletes. We understand that repetition is an important principle of learning, and that young athletes have to repetitively practice skills and tactics to overlearn them so they become automatic for competition. However, effective practice management means that coaches keep athletes engaged and active and use a variety of drills to automate skills.

The last point on the checklist emphasizes that evaluation can disrupt flow. So the last thing you want to do to an athlete in the middle of a great performance is to call his attention to his performance. Remember that flow occurs when we're so inside of playing that we're not distracted by evaluating how we're doing. When an athlete is playing great, just continue coaching in your typical manner as though this is an everyday occurrence. Avoid such distracting comments as "You're two innings away from a no-hitter!" or "You haven't missed a free throw all night!" When athletes are in that cocoon of flow, don't disturb it by calling their attention to it.

BURNOUT IN YOUTH SPORT

"I don't know, Mom, I just feel burned out." As a parent, what would you do if you heard this? We all have a vague understanding of burnout, but should we advise our kids to drop out, take a break, make some changes, or suck it up? Because *burnout* is a popular term, we need to carefully consider what is true and not true about burnout in youth athletes.

What Is Burnout?

Burnout is a negative psychological and physical state in which young athletes feel tired, less able to perform well, and less interested in playing their sports. Three symptoms characterize burnout.

Physical and Emotional Exhaustion

Although it is common for athletes to get tired after training sessions or competitions, the exhaustion associated with burnout involves the depletion of emotional and physical resources beyond the typical tiredness that comes and goes throughout a sport season. Parents may notice kids feeling too tired to do things outside their sport, feeling emotionally drained and lethargic, and wanting to take a break from sport.

Reduced Sport Accomplishment

The second symptom can be a lack of performance success or inconsistent performance, or it can be more about the perception on the part of the athlete that she is not playing up to her potential. The athlete may feel that she's not getting anywhere—for example, not improving or moving forward.

Devaluation of Sport

Devaluation means a reduction in value: The athlete doesn't care as much about his sport. Athletes may say "I'm sick of doing this"; "I don't care about playing anymore"; or "It's just not fun anymore." Another common symptom is questioning things—for example, "Why am I doing this?"

How Prevalent Is Burnout in Youth Sport?

Many popular media stories warn of an impending burnout epidemic in youth sport. However, research has identified only a very small percentage (1-2%) of adolescent athletes who have experienced severe burnout. It is true, though, that the majority of youth athletes surveyed admitted to having experienced low to moderate levels of burnout (Gustafsson, Kentta, Hassmen, & Lundqvist, 2007; Raedeke & Smith, 2004). Athletes report more burnout as they increase in age from 7 to 17 years (Harris & Watson, 2014).

What Causes Burnout in Youth Athletes?

Several factors contribute to burnout in youth athletes. We've categorized them into three groups: overload factors, social climate factors, and personality factors (see table 11.1).

Overload Factors

Overload factors represent what people usually think about when they hear that someone is burned out. Previously in this chapter, you learned that overstress involves demand that exceeds athletes' abilities to cope, such as when they are overloaded without adequate physical and mental recovery. As discussed in chapter 9, overtraining is the result of excessive training and inadequate recovery, which typically leads to decreased performance and psychological distress (Richardson, Andersen, & Morris, 2008). The difficulty for coaches is determining how much overload (an essential, useful aspect of sport training) is appropriate for their athletes. Some overload is needed to induce a training effect and improved performance, but too much overload without adequate recovery results in decreased performance (called staleness), exhaustion, decreased interest in training, and negative moods (burnout). To clarify, **staleness** is the term typically used to describe impaired performance as the result of overtraining; burnout is a broader concept that focuses on psychological distress and decreased

motivation in a previously enjoyed activity (Kentta & Hassmen, 1998) as a result of overload without adequate recovery.

Social Climate Factors

Social climate contributors to burnout are those negative aspects of the youth sport culture that are harmful to the psychological development and well-being of kids. These include pressure from parents to perform or achieve certain outcomes (e.g., winning, making the varsity team, gaining a college scholarship) and negative coaching behaviors, such as extreme controlling behaviors and developmentally inappropriate training and performance expectations. Athletes who feel trapped in their sport participation tend to be higher in burnout than athletes who were personally invested in and enthusiastic about swimming (Raedeke, 1997). This occurs when athletes do not really want to participate but feel they have to maintain their involvement in sport based on social pressure from others.

It has been argued that burnout is not a response to stress but rather a response to the social climate of highly organized youth sport, in which young athletes are highly controlled and inhibited in their identity development (Coakley, 1992). According to this perspective, stress is a symptom of burnout, but not the cause. Interviews with 15 elite youth swimmers who experienced burnout indicated that these athletes became powerless to control what was happening in their lives and their personal development.

Table 11.1 Factors Related to Burnout in Youth Athletes

Overload factors	Social climate factors	Personality factors
Overstress	Pressure from parents	Trait anxiety
Overtraining	Negative coaching behaviors	Weak coping skills
Staleness	Feeling trapped in sport participation	Negative perfectionism
	Lack of personal control	Obsessive passion
		Unidimensional identity

The result of this highly controlling, over-structured quality of youth sport was burnout. This explanation for burnout is important because it identifies the roots of burnout as the youth sport culture, as opposed to some personal failure or lack of competence (e.g., toughness) in young athletes.

Personality Factors

Although the structure of youth sport and the behavior of coaches and parents are critical in influencing burnout, several personality factors have been related to burnout in youth athletes. Trait anxiety and weak coping skills are obvious factors, based on their importance in the stress process discussed previously. Negative perfectionism (Hill, 2013) and obsessive passion (Martin & Horn, 2013) are examples of personality factors that create extreme aspirations and irrational needs (inability to accept mistakes, inflexible goals, compelling pressure to participate) in relation to one's sport participation. Interestingly, positive or adaptive perfectionism (high standards, organizational skill, achievement orientation) and harmonious passion (loving one's sport without feeling controlled by it) is related to lower levels of burnout. Unidimensional identity, also related to burnout, was identified in chapter 10 as a dangerous narrowing of a child's self-concept based on overexclusive specialization in sport. Youth sport athletes should protect themselves from burnout by engaging in different types of activities to define themselves in multidimensional ways.

Strategies to Help Athletes Avoid and Deal With Burnout

1. Although definitiveness is lacking, it is thought that physical and emotional exhaustion serves as a first indicator of developing burnout in young athletes. Observing these symptoms should prompt adult coaches and parents to intervene immediately and work with the athlete to find the best strategy to ensure some rest, recovery, and mental rejuvenation.

2. Identify athletes whose personalities or life situations predispose them to burnout, and make it a point to intervene with guidance and suggestions to help them achieve without crossing the line into harmful training behaviors. One recommendation is to identify a sport psychology consultant who can work with youth athletes to enhance their mental approaches to competition. Gaining perspective and developing skills to move from negative types of passion and perfectionism toward more adaptive forms of these characteristics would be useful.

3. Anyone (parent or coach) can help young athletes learn active coping skills. Better lifestyle management, healthier decisions, more rational perspectives on competition, and skill in identifying and pursuing personal mastery goals are all coping skills that can be learned by young athletes.

4. Guide young people in adopting multiple areas of interest and achievement. Such variety and multidimensionality guard against burnout that occurs from a single-minded obsession gone awry.

Personal Plug-In

Have You Been Burned Out?

Did you ever experience burnout as a youth athlete? Describe how it felt: Were all three burnout symptoms present? Consider the specific factors that led to this experience of burnout for you. Why do you think it happened? How did it affect your sport experience, particularly your motivation and choices about staying in sport

5. Listen to your kids, and clarify whether they want to continue in a sport. This is difficult for parents, especially when they observe the special talent a young athlete has in a particular sport only to see him decide to give it up. Although we agree that parents have an initial role in getting kids to try different sports, it doesn't work for athletes to feel compelled to stay in a sport only because of their parents.

6. Parents know best the vast array of stressors operating in a young athlete's life, so it's up to parents to hold the line in staking out recovery time for their children (often despite coaches' and the young athletes' protests). Someone has to be in charge and protect the health and well-being of the athletes, particularly since they're young.

7. Lead the charge for developmentally appropriate practice in youth sport. The excessive control and exploitation of youth athletes to pursue adult-mandated goals such as early specialization, as well as an emphasis on winning over athlete development, lead to burnout and dropping out. Follow the guidelines in the long-term athlete development model (Balyi, Way, & Higgs, 2013) presented in chapter 5 so that the emphasis is on a progressive development of skills, a gradual introduction to competition, a focus on enjoyment and the nurturing of motivation, and a lifelong commitment to physical activity.

WRAP-UP

Everything discussed in this chapter is about balance. Stress is an important stimulant for personal growth, but when it turns to over-stress, children's health and performance get out of balance. Flow occurs when young athletes find the "sweet spot" in balancing their skills with selected challenges, and experiencing that sweet spot is what hooks them on sport. Burnout occurs when kids' training and recovery become imbalanced, their mental approach to sport gets skewed, or they lack needed social support.

This doesn't mean that young athletes can't fall so much in love with their sport that their commitment to training far exceeds what others think of as normal training regimens. Rory McIlroy, David Beckham, and Chris Evert are amazing examples of the commitment to achieve elite status as one of the best in the world. But this was their dream, their choice, and their goal because of their love of what they were doing. They didn't feel trapped or pressured to pursue their dreams, and although they were and are not immune to stress and burnout, their deep commitment to their sports provided them a safety net. Most youth athletes won't become international sport stars, but hopefully they too can have the freedom to pursue sport on their own terms. Let's do the best we can to offer them the challenges they need to grow and the support they need to meet those challenges.

LEARNING AIDS

Key Terms

active coping—Strategies that help athletes solve problems or reduce and manage stressors.

anxiety—Unpleasant emotional state characterized by nervousness, worry, or both.

arousal—A state of physical and mental readiness.

burnout—A negative psychological and physical state in which young athletes feel tired, less able to perform well, and less interested in playing their sports.

coping—Conscious attempts individuals make to manage situations that they perceive as stressful and as a danger to their well-being.

flow—An optimal mental state characterized by total absorption in the task.

overstress—Stress without adequate recovery or stress in amounts that are too great.

social evaluation—Being publicly judged for the quality of one's performance.

staleness—Impaired performance as the result of overtraining.

stress—A demand placed on a person.

stressor—Something that causes stress.

trait anxiety—A personality characteristic that predisposes people to view competition and social evaluation as threatening.

Summary Points

1. Stress is useful when applied in the right amounts, but overstress creates adverse health consequences.

2. Young athletes need small doses of stress over time as "inoculation" that will stimulate the development of resources to deal with higher doses of stress when they're older.

3. Stress is a four-stage process that involves a demand or stressor, the athlete's assessment of the demand, the athlete's responses to the demand, and the outcomes of the process.

4. Social evaluation, importance, and uncertainty are the three fundamental sources of stress inherent in competitive youth sport.

5. Active coping is associated with better adjustment as compared to avoidance, withdrawal, and the soothing of negative emotions.

6. Youth athletes who are high in trait anxiety, negative perfectionism, and fear of failure, and who view competitive anxiety as harmful, perceive greater threat in sport.

7. High levels of arousal, attentional distraction, and self-focus are negative responses to stress.

8. Flow occurs when athletes experience balance between their skills and the challenges of the situation.

9. Coaches can enhance flow by providing variety in training, optimal challenge, and time for play without evaluation and instruction and by avoiding distracting comments.

10. Burnout includes the symptoms of physical and emotional exhaustion, reduced sport accomplishment, and devaluation of sport.

11. Burnout is associated with overload factors, social climate factors, and personality factors.

Study Questions

1. Explain why stress can be good as well as bad, using examples of each and working through the four stages of the stress process.

2. Identify the three underlying sources of stress inherent in competitive youth sport, and provide two examples for each source.

3. Explain four strategies to reduce or optimize stressors faced by youth athletes.

4. What types of youth athletes tend to perceive threat instead of challenge when confronted by demands?

5. What are some strategies to enhance youth athletes' abilities to perceive stress more productively?

6. Explain what coping is and why active coping is preferred as a coping strategy.

7. Explain the concept of flow and several characteristics of the flow state. How can youth sport coaches help their athletes achieve flow?

8. Identify the three main symptoms of burnout, and provide examples from the three categories of factors that lead to burnout in youth athletes.

Reflective Learning Activities

1. Recall a stressful situation that you experienced in your youth sport career. Work through the four stages of the stress process, describing the stressor(s), your assessment of it and responses to it, and the outcomes of the process for you. What types of coping strategies did you use, and were they effective? Was the outcome a growth or learning experience for you? Why or why not? What can or did you learn in retrospect from this experience?

2. Using the Sport Anxiety Scale-2 in appendix I, assess the trait anxiety of a youth athlete (9 years or older). Then, develop interview questions and arrange an interview with the athlete to examine his or her perceived stressors, what he or she thinks about and how he or she feels about competition, things that create anxiety for this person, how she or he deals with the anxiety and stressors, typically how she or he feels after competition, and anything else you think is important. Write up a case description for this athlete in terms of her or his approach and response to stress in youth sport.

3. Develop an active coping plan for a youth athlete in a particular sport. This could include mental strategies and techniques, lifestyle management ideas, physical training ideas, and any other coping resources you think could be helpful. Make the plan brief, simple, practical, and easy for a youth athlete to follow.

Resource Guide

Avoiding Athlete Burnout in Youth Sports (YouTube) (www.youtube.com/watch?v=JHeJlmVSPbw).

How to Calm Oneself in Sport (YouTube) (www.youtube.com/watch?v=9Ij7rSykFoY).

How to Energize Oneself in Sport (YouTube) (www.youtube.com/watch?v=36023iyDIDg).

How to Manage Stress in Youth Sport Part 1 (YouTube) (www.youtube.com/watch?v=0kYNSNqeBcE).

chapter 12

INJURIES IN YOUTH SPORT

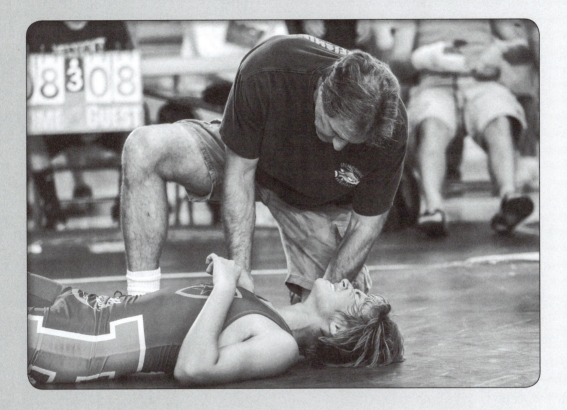

CHAPTER PREVIEW

In this chapter, you'll learn

- » the multiple causes of overuse injuries in sport;
- » about physeal, or growth plate, injuries;
- » that anterior cruciate ligament injuries are epidemic in female athletes; and
- » about concussions in youth athletes.

In a classic scene from the movie *Jaws*, two embattled shark hunters amusingly compare scars representing multiple injuries they sustained over their years of pursuing sharks. Those of us who grew up playing sport could do the same thing. Most of us experienced multiple injuries throughout our sport careers, because sport involves moving our bodies in forceful ways and attempting to stretch the limits of our abilities to perform well.

Unfortunately, injuries are part of sport, including youth sport. Parents should understand that minor injuries, such as sprains and strains, are common. However, all adult stakeholders in youth sport should be particularly concerned about three main aspects of injury in youth sport:

1. The increasing incidence of injuries that occur because of developmentally inappropriate practices in youth sport, which could be prevented (e.g., overuse injuries)
2. The particular vulnerability of children and adolescents to certain types of injuries (growth plate and head injuries)
3. The increase in catastrophic injuries, particularly concussions and anterior cruciate ligament (ACL) injuries

Our intent in this chapter is to raise your awareness of how and why certain injuries occur in youth sport, and help you understand ways in which you can prevent and identify them. (Exertional heat illness, discussed in chapter 9 in relation to physical training issues, should be considered by youth sport coaches and parents as a serious yet preventable "injury" or health risk to kids.) This chapter is not designed as a comprehensive sport first-aid course, and we strongly urge all youth sport practitioners to become certified in such a program (e.g., Sport First Aid course offered by the Human Kinetics Coach Education, www.HumanKineticsCoachEducationCenter.com).

YOUTH SPORT INJURY BASICS

Let's begin by identifying some general aspects of youth sport injuries as background for our later discussion of specific injuries.

Characteristics of Youth Athletes That Influence Injuries

Certain physical differences between youth and adult athletes make kids more vulnerable to injury (Adirim & Cheng, 2003). They have larger heads compared with the rest of their bodies, which makes them more prone to head injuries. Because children are smaller and vary in size, protective equipment may not fit them appropriately. Children's skeletons are growing, and the growth plates on their long bones are vulnerable to fractures and overuse injuries. Prepubescent athletes are more at risk for heat injuries due to their higher threshold for sweating and lower sweat rate.

Children's lack of mature motor skills may place them at greater risk of injury in some sports. The impulsiveness and recklessness associated with brain immaturity in teenagers may increase the likelihood of injury. And unfortunately, children are dependent minors who follow the direction of parents and coaches without question, even if this direction is misguided. Less knowledgeable volunteer coaches, which is common in youth sport, may put children more at risk for injury. Coaches are not expected to be medical experts, but they should be educated about both the nature and risks of injury in the sports they are coaching and developmentally appropriate practices to prevent and respond to sport-specific injuries.

Injury Occurrence in Youth Sport

About 4 million kids under age 14 receive medical treatment for sport injuries each year. Here are some basic points about injury occurrence in youth sport:

1. About half of all youth sport injuries are caused by overuse.

2. Generally, the rate and severity of injury increase with age. Prepubescent children are less likely to sustain injuries because they have less speed, mass, and strength (thus generate less force) compared to older athletes.

3. More than half of all youth sport injuries are preventable.

4. **Contusions** (bruises), **sprains** (overstressing ligaments), and **strains** (exerting a muscle beyond its limit) are the most common injuries to youth sport athletes.

5. Youth sports with the highest frequencies of injury are football, wrestling, gymnastics, basketball, and ice hockey.

6. When athletes are matched by size and skill level, injury rates decrease.

7. Sport-related injuries occur in youth athletes in two different ways:

    a. Sudden macrotrauma, which is a single application of major force applied to a body part, such as an ankle sprain from landing on an opponent's foot after jumping in basketball or a dislocated shoulder from sliding into second base in softball

    b. Repetitive microtrauma, in which repeated stress on a body part over a prolonged period of time overwhelms the body's ability to recover and repair itself (e.g., overuse shoulder injuries in swimmers, Little League elbow, stress fractures)

The "Shaking It Off" and "Toughing It Out" Injury Ethos of Sport

The headline proclaimed: "Kerri Strug Fights Off Pain, Helps U.S. Win Gold." The story captured the moment in the 1996 Olympic Games when 18-year-old Kerri Strug courageously performed her second vault movements after tearing two ligaments in her ankle on her first vault. Young athletes hear such stories as this and assume that "playing with pain" is what you're supposed to do in sport. A former star Little League pitcher recalls his coach directing him to hold his pitching arm in the freezer next to the ice pops so it would become numb enough for him to pitch the next game despite the pain (Hyman, 2009). This is the "shaking it off" and "toughing it out" ethos perpetuated by some adults and accepted, even embraced, by youth athletes (Malcom, 2006). Not only does this ethos

---

Personal Plug-In

Cultural Messages About Sport Injuries

Were you expected to play with pain or shake off what may have been a serious injury as a youth athlete? What was your youth sport culture like with regard to injury? How did you respond to this, and how do you feel about it now?

lead to severe injuries; it can also have life-threatening consequences.

OVERUSE INJURIES

Overuse injuries became the most common injury in youth sport, beginning with the late 1980s surge in club sports, year-round participation, and sport specialization. An **overuse injury** is microtraumatic damage to a body part (e.g., bone, muscle, tendon) that has been subjected to repetitive stress without sufficient time to heal or recover (Brenner, 2007).

Causes of Overuse Injuries

It doesn't take a genius to identify the main cause of overuse injuries: overuse. However, there is often a combination of factors that increase a young athlete's susceptibility to overuse injuries. As shown in table 12.1, these risk factors exist in the sport environment as well as within athletes themselves.

Sport Environment Factors

The sheer volume of training and competing is the most consistent predictor of overuse injuries. The excessive repetition inherent in sport training is the main culprit—number of pitches in baseball or softball, number of strokes in swimming, number of foot strikes in running, or number of jumps in volleyball. Young athletes who spent more hours per week than their age in years playing one sport—such as a 12-year-old

who played tennis 13 or more hours per week—were 70% more likely to experience serious overuse injuries than other athletes (Loyola University Health System, 2013). An unrealistic training progression beyond the recommended 10% per week, as well as a lack of appropriate rest and recovery periods, also contributes to overuse injuries.

Running and playing on hard surfaces may contribute to overuse injuries, as does ill-fitting equipment, especially shoes. Parents should buy footwear that is particularly designed for specific sports and is properly fitted for each athlete's unique needs. The final sport environment factor that predisposes kids to overuse injuries is pressure to train excessively and be "tough" in shaking off injuries to train through pain. Young athletes need to be specifically educated as to how minor pain in certain parts of their bodies is a warning sign that more severe overuse injuries could occur.

Athlete Factors

Along with environmental factors, several characteristics of athletes contribute to the overuse injury profile. Inappropriate technique in performing sport movements—as might be expected in young athletes—can easily lead to overuse injury. For example, poor form in throwing (e.g., baseball pitching, throwing the javelin) risks shoulder and elbow injuries. A volleyball coach pointed out to me (first author) how one of her hitters tended to land on one foot after

Table 12.1   Risk Factors for Overuse Injuries in Youth Athletes

Sport environment factors	Athlete factors
Excess repetition and training volume	Inappropriate technique
Accelerated physical training progression	Anatomical misalignment or imbalance
Lack of recovery or rest periods	Prior injury
Inappropriate surface for activity	Poor fitness or conditioning
Inappropriate equipment (particularly shoes)	Growth
Excessive pressure from parents, coaches, peers	Unhealthy female athlete triad
	Perfectionistic or obsessive personality

spiking the ball, which predisposed her to a stress fracture or ligament injury from an off-balance landing. Coaches should be mindful of teaching correct technique, not only for performance improvement but also to reduce injuries.

Certain types of anatomical misalignment or imbalances create more wear and tear than normal on body parts, such as discrepancies in leg length, flat or high-arched feet, excessive pronation, knock-knee, and bowleg. Prior injury may predispose athletes to additional injury, and the poor conditioning of many young athletes who show up to train with a youth sport team puts them at risk of injury. The growing bones of young athletes cannot handle as much training stress as the mature bones of adult athletes. As discussed in chapter 9, the unhealthy female athlete triad of disordered eating, menstrual dysfunction, and osteoporosis (poor bone health) predisposes these athletes to overuse injuries. Eating disorders and amenorrhea increase female athletes' risk for stress fractures (Loud, Gordon, Micheli, & Field, 2005). Finally, certain personality characteristics, such as perfectionism and obsessive passion, may lead youth athletes to engage in excessive training, forego needed rest and recovery, and continue participation despite pain.

Examples of Common Overuse Injuries in Youth Sport

As you might expect, different types of overuse injuries are associated with specific types of sports. Stress fractures occur more in the ribs of rowers and in the tibias (lower leg) and feet of runners and tennis, basketball, and volleyball players. **Stress fractures** are skeletal defects (usually hairline cracks) that result from the repeated application of a stress lower than that required to fracture a bone in a single blow or loading (Loud et al., 2005). Shoulder injuries occur more in swimming, baseball, tennis, softball, and volleyball because of the nature of arm movements in those sports.

We want to focus on three overuse-type injuries related to growth in youth athletes. All three of these injuries involve apophysitis. An **apophysis** is an outgrowth where a tendon inserts on a growing bone. The apophysis (a type of growth plate) contributes to growth in bone shape, but not to longitudinal growth. So **apophysitis** is inflammation (as the suffix *-itis* indicates) in the area of the growing bone where the tendon attaches. It occurs due to repetitive motion and overuse during periods of rapid growth. The most common sites for apophysitis in young athletes are the knee, heel, and elbow.

Osgood-Schlatter Disease

Despite its ominous-sounding name, **Osgood-Schlatter** is not really a disease. It is apophysitis of the knee that occurs in young athletes during their adolescent growth spurt. The rapid growth or lengthening of the bone leads to tightness in the muscle–tendon units spanning the knee. Picture a rubber band that is stretched tight enough to rub across the bone, irritating it and in some cases pulling or chipping off pieces of it (avulsion fractures). The youth athlete feels a lot of pain and soreness in the front of the knee. The condition is typically not serious, and the symptoms disappear once bone growth stops. Athletes do not necessarily have to quit the activity, although they may want to rest, ice the affected area, and take anti-inflammatory drugs, like ibuprofen, to lessen the pain. Often, people who had Osgood-Schlatter as a child retain a bump on their knee at the apophyseal site. Because apophyses are not involved in longitudinal bone growth, Osgood-Schlatter disease is not a threat to normal growth.

Sever's Disease

Sever's disease also involves apophysitis of the heel, caused by repetitive stress on the Achilles tendon. The heel bone grows faster

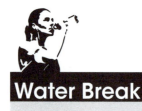
Are We Losing the Youth Baseball Arms Race?

The arms race in youth baseball isn't about nuclear weapons. It's about misguided adults who value winning games over the well-being of kids. The overuse and misuse of youth baseball pitchers have led to an epic rise in arm injuries. Beyond the inflammation of Little League elbow, young pitchers experience growth plate fractures, growth abnormalities, strains and tears of rotator muscles and tendons, cartilage tears, bone breakdown, and the classic tear of the ulnar collateral ligament in the elbow. This last injury leads to Tommy John surgery, named after the Major League Baseball pitcher who first had the surgery in 1974.

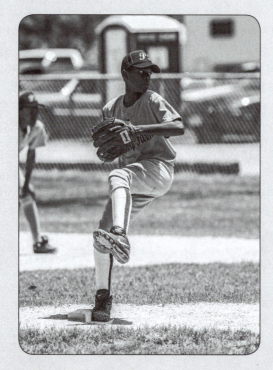

The overuse and misuse of youth baseball pitchers has led to an epic rise in arm injuries.

Multiple research studies show that the number of pitches thrown is the main cause of arm injuries in young pitchers. Dr. Joseph Chandler, former orthopedic surgeon for the Atlanta Braves, examined numbers of pitches thrown by pitchers in the Little League World Series over several years (Chandler, 2011). He became interested after marveling at the skill of Little League pitchers but wondered why none ever went on to star in Major League Baseball. His research showed that starting pitchers (11-13 years old) on average pitched as much as or more than pitchers starting in the adult version of the World Series (around 90 pitches). Adult pitchers who throw more than 80 pitches in a game have four times the risk of injury leading to surgery compared to pitchers who throw less.

Chandler's other finding was that the throwing of breaking balls (curveballs and sliders) had increased substantially since 1990. These types of pitches have been historically implicated as causes of arm injuries, although recent research has suggested that overuse or the sheer number of pitches is a stronger predictor of arm injuries than the throwing of breaking balls (Valovich McLeod et al., 2011). However, these more advanced pitches require knowledgeable coaches to teach correct technique. Inappropriate throwing technique exacerbates the stress on the arm and predisposes kids to injury. Research shows that professional pitchers first threw curveballs at age 14, compared to the 11.6-year-old average of today (Chandler, 2011). They first threw sliders at 17.8 years, compared to 14.5 years today. The pros did not throw more than 75 pitches per game and did not play year-round baseball. They stated that they would not allow their sons to throw a curveball until age 15 or a slider until age 17.

Because some baseball pitchers believe they can throw harder after Tommy John surgery than before, some parents have pushed their children to have the surgery to enhance their throwing ability. This is absurd. Surgery is an extremely invasive process, with the possibility of many complications (e.g., scar tissue, arthritis, infection). Dr. Frank Jobe, who invented the Tommy John procedure (replacing the torn ligament with a tendon taken from somewhere else in the body), has emphatically stated that improved performance is not the goal of the surgery, and research evidence has shown that the surgery does not boost performance (Alexander, 2014).

Let's get out of the inappropriate arms race in youth baseball, which is costing young pitchers their health and their ability to play the game they love. We urge youth program leaders to implement developmentally appropriate rules to safeguard young pitchers' arms and well-being (see recommendations in table 12.2).

Table 12.2 Suggested Guidelines to Prevent Arm Injuries in Youth Baseball

Age	MAXIMUM NUMBER OF PITCHES			
	Per game	Per week	Per season	Per year
8-10	50	75	600	1,500
11-12	75	100	800	2,000
13-14	75	125	1,000	3,000
15-16	90	150	1,500	3,500
17-18	100	150	1,500	3,500

1. Children should not throw curveballs until age 14 (or not until they begin shaving!).

2. Children should not throw sliders until age 18.

3. Pitchers should not compete for more than eight months per year and should avoid overhead activities during the four months of rest.

4. At least a two-day rest is recommended between a series of competitive pitches.

5. Pitchers should avoid pitching with arm fatigue and arm pain.

6. Coaches or parents or both should systematically use pitch-count tracking sheets, available online from Little League Baseball.

7. Lighter baseballs may be used with younger pitchers.

8. Proper throwing mechanics must be emphasized and enforced by coaches to create a kinetic (movement) sequence by the entire body to transfer force in an efficient way.

9. Avoid backyard pitching after a pitched game or excessive practice between starts.

10. Avoid pitching on multiple teams with overlapping seasons.

11. Never use a radar gun, as it encourages overthrowing. Emphasize control, accuracy, and good mechanics.

Adapted from Magra, Caine, and Maffulli 2007; Valovich et al. 2011.

than the ligaments in the leg, which become tight and overstretched, causing inflammation and pain. The heel is especially susceptible to injury since the foot is one of the first parts of the body to grow to full size and the heel area is not very flexible. Again, no long-lasting damage typically occurs with Sever's disease, and young athletes can take time off depending on how much pain they're experiencing, and also use ice to reduce pain and swelling.

Little League Elbow

The term **Little League elbow** refers to apophysitis (inflammation) on the medial side (inside) of the elbow (you can feel the bony bump on the inside of the elbow, called epicondyle). This injury is named for Little League because it occurs predominately in youth baseball pitchers. Along with apophysitis, Little League elbow may involve avulsion fractures, with fragments or the entire epicondyle chipped off due to overuse. Avulsion of the medial epicondyle is the most common fracture in adolescent and preadolescent overhead throwing athletes (Magra & Maffulli, 2005).

Little League elbow is caused by throwing too much, which overstresses the muscles that bend the wrist, where they attach to the inner side of the elbow. The young athlete experiences pain, and perhaps swelling, on the inside of the elbow. Once the athlete (typically a baseball pitcher) experiences pain (even minimal pain), parents and coaches should immediately remove him from activity, apply ice, and ensure that a physician examines the child's arm and elbow. Remember that injuries to growing skeletons have the potential to be much more serious than in adults. Overuse in the form of too many overarm throws can have serious health consequences for youth athletes.

Strategies to Prevent Overuse Injuries in Youth Sport

Parents and coaches can find sport-specific guidelines similar to those in our baseball example in table 12.2 to prevent overuse injuries. For example, the U.S. Cycling Federation provides gear ratio limits for youth athletes; running organizations recommend maximum training distances for different age groups; and U.S. Swimming recommends numbers and lengths of sessions per week for various levels of age-group swimming. In addition, these are some general strategies to prevent overuse injuries in youth sport:

1. Teach young athletes to recognize and report even low-level aches and pains that are warning signs of possible overuse injuries in their specific sports.

2. Youth athletes should have at least one or two days per week off from organized physical training or competition. They should also have at least two to three months off per year from their particular sport. During this time, they may engage in cross-training in other sports and in fitness activities as a change of pace.

3. Coaches and parents should consider the practice in certain youth sports (volleyball, soccer, softball, baseball) of participating in weekend tournaments. In an attempt to maximize participation, young athletes often compete in these tournaments without adequate rest and recovery, which increases their risk of injuries. We worked with our daughter's soccer club to schedule mostly single games, keeping tournament play to a minimum. Everyone preferred this format, even the players.

4. Overuse injuries have been shown to decline in programs that incorporate structured warm-ups, including dynamic stretching, balance, and coordination exercises.

5. Use variety in practice to tax different skills and muscle groups, and use intervals of hard and easy activity to allow athletes to recover during training sessions.

6. Search the Internet for information related to training and injury occurrence in your sport. Incorrect information is often accepted as fact. For example, a common belief is that the windmill underarm pitching technique in softball is a natural motion that places little stress on the pitcher's arm. However, recent research has shown that this style of pitching adds as much stress and torque to the elbow and shoulder as does overarm pitching. Anterior (front) shoulder pain is a common overuse injury in female softball players.

PHYSEAL INJURIES

Because youth athletes are growing, it is particularly scary when sport injuries affect the longitudinal growth centers of the long bones (arm and leg bones). These are popularly called growth plate injuries, with the threatening outcome of interrupted growth or bone deformity. Although growth plate injuries are serious, the majority of them do not result in growth arrest.

Anatomy of a Growing Bone

All long bones have an area called the **epiphysis,** which is the rounded end of the bone (see figure 12.1). The long, middle part (or shaft) of the bone is the **diaphysis,** and the area where the bone gets wider at its end is the **metaphysis.** The growth plate, or **physis,** is located between the epiphysis and metaphysis in a growing child. The physis is made up of cartilage, a rubbery, flexible material that elongates as new bone tissue is produced.

When a child's bones have completed growing (or reached skeletal maturity), the growth plates ossify (harden) and the epiphysis fuses with the metaphysis to form a complete ossified bone. Longitudinal bone growth occurs in a complex biological

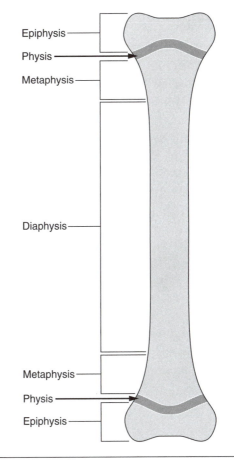

Epiphysis

Physis

Metaphysis

Diaphysis

Metaphysis

Physis

Epiphysis

Figure 12.1 Anatomy of a growing long bone.

process, in which special cells in the physeal plate proliferate, line up, and divide to lengthen the bone. Injuries that damage these cells are the most dangerous and may interrupt the normal growth process. (Note: The entire growth area is sometimes referred to as the epiphyseal plate, including the physis and epiphysis.)

Types of Physeal Injuries

Like other parts of the body, growth plates can be injured by acute trauma (e.g., fractures) or chronically through overuse. Generally, the physeal–epiphyseal area is more susceptible to acute injuries such as fractures, while the apophyses (tendon attachment sites discussed previously) typically incur more stress or overuse injuries.

Acute Physeal Injuries

A popular system for classifying acute physeal injuries was designed by Salter and Harris (1963) (shown in figure 12.2). Salter-Harris injuries are classified into five types on a scale of increasing seriousness. A useful way to remember these using the acronym SALTER is as follows.

Type I injuries ("S" for "straight across") involve a lateral fracture across the physis or a separation that increases the width of the physis (more space between the epiphysis

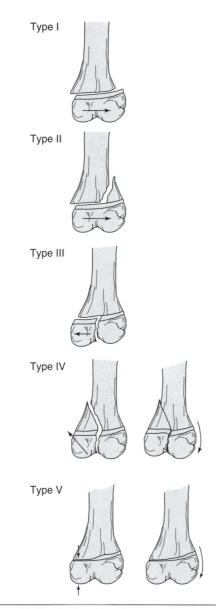

Type I

Type II

Type III

Type IV

Type V

Figure 12.2   Salter-Harris classification of physeal fractures.

and metaphysis). No ossified bone is fractured, and the growth cells within the physis are undisturbed. Healing of type I injuries is rapid, with rare complications; these injuries are often treated with a casting of the joint. However, this is a difficult injury to see on an X ray because it is across the cartilage area; thus it is often diagnosed clinically. Type I injuries tend to occur in younger children.

Type II injuries ("A" for "above"), the most common, include the separation in the physis as in type I injuries and a fracture out into the metaphysis of the bone. The triangular fracture of the metaphysis is what is seen on X rays. The epiphysis is not involved in the injury; thus type II injuries are usually not serious.

Type III injuries ("L" for "lower") are intra-articular (within the joint) fractures, through the physis and epiphysis. The site of these injuries makes them more serious, as fractures within the joint must be reduced (realigned by an orthopedic physician) perfectly and often require surgery.

Type IV injuries ("T" for "two" or "through") are even more serious because these fractures run through the metaphysis, physis, and epiphysis. Because the fracture is through the entire growth area and the joint, proper positioning (reduction) is essential, typically through surgery.

Type V injuries ("ER" for "erasure of the growth plate") are drastic compression injuries (e.g., from a fall from a significant height onto one's leg or from running into a wall or the hockey boards with the arm extended). There is a strong risk of growth arrest and bone deformity in type V injuries due to the crushing and destruction of the physeal growth plate.

When youth athletes complain of a sprain, parents and coaches should be mindful that a growth injury, even a fracture, is possible. Growth plates in kids are their weak links, and typical ankle injuries that result in sprains in adults often become fractures in kids. We want you to understand the different Salter-Harris types of injuries, but we urge you to be conservative and have even what seems to be a minor sprain in a young athlete examined by a physician. It is especially advantageous to see a pediatric orthopedist, who specializes in children's musculoskeletal injuries and who can more easily diagnose the problem. When our son broke his femur as a 2-year-old, we immediately sought treatment at a specialized children's hospital with pediatric orthopedic experts and received outstanding care and a positive outcome for our son.

Overuse Physeal Injuries

We've already discussed apophyseal injuries that occur on the bones' tendon attachment sites as the result of overuse. Physeal growth plates may also be damaged from chronic repetitive trauma that disrupts the growth cells in the physis. Widening as well as premature closure of growth plates of the wrist has been observed in youth gymnasts as a result of overuse.

Physeal injuries do occur in sport, ranging from 1% to 12% of injuries depending on the sport. Growth disturbances are rare, but possible; thus orthopedic injuries to growing children require special consideration by medical experts with experience in pediatric injuries. When fractures do occur, particularly at higher levels of the Salter-Harris scale, meticulous anatomical alignment and casting are needed to maintain the integrity of the bone and joint.

ANTERIOR CRUCIATE LIGAMENT INJURIES IN FEMALE ATHLETES

In the book *Warrior Girls*, Michael Sokolove (2008) chronicles the rise of anterior cruciate ligament (ACL) injuries in female athletes over the past few decades. He describes the career of Amy Steadman, who as a youth sport soccer phenom was destined to be one of the best soccer players of her generation

and a stalwart on the U.S. national team. The top high school defensive player in the United States and captain of the U.S. under-19 team, Steadman repeatedly battled knee injuries. By the age of 21, she had torn the ACL in her right knee three times and had undergone eight surgeries. Her career was over. And her future physical well-being was significantly altered. Individuals with injured ACLs have 10 times the risk of early-onset osteoarthritis compared to noninjured persons. Adolescents with ACL injuries have a high risk of suffering chronic pain and limitations from knee osteoarthritis by their 20s or 30s (Lohmander, Englund, Dahl, & Roos, 2007).

Anatomy and Role of the ACL

The ACL is one of two ligaments that form a cross (hence the term *cruciate*) under the kneecap. **Ligaments** are connective tissue that fasten bone to bone and stabilize a joint. As the *anterior* cruciate ligament, the ACL is in the front of the knee. The job of the ACL is to stabilize the knee by preventing the tibia (lower leg bone) from sliding forward beneath the femur (thigh bone), and it also limits rotational movements of the knee. It provides approximately 90% of the stability of the knee joint. This is a pretty big job for such a small body part. The ACL is smaller than a pinkie finger and is rectangular in shape, similar to a smoothed-out section of rubber band. When injuring an ACL, athletes feel pain and instability in the knee, giving rise, for example, to the sensation that the knee is giving out. When the ACL is torn, it cannot be sewn back together. Rather, a replacement graft is used, such as a tendon from somewhere else in the body, to construct a new ACL.

How ACL Injuries Occur

Although ACL injuries can occur through contact (e.g., hyperextension or buckling of the knee when a player is being tackled in football), 80% of these injuries occur in noncontact situations. Typical movements leading to the injury are planting and cutting, pivoting to change direction, suddenly decelerating, and landing from a jump.

A common body position noted in many ACL injuries is the *dynamic knee valgus,* which means the leg is moving toward a knock-kneed position and the foot pointed slightly outward (see the valgus position in figure 12.3). So such a movement is a risk factor for ACL injuries, as is individual anatomy or postural habits that create this position of the knee.

Who Gets ACL Injuries?

Anyone can experience an ACL tear, but certain people are more predisposed than others to the injury. Certainly, there are anatomical factors that contribute to this injury, based on the mechanisms of the injury as just discussed (e.g., greater knee valgus, or knock-knees). Anterior cruciate ligament injuries are rare in children younger than 12. Skeletally immature children are more likely to sustain fractures than ligament sprains or tears because their ligaments are stronger than their growing bones. Anterior cruciate ligament injury rates increase at age 12 for girls and 14 for boys.

Anterior cruciate ligament injuries are much more common in female athletes, with female athletes eight times more likely to tear their ACL than males. One in 10 female basketball and soccer players will tear an ACL. Sports medicine professionals have labeled this phenomenon an epidemic and have engaged in a great deal of research to ascertain why females are at such higher risk for ACL injuries.

Why Are Females at Greater Risk for ACL Injuries?

Several factors have been identified that predispose female athletes to ACL tears more than they do males.

Anatomic and Hormonal Reasons

In the knee joint, an intercondylar notch (or space) lies between the two rounded ends of the thigh bone. The ACL moves within this notch, connecting the thigh and shin bones. Females typically have narrower notches than males, providing more limited space for the ACL and a greater tendency for the ligament to be pinched during movement. Females also tend to have wider Q angles; the Q angle is a measure of knee alignment from the middle of the kneecap to the center of the hip. Often, the relatively wider hips and shorter femurs of females increase their Q angles, which has been linked to knee problems. Wider Q angles also lead to greater knee valgus (knees pointing inward or knock-knees), which has been linked to ACL injuries.

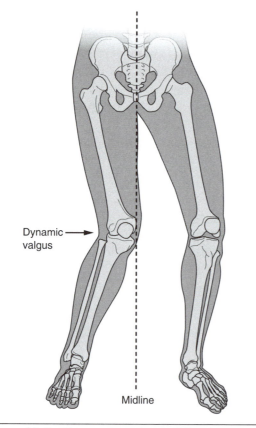

Dynamic valgus

Midline

Figure 12.3 Dynamic valgus of the knee, which increases vulnerability to anterior cruciate ligament injuries.

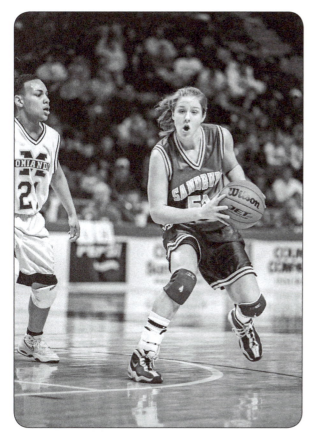

Female athletes are eight times more likely to tear their ACLs than male athletes.

Compared to males, females have a greater range of motion and "looser" knees. Research has also shown that the laxity of the ACL is related to changing hormone levels in females. For example, females are at greater risk for ACL injuries during the ovulatory phase of their menstrual cycle (Zazulak, Paterno, Myer, Romani, & Hewett, 2006).

Neuromuscular and Biomechanical Reasons

The anatomical differences that may predispose females to ACL injuries are interesting, but they're unchangeable. On the other hand, the neuromuscular and biomechanical factors that influence ACL injuries in female athletes may be addressed during training. Thus, we want you to understand these factors and consider ways you can help young female athletes avoid knee injuries, including ACL tears. Compared to males, females typically have less muscular strength, use the muscles in the front of the thighs (quadriceps) more for stability, and take a longer time to develop muscular force at a given moment. These factors result in greater stress on the ACL.

Incorrect or poor motor skill patterns have been shown to lead to ACL injuries. Less mature jumping patterns (less knee bend during landing from a jump, landing on flat feet vs. the toes or balls of the feet) expose the knee to more pressure and force. Sixty percent of ACL injuries in female basketball players occur during landing from a jump. Girls are less apt to reach the most mature stage of jumping compared to boys, as girls tend to use less knee flexion and more knee valgus when landing from jumps. Another immature motor pattern related to ACL tears is turning or pivoting in an upright position, and female athletes again show less knee flexion and more knee valgus when cutting and pivoting. Biomechanics experts have found that many girls run differently from boys, with less knee bend and an upright gait. They land harder from jumps and fail to decelerate as safely when slowing down to cut. These are motor skills that can be taught, practiced, and learned. The focus of youth sport practitioners (coaches, athletic trainers, strength and conditioning specialists), particularly in sports like basketball and soccer, should be to incorporate the training of fundamental movement skills and neuromuscular development designed to prevent ACL injuries.

Strategies to Prevent ACL Injuries

We can't say that the higher incidence of ACL injuries occurring in female athletes is based solely on anatomical differences. As with overuse injuries, it's often a combination of at-risk anatomical features and at-risk movement patterns. Neuromuscular and fundamental motor skill training programs designed to prevent ACL injuries in female athletes have been highly successful. Prevention programs in skiing, basketball, soccer, and team handball have shown a reduction in ACL injuries ranging from 60% to 89% (Silvers & Mandelbaum, 2007). For adolescent female athletes, prevention programs have reduced ACL injuries by 72% (Dharamsi & LaBella, 2013). These programs include a combination of warm-up, stretching, strengthening, plyometrics (repetitive explosive jumps), sport-specific agilities, and cool-down. An example is the Santa Monica PEP ACL Injury Prevention Program (http://smsmf.org/pep-program); other programs and sample training exercises are available on the Internet.

The emphasis in all these training programs is appropriate technique. During a jogging warm-up, girls should be told to keep their hips, knees, and ankles in straight alignment, without their knees caving in (valgus) or their feet whipping out to the side. In walking lunges to build strength, athletes are instructed to keep their front knee over their ankle and to avoid allowing their front knee to cave inward (valgus). The focus in the repetitive jumping activities (e.g., side to side, over lines or cones) is to land softly on the balls of the feet with flexed knees directly over their hips. If the athletes become fatigued and cannot perform the exercise with near-perfect technique, the exercise should be stopped. Proper technique is the goal.

With children under 12, continuous jumps should be over lines on the court or flat cones, emphasizing landing technique, not height of jump. Younger children should also do two-legged landings, with single leg jumps added after puberty. Adults should use verbal cues to familiarize young athletes with the desired movement, such as "knees over toes" or "light as a feather" (during landing). Provide feedback to athletes so they become aware of the feel of biomechanically efficient positions versus unsound body positions that put them at risk for injury.

A good basic posture to teach youth athletes is the *athletic position* (see figure 12.4)

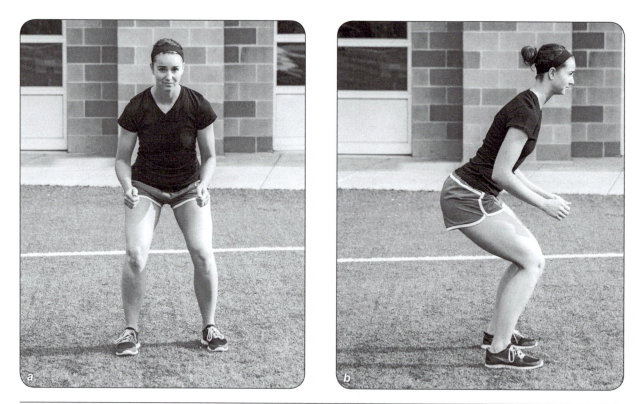

Figure 12.4   The athletic position: (*a*) front view and (*b*) side view.

(Myer, Ford, & Hewett, 2004). This is a stable, balanced position with knees flexed, eyes up, feet about shoulder-width apart, and body mass balanced over the balls of the feet. The knees should be over the balls of the feet, and the chest should be over the knees. Throughout training sessions, athletes can be repeatedly directed to take the athletic position so that over time it becomes habitual. Coaches can extend the standing athletic position by having athletes practice cutting and pivoting while maintaining this position. Coaches should incorporate such basic neuromuscular drills and training methods into daily practice sessions in sports that require cutting, jumping, running, and pivoting.

CONCUSSION IN YOUTH SPORT

Overuse, growth plate, and ACL injuries in children require our concern and attention. However, these injuries pale in comparison to the specter of traumatic brain injuries in young athletes. We are our brains; they are the control center for all aspects of our being, and unlike knees and elbows and other body parts, our brains are unfixable. They can't be cast, sutured, iced, taped, or replaced with a tendon—they can only be rested in hopes that they will heal on their own. And sometimes they don't. Eight high school football players died from traumatic brain injuries while playing the game in 2013 (Gregory, 2014).

How Concussions Occur in Sport

The term **concussion** comes from the Latin *concussus* ("striking together"). A concussion is an injury to the brain from a hit, tackle, fall, or impact that results in a period of neurological impairment (Moser, 2012). In the past 10 years, the number of 8- to 13-year-olds sustaining sport-related concussions has

doubled, while the number of 14- to 19-year-olds seeking treatment for head injuries has increased by more than 200%. The sport with the highest risk of concussion in high school is football. In girls' sports, the rate of concussion is highest in soccer and basketball. Rugby, ice hockey, and lacrosse also have higher rates of concussion compared to other youth sports.

Sport-related concussions are typically caused by acceleration and deceleration. Blows to the head are acceleration examples, as when an American football player is tackled with a vicious hit to the head. Deceleration occurs when athletes strike their head against a relatively stationary object, as in when players are slammed onto the floor in basketball, when they make a helmet-first tackle in American football, or when they smash heads with a soccer opponent going up for a header. Concussions are also caused by violent rotation of the head in reaction to a blow—for example, when a player is body-checked from the blind side in ice hockey.

Inside the skull, the brain floats in a cushion of cerebrospinal fluid. When a blow or strong force is applied—for example, when helmets clash in football—the head decelerates instantly, but the brain keeps traveling inside the skull and slams into the side of the skull. (This is why helmets do not protect American football players from concussion. Helmets prevent scalp lacerations and skull fractures, but not concussions.) This impact causes bruising of the brain and the neurological impairment of concussion. The twisting motion stretches and strains nerve cells in the brain so that their ability to send and receive messages from the rest of the body is disrupted.

The impact disrupts the brain's delicate electrochemical balance, causing it to go into crisis mode. Crisis mode means that the brain, a pretty smart organ, immediately directs all its energy (glucose) toward protecting itself and attempting to heal the injury. As this happens, energy needed for other regular brain functions (memory, concentration, motor control) is not available, so these processes are impaired. Throughout the recovery process—which may be days or weeks or even longer—the brain remains in a state of metabolic depression, as the injury exhausts the brain's ability to function (Moser, 2012). This is why complete mental and physical rest is critical to allow the brain to heal itself. This often means no text messaging, video games, computer use, homework, reading, and even limited television in an effort to completely rest the brain after a concussion (Moser, 2012). Of course, a physician should prescribe activity limits and amount of rest for youth athletes who have suffered a concussion.

Vulnerability to Concussion

Children's and adolescents' brains are more vulnerable to concussion than adults'. Youth athletes have incomplete myelination of brain axons, relatively bigger heads and smaller neck muscles, thinner cranial bones, and less efficient motor skills and body control as compared to adult athletes. High school football players are at three times greater risk for catastrophic head injuries than college players. Children's concussion symptoms are often delayed so that the severity of the injury is not apparent until days later. Complicating the matter, children may be more unaware of symptoms of what can be a life-threatening injury; and when made aware, they often hide their symptoms to avoid having to miss competition. When asked why they didn't report concussion symptoms, high school athletes said they didn't think the symptoms were serious enough to bring up (66%), didn't want to leave the game (44%), and didn't want to let their team down (22%) (Gregory, 2010).

Mounting evidence indicates that females are more susceptible to concussion than males; and when compared to males, females experience more severe and long-lasting symptoms (Moser, 2012). Among soccer players, girls are 68% more likely than boys

to sustain concussions. Various reasons are offered (differences in brain anatomy, hormones, neck musculature, more honesty in reporting symptoms), but no conclusive explanations have been established.

Youth who've already had a concussion are four to six times more likely to get another than they would be otherwise. Youth athletes are particularly vulnerable to **second impact syndrome** (SIS), a catastrophic brain injury that occurs when an athlete suffers a second head injury before fully recovering from the first. Second impact syndrome causes severe and irreversible brain damage and is fatal in about half of the cases.

Signs of Concussion in Youth Athletes

Parents and coaches may observe several signs that an athlete has been concussed, which fall into four categories: physical, cognitive, emotional, and sleep. Headache is the most frequently reported symptom, yet any one of these signs may be indicative of concussion. Loss of consciousness occurs in less than 10% of concussions. Other physical symptoms include nausea, vomiting, balance and visual problems, fatigue, sensitivity to light, and feeling dazed or stunned. Cognitive symptoms include feeling mentally foggy or slowed down, difficulty concentrating and remembering, confusion about recent events, and answering questions slowly or repeating them. Emotional symptoms include irritability, sadness, nervousness, and feeling more emotional. Sleep can also be affected by concussion, and drowsiness, difficulty falling asleep, and sleeping more or less than usual can be symptoms (Halstead & Walter, 2010).

Sideline Assessment

If a young athlete is involved in a concussion-like situation, a responsible adult should assess on the sideline for immediate symptoms. This involves asking questions to see how well oriented the athlete is and also how he is feeling at the moment. The best-case scenario is for a certified athletic trainer to do the assessment. Certified health professionals may use one of several available sideline assessment tools that include questions to evaluate an athlete's orientation and memory and assessments of their postural stability in different positions (Halstead & Walter, 2010).

Because most youth sport teams don't have athletic trainers, coaches, parents, or both should be able to do a cursory assessment by observing behavior and asking simple questions. Remember that this initial assessment is only to verify whether a concussion may have occurred—it cannot determine the severity of the concussion. If a concussion is suspected, the athlete should immediately be removed from activity and prompt medical attention should be obtained (e.g., hospital emergency care).

Decisions About Return to Play

Symptoms may linger for weeks or even months. No athlete should ever be allowed to return to play if she is experiencing any symptoms. It doesn't matter how severe the symptoms are; the presence of any symptoms indicates that the brain is still recovering. Concussion experts warn against arbitrary rules, like being allowed to return 24 hours or three days after the injury. Concussions must be managed on a case-by-case basis, and return-to-play decisions should be made by medical doctors. When in doubt, sit them out!

Long-Term Consequences of Concussion

High school athletes with a history of two or more concussions experience more cognitive (academic) and emotional problems than athletes without any concussion history (Moser, 2012). Concussed athletes who previously were good students may struggle with grades and have lingering physical symptoms such as headaches, dizziness, and blurred vision. In addition, emerging evidence is painting a sobering picture of the long-term effects of concussion.

In 2011, 75 former professional football players, along with some former players' wives, sued the National Football League (NFL). The suit stated that the league knew about the long-term effects of multiple concussions, including brain damage, dementia, and depression, but kept this information from the players. A growing number (over 40) of former football players' brains, examined after their death, have shown signs of a degenerative brain disease known as chronic traumatic encephalopathy (CTE). Although most of the brains examined were of older, retired athletes, brain autopsies of football players who died in their 20s have shown early stages of CTE. A typical person aged 30 to 49 has a 1 in 1,000 chance of suffering dementia or Alzheimer's disease. A retired NFL player in the same age range has a 1 in 53 chance of getting the same diagnosis (Gregory, 2010). Depression and suicide in former NFL and National Hockey League players have been associated with multiple concussions (Caron, Bloom, Johnston, & Sabiston, 2013).

Why are we presenting these statistics in a book about youth sport? We do it to open the eyes of a culture that resists change in traditional sporting activities that literally destroy the lives of many of their participants. In a 2013 national poll, one-third of Americans said they were hesitant to allow their children to play football because of the risk of concussion. Although there is always a risk of injury in sport, particularly in collision sports like American football, the growing concern about brain injuries may serve to change participation patterns in sport in the United States. From 2007 to 2013, tackle football participation fell 26.5% among U.S. kids ages 6 to 12 (Gregory, 2014). A September 2014 cover of *Time* magazine posed the question "Is football worth it?" alongside a picture of 16-year-old Chad Stover, who died of a traumatic brain injury in a high school game in Missouri. We offer sincere condolences to the Stover family.

Strategies to Prevent and Effectively Respond to Concussion in Youth Sport

1. Parents, coaches, or both should talk directly with youth athletes about the dangers and symptoms of concussion. Be frank, even severe, about the dangers of head injuries, including death if the injuries are unreported. Go over the symptoms of concussion, and ask the athletes to commit to fully disclosing symptoms. Address the harmful cultural practice of hiding or playing with injuries, and perhaps invite a well-known athlete to speak with athletes about concussion. Reported concussion rates doubled for high school football players from 2005 through the 2013-2014 school year (Gregory, 2014). This increase suggests that there is more awareness and honest reporting of concussion symptoms by athletes, parents, and coaches.

2. If possible, implement neurocognitive baseline testing with athletes, such as the Immediate Post-Concussion Assessment and Cognitive Test (ImPACT), which is used by many professional and college athletic programs. These computerized programs assess athletes in the preseason (baseline) on different aspects of cognitive function, such as attention, memory, processing speed, and reaction time. If and when an athlete sustains a concussion, he is retested and scores are compared. Athletes must perform at their baseline measure level before being allowed to return to play.

3. Require that coaches become educated and advocate that parents educate themselves about concussion in youth sport. The National Federation of High School Athletic Associations offers an online program,

Concussion in Sports (www.nfhslearn.com/courses/38000). This free online course includes the return-to-play guidelines required in each state for middle and high schools. Forty-seven states and the District of Columbia have enacted strong youth sport concussion safety laws since 2009.

4. Provide parents and coaches with fact sheets about concussion, such as "Heads Up: Concussion in High School Sports," available from the Centers for Disease Control and Prevention (CDC), or information on state programs (www.healthyohioprogram.org/concussion).

5. Youth sport leaders and coaches should proactively consider important changes in rules, policies, and sport techniques to help protect youth athletes from head injuries. For example, the 1976 rule change in college and high school football to disallow spearing, or deliberate use of the helmet as the initial point of contact with opponents, resulted in an 87% decrease in catastrophic cervical spine injuries (causing quadriplegia). The old teaching technique "face in the numbers" was replaced with "see what you hit" to protect players from these injuries. USA Football offers the Heads Up football education–certification program that includes concussion awareness and heads-up tackling information (usafootball.com).

Pop Warner youth football responded to growing concussion concerns by limiting contact during practices. No full-speed head-on blocking or tackling drills are allowed when the players are lined up more than 3 yards (2.7 meters) apart. Also, the amount of contact at each practice was reduced to a maximum of one-third of practice time, including any drills or scrimmages. USA Hockey increased the checking age in ice hockey from 11 to 13 years. And U.S. Lacrosse introduced rule changes at the high school and college levels to prohibit any contact to an opponent's head, also outlining a progressive introduction of body contact at younger levels based on developmental levels of the players. Although preventing all concussions is impossible in sport, these rule changes are significant steps toward reducing the risk of concussion for youth athletes.

LEGAL DUTIES AND THE EMERGENCY ACTION PLAN

Managing injuries in youth sport starts with comprehensive planning and the implementation of policies and procedures before training and competition begins. Youth sport leaders should understand their legal duties in relation to injuries and the importance of developing a practical emergency action plan in response to serious injuries.

Legal Duties Related to Injury Prevention and Management

To avoid claims of negligence, youth sport directors and coaches must fulfill several legal duties to prevent and manage injuries. Negligence may occur because of an inappropriate act (requiring full-pads football practice on an extremely hot and humid day without adequate breaks and hydration) or failure to act (not teaching appropriate football tackling technique). The legal duties of coaches are specifically outlined in chapter 14 as a part of the managerial responsibilities of youth coaches (also see Martens, 2012).

Youth sport leaders must be acutely aware of these duties, particularly in relation to the prevention and management of injuries. Providing appropriate emergency assistance, evaluating athletes for injury and capacity, providing proper instruction, warning of inherent injury risks (e.g., what can happen if you tackle with your head down in football), and providing safe physical environments and equipment are critical duties related to preventing and responding to injuries.

For example, teaching outdated tackling technique in football (e.g., spearing or leading with the helmet) is negligent because it fails to fulfill the legal duty of providing proper instruction. If a young baseball player launches himself into a headfirst dive at the catcher at home plate and incurs a traumatic brain injury or spinal cord injury, the coach could be found negligent for not warning players that this action could result in serious injury. So coaches should not only teach and emphasize the use of proper technique; they should also repeatedly warn young athletes about the dangers of certain actions that could lead to serious injury.

The Emergency Action Plan

The duty of providing appropriate medical assistance to injured athletes requires youth sport programs to develop and rehearse emergency action plans (EAPs). The EAP is an established procedure for dealing with serious injuries that occur in a youth sport event. Specific examples of EAPs are plentiful on the Internet, and EAP templates and forms are also available (e.g., at www.nays.org/resources/emergency-action-plan.cfm). A sample EAP template is provided in appendix K. The following are the primary areas of preparation and information needed in an EAP.

Personnel

Designate specific adults who will definitely be present at the site for required EAP duties. There are various ways you can divide up duties, and we provide one example here. Remember that these individuals must be designated to fulfill these duties in advance. That's why the plan is called an emergency action plan. When a medical emergency occurs, everyone should be aware of her specific duties in the situation and immediately act in fulfilling her prescribed responsibilities.

One adult is designated as the care person—he attends to the injured athlete and provides appropriate first aid and care. Obviously, this person should be certified in first aid and cardiopulmonary resuscitation (CPR). In the best case this would be a certified athletic trainer, but in many youth sport situations it will have to be a coach.

The second designee is the communications person—she makes the telephone call for emergency assistance, explains the situation, and provides directions to the site to the emergency medical services (EMS) crew; guides the ambulance or health care professionals in and out of the facility; and contacts and continues to communicate with parents or the athlete's designated emergency contact.

The third designee is the charge person—he secures a calm and controlled environment by controlling bystanders and those who have access to the injured athlete, and works with officials, coaches, and players to explain the situation and decide whether the event should continue. The charge person may also be tasked with contacting supervisors, athletic directors, or other people in the program who should be aware of the situation. This allows the communications person to focus specifically on medical assistance for the injured athlete and support for the athlete's family.

One person should be responsible for the team first-aid kit and any other emergency equipment for the site (e.g., ice). One person should also be responsible for the athlete medical emergency forms that should be on-site for every event.

Information on Participants

An athlete medical emergency card or roster should be on-site for every event. This should include the name and phone numbers for an emergency contact person (typically parents), any preexisting medical conditions (e.g., epilepsy, diabetes, asthma), and current prescription medication. Copies of this form should be available to the care and communication persons and made available to the EMS responders if needed. This information is confidential and should not be made public or shared with other parents or athletes on the team.

Phones Numbers and Site Addresses and Directions

Cell phones with service should be on-site and immediately available to the communications person. Additionally, the EAP should include a list of important phone numbers, such as those of EMS, head and assistant coaches, park supervisor, director of athletics, a consulting physician on call, and the nearest hospital emergency room. All facility addresses should be on the EAP; this may require multiple addresses—for example, in recreational league basketball where games are scheduled in different gyms throughout the season.

Directions to every site should be prepared and provided in the EAP. These can be communicated to the EMS personnel to ensure their immediate arrival. The opening of locked gates and clearing of other obstacles to access for the EMS crew should be part of the EAP as well. In our EAP example, this would be the responsibility of the communications person.

The responsibilities and procedures outlined here can and should be customized for each youth sport situation. However, these basic elements of an EAP should be included. Appendix K illustrates how an EAP might look in written form.

WRAP-UP

Injuries are a part of youth sport. We can't eradicate them—even severe injuries happen despite developmentally appropriate training and coaching. We can focus on the "controllables": effective instruction, injury prevention activities and training for specific sports, an EAP with clear responsibilities that have been rehearsed, and coaching education and certification. And we can continue to advocate for developmentally appropriate rule changes and cultural shifts in attitudes to move beyond the "shake it off, tough it out" ethos that places children at risk for disabling and even life-threatening injuries.

LEARNING AIDS

Key Terms

apophysis—Where a tendon inserts on a growing bone.

apophysitis—Inflammation on the area of the growing bone where the tendon attaches.

concussion—An injury to the brain from a hit, tackle, fall, or impact that results in a period of neurological impairment.

contusion—Bruise.

diaphysis—The long, middle part (or shaft) of the bone.

epiphysis—The rounded end of the bone.

ligament—Connective tissue that fastens bone to bone.

Little League elbow—Apophysitis (inflammation) on the medial side (inside) of the elbow.

metaphysis—The area where the bone gets wider at its end.

Osgood-Schlatter disease—Apophysitis of the knee that occurs in young athletes during their adolescent growth spurt.

overuse injury—Microtraumatic damage to a body part (e.g., bone, muscle, tendon) that has been subjected to repetitive stress without sufficient time to heal or recover.

physis—The growth plate located between the epiphysis and metaphysis in a growing long bone.

second impact syndrome—A catastrophic brain injury that occurs when a young athlete suffers a second head injury before fully recovering from the first.

Sever's disease—Apophysitis of the heel, caused by repetitive stress on the Achilles tendon.

sprain—Overstressing a ligament.

strain—Exerting a muscle beyond its limit.

stress fractures—Skeletal defects (usually hairline cracks) that result from the repeated application of a stress lower than that required to fracture a bone in a single blow or loading.

Summary Points

1. Several physical differences between youth and adult athletes make kids more vulnerable to injury.

2. About half of all youth sport injuries are caused by overuse, and more than half of all youth sport injuries are preventable.

3. Overuse injuries are caused by a combination of environmental and athlete factors.

4. Three overuse-type injuries that affect the apophyses of growing bones are Osgood-Schlatter disease, Sever's disease, and Little League elbow.

5. Overuse of young baseball pitchers has led to a large increase in elbow injuries, including tears of the ulnar collateral ligament, resulting in Tommy John surgery.

6. Physeal, or growth plate, injuries may be classified into five types, from most benign to most serious.

7. Female athletes in sports that emphasize planting and cutting (soccer, basketball) are more susceptible than others to knee injuries, including tears of the anterior cruciate ligament (ACL).

8. Youth coaches and strength and conditioning specialists can reduce knee injuries in girls' sports through neuromuscular and fundamental motor skill training.

9. Sport concussions result from acceleration and deceleration, which cause the brain to slam into the side of the skull.

10. Neurocognitive tests are used by many colleges and some high schools as an assessment method to determine when an athlete may return to activity.

Study Questions

1. Identify several characteristics of youth athletes that make them more vulnerable to injuries than adults.

2. List the multiple environmental and personal factors that cause overuse injuries in youth athletes.

3. What is apophysitis, and why is it a type of overuse injury in kids? Give three examples of where it commonly occurs in youth athletes.

4. Describe anatomically how long bones grow in children and provide some examples of how injuries can damage the growth plate area. What types of growth plate injuries are more serious and why?

5. Explain the various reasons female athletes in basketball and soccer tend to tear their anterior cruciate ligament more than male athletes in similar sports.

6. Provide specific examples of what youth sport coaches can do to help young girls protect against knee injuries.

7. Why do American football or hockey helmets not prevent concussions? In your answer, explain anatomically and physiologically how concussions occur and how the brain responds to concussion.

8. Why are youth athletes more vulnerable to concussion than adult athletes?

9. Identify several concussion symptoms, and explain how coaches or parents can immediately assess for symptoms when a concussion is suspected.

10. What strategies would you use as a youth sport coach to attempt to deal with concussions in your sport?

Reflective Learning Activities

1. Choose a specific sport. Research the injury epidemiology for youth in this sport, and describe the types of injuries common in the sport. Based on the nature of injuries in the sport, identify several ideas about injury prevention that could be implemented.

2. Design a 15- to 20-minute prepractice program that could be implemented with female youth soccer players to prevent ACL injuries. You should engage in some independent research to find examples of these types of programs. Illustrate how you would set up a field area for a group of girls to do this program each day at the start of soccer practice.

3. What is your prediction for the future of American football given the concussion epidemic and emerging data showing long-term brain degeneration in football players?

Resource Guide

Flegel, M.J. (2014). *Sport first aid* (5th ed.). Champaign, IL: Human Kinetics.

Moser, R.S. (2012). *Ahead of the game: The parents' guide to youth sports concussion.* Hanover, NH: Dartmouth College.

Concussion in Sports, NFHS free online course (www.nfhslearn.com).

First Aid, Health and Safety for Coaches, NFHS certification course (www.nfhslearn.com).

Heads Up: Concussion in Youth Sports, online training course and fact sheets (www.cdc.gov/concussion/pdf/Coach_Guide-a.pdf).

Sport First Aid, Human Kinetics Coach Education, online course (www.HumanKineticsCoachEducationCenter.com).

part IV

Social Considerations in Youth Sport

Welcome to part IV of *Best Practice for Youth Sport,* in which you'll find out about different social influences on youth sport. Here's a sampling of things you'll learn in the next four chapters:

- The harmful effects of rigid stereotypes, such as gender and racial stereotypes, on youth sport
- How you can increase your cultural competence as a youth sport leader
- Why sport doesn't build character, but how coaches and parents can help youth athletes develop life skills and higher levels of moral reasoning
- The skill sets needed by youth sport coaches
- How parents influence youth athletes

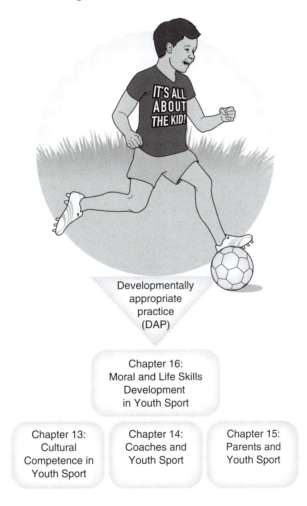

Developmentally
appropriate
practice
(DAP)

Chapter 16:
Moral and Life Skills
Development
in Youth Sport

Chapter 13:
Cultural
Competence in
Youth Sport

Chapter 14:
Coaches and
Youth Sport

Chapter 15:
Parents and
Youth Sport

The chapters in this section help you understand the constellation of social influences swirling around youth sport. Our job is to help align all the stars in this constellation to ensure a just and supportive social environment so that kids enjoy and benefit from youth sport.

CULTURAL COMPETENCE IN YOUTH SPORT

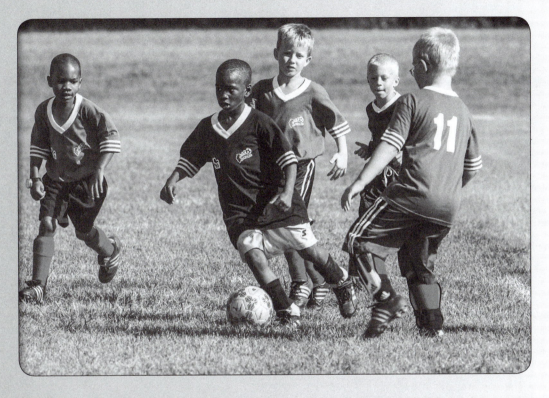

CHAPTER PREVIEW

In this chapter, you'll learn

> » that males and females are more alike than different,
>
> » how gender and racial stereotyping damages youth sport participants, and
>
> » ways to become more culturally competent as a youth sport leader.

Two wrestlers on your middle school team refuse to wrestle in an upcoming meet because they are slated to compete against girls in their weight classes. Or, you're a high school basketball coach, and a young athlete discloses to you that he is gay and would like your support and guidance in talking to teammates about his sexuality. Or, some white players on your 7- and 8-year-old girls' soccer team start calling two African American teammates nappy-heads, which they think of as friendly fun, because they heard this term from an adult. Or, a Muslim girl joins your club tennis team, and other members of the team ask you why she has to wear a hijab and long sleeves on hot training days.

Do you feel prepared to handle these situations? Don't worry if your answer is no, because these would be challenging situations for all of us. Responding effectively in such situations requires **cultural competence,** which is our ability to interact effectively with people of different cultures, subcultures, and backgrounds. Cultural competence also involves being aware of our own cultural identity and personal views about difference. All of us working in youth sport need to enhance our cultural competence. Our culture continues to become more diverse, challenging us to broaden our understanding of subcultural groups different from ours.

CONTINUUM OF CULTURAL COMPETENCE

One's level of cultural competence may be thought of as falling on a continuum as shown in table 13.1 (adapted from Cross, Bazron, Dennis, & Isaacs, 1999). Although our goal is to be culturally competent, many of us fall into the categories of cultural precompetence, cultural blindness, or cultural incapacity. Those of us at the cultural precompetence level would like to be more competent, but we fail to engage in the education and self-reflection needed to become more culturally aware. At this level, people often engage in **tokenism,** which is a superficial action, similar to "going through the motions," to be inclusive of members of different groups. The tokenism example in table 13.1 is inviting a woman to be an assistant coach just to have a female coach but not including her in any significant planning or decision making.

Table 13.1   Continuum of Cultural Competence

Level	Description	Examples
Cultural competence	Acceptance of and respect for difference; continuing self-assessment regarding cultural understanding; careful attention to the dynamics of difference	Intolerance of sexist comments made by boys (and teaching them why this is inappropriate); learning some basic sign language to communicate with a hearing-impaired athlete
Cultural precompetence	Desire but no clear plan or behavioral intention to achieve cultural competence; tokenism	Inviting a female to be assistant coach but not incorporating her into team planning or involving her in any decision making
Cultural blindness	Perception of oneself as totally unbiased and that all people are the same; encourages assimilation; ignores cultural strengths and advantages of diversity	"I don't see color. I treat everyone the same"; expecting all athletes to wear clothes and hairstyles of the dominant culture
Cultural incapacity	No intention to be culturally destructive but lacking the ability to respond effectively to diverse people	Lower effort or performance standards for female athletes; stereotyping African American athletes to play certain sport positions
Cultural destructiveness	Beliefs, actions, and policies that are damaging to cultures	Exclusion of girls from sport; ridiculing gay and lesbian athletes; making racist, sexist, or homophobic comments

Cultural blindness is seen when people invoke the classic "I don't see color. I treat everyone the same." Youth athletes are not all the same—they have different needs, personalities, motivation, faiths, beliefs, and backgrounds. Treating everyone the same typically means assuming that everyone fits with the dominant cultural practices of the day. Telling your 7- and 8-year-old soccer players to kick the ball around at home with their dads assumes that everyone has a father at home (and that moms can't pass soccer balls!). Asking members of a female high school swim team not to spend the meet texting with their boyfriends assumes that they're all heterosexual. Sameness is not fairness, and actually, treating everyone the same is unfair. Would you penalize one of your field hockey players for not attending practice on Yom Kippur, the holiest day of the year for Jewish people? We hope not. Embracing cultural diversity and uniqueness takes more work because it makes us move outside our cultural comfort zones, but the message of acceptance and support has a powerful effect on the well-being of kids in sport and our society as a whole.

Cultural incapacity involves behaviors that are not intended to be destructive but that are destructive in subtle ways. By assuming that girls are not as serious, motivated, and skilled as boys, coaches are cheating them of the challenge and skill development they need. A golf instructor who tells an African American youth "Not many African Americans play golf and you don't see many on the pro tour" could certainly affect the child's level of aspiration or even how appropriate and comfortable he feels in taking lessons.

Cultural destructiveness damages our culture and all the people in it by deliberately discriminating against people of different subcultures. It took the passage of Title IX of the Educational Amendments Act (discussed in chapter 2) and years of lawsuits and dogged advocacy to open up sport opportunities for girls and women. The derogation of females, as well as of gay and lesbian athletes, is common in the masculine culture of competitive sport (Woods, 2011). Even tacit acceptance of (or ignoring) sexist, racist, and homophobic comments and "jokes" is culturally destructive. We can't ignore our responsibility for cultural competence. All of us can improve our cultural competence to make youth sport more inclusive, open, and accepting.

Many aspects of cultural understanding are important in youth sport, but to explore all of them is beyond the scope of this book. We will at least identify what we view as important areas of cultural competence for youth sport professionals, and we urge you to seek out additional information to help you on your continued journey toward cultural competence. In chapter 1, we identified several barriers to youth sport participation, including sex, race, ethnicity, socioeconomic status, and disabilities. The purpose of the information in chapter 1 was to introduce you to the "face" of youth sport, including barriers to participation for certain types

Personal Plug-In

How Culturally Competent Are You?

Look over the levels of the continuum of cultural competence. Reflect on your personal cultural competence in relation to the scenarios presented at the beginning of the chapter. What level are you at right now? Has your cultural competence changed over time, and if so, what contributed to this change? It's okay if you don't feel culturally competent in all situations. The important thing is to increase your awareness about cultural competence—to commit to enhance your competence in relation to specific cultural challenges.

of kids. In this chapter, the focus is more on increasing your awareness of and ability to understand cultural and subcultural differences to enhance the experience of youth sport for all participants (as well as to enhance the culture as a whole). The area that we give the most attention to in this chapter is gender, due to its critical influence on youth sport (e.g., gender equity, gender stereotyping in sport).

GENDER AND YOUTH SPORT

No subcultural group that we belong to affects us more than gender. From the moment of birth (and even beforehand, as parents and families prepare for a baby girl or boy), females and males are talked to, handled, and viewed differently by adults. **Gender** refers to the characteristics, behaviors, and activities that society considers appropriate for females and males, typically labeled as feminine and masculine. **Sex,** as in sex differences reported in the news or research, is a biological characteristic based on a person's chromosomes, hormonal profiles, and internal and external reproductive organs.

So, sex is biological and fixed, whereas gender is culturally constructed and fluid. For example, that there are more male than female high school wrestlers in the United States is a gender difference. That the average height of adult males is greater than the average height of adult females is a sex difference. This distinction is important, because when certain differences are erroneously labeled sex differences (but are really gender differences), we tend to assume that males and females biologically differ on culturally constructed characteristics. Some males who battled the implementation of gender equity policies after the passage of Title IX (discussed in chapter 2) argued that females were not as interested in participating in sport as males. This argument incorrectly presumed that females were

biologically different from males in the types of activities they became interested in participating in. Clearly, the cultural history of sport as a masculine activity created a huge gender difference in opportunities for girls to participate in sport.

More Similar Than Different: Sex and Gender Overlap

When you read a magazine article stating that girls are more flexible than boys or that boys are stronger than girls, it is often assumed this means that all girls are more flexible than all boys and that all boys are stronger than all girls. Of course this isn't true. What these articles are referring to are average differences for a certain group or population (or statistical differences between means). The problem is that when we read about these averages, we often simplistically infer that these differences apply to all people. They don't. There are more similarities than differences between males and females (Horn et al., 2015; Hyde, 2005).

To understand sex and gender differences and similarities, it's helpful to visualize how various characteristics are spread across entire groups of males and females (Hyde, 2005; Ulrich, 1987). The five sets of lines shown in figure 13.1 represent sex or gender similarities and differences. Males and females are more or less similar or different based on each set of lines. Each set has a male (M) and a female (F) line, and each line is marked at its highest, average, and lowest point. To help you understand the concept of overlapping lines, let's identify physical or motor performance characteristics that fit each set of lines.

Total Overlap

The A set of lines represents total overlap, or no differences, between males and females. The age at which babies achieve the various motor milestones of infancy (rolling over, turning head, pulling up, crawling, walking) does not differ between girls and boys. It's

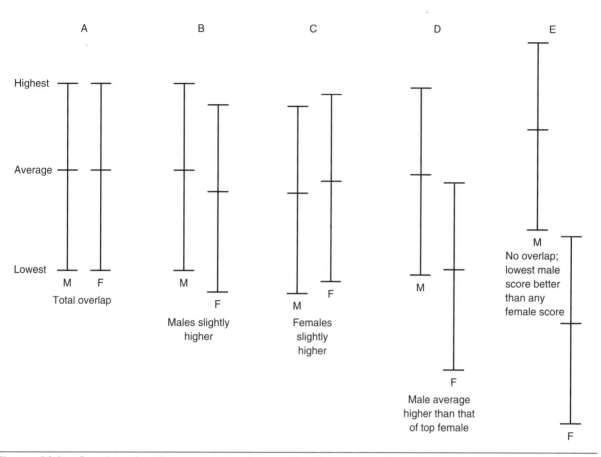

Figure 13.1 Overlapping lines representing similarities and differences based on sex or gender.

noteworthy that many characteristics of newborns and infants completely overlap. Another characteristic shared by males and females is their gain in weight and height from infancy to puberty. Even though our society often chooses to separate prepubescent boys and girls in youth sport programs, there are no physical reasons to do so.

Males Slightly Higher

The B set of lines represents characteristics on which males are slighter higher than females. Height at adulthood is a good example (5 feet, 9 inches [175 centimeters] average for males and 5 feet, 4 inches [163 centimeters] average for females). Postpubescent upper-body strength would also fit this set of lines, as would proficiency in throwing and catching in childhood. However, even though males on average are taller than females in adulthood, many

adult women are taller than adult men (as represented by the upper part of the female line in the B set of lines). The same is true for postpubescent upper-body strength. On average, postpubescent males are stronger in their upper body than females, yet the overlap between the lines indicates that a lot of women are stronger than a lot of men. Even though the average or mean for males is higher in the B set of lines, there are many females who score higher than men on these characteristics. The overlapping lines remind us that gender and sex differences are based on averages and that there is great variability (and similarity) beyond the basic mean differences between the sexes.

Females Slightly Higher

The C set of lines represents characteristics on which females are slightly higher or ahead of males. Characteristics that fit this set of lines include flexibility, fine motor skills during childhood, amount of body fat after puberty, and the timing of biological maturation (girls mature at an earlier age). But again, remember that there is a lot of overlap—these lines are not that different. Many males are more flexible as compared to females, have better fine motor skills during childhood, have more body fat after puberty, and mature at an earlier age. The lines show us that on average, females are ahead; but don't make the mistake of assuming that all females are higher in these characteristics. That assumption is untrue and is illustrated quite clearly in the amount of overlap in the two lines.

Male Average Higher Than That of Top Female

Now it gets harder. The D set of lines represents characteristics on which the average male score is higher than that of the top female. Many times students in our classes use examples like driving distance in golf or sprinting speed for this set of lines. But think about it. Across the population (let's choose teenagers in the United States), could the average teenage boy drive a golf ball farther than the best teenage girl golf driver in the country? Would the average 100-meter sprint time of all teenage boys be faster than that of the fastest teenage girl in the United States? Of course not.

The trick in identifying characteristics for the D lines is that you have to narrow your sample and not include the entire population. For example, let's choose the top 300 male and female golf professionals to examine driving distance. The average driving distance of the top 300 male professional golfers is the same as that of the top female golf professionals (about 275 yards, or about 251 meters). However, there are still some female professionals who drive the ball farther than some male professionals, as illustrated by the overlap in the gender lines. Most examples that fit the D set of

lines involve smaller samples of physically trained postpubescent athletes.

No Overlap at All

The E set of lines illustrates no overlap at all between males and females, with the lowest male score better than any female score. The easiest examples of this are biological ones, such as sperm production or size of reproductive organs. You could also choose elite, trained athletes, such as 100-meter sprinters competing in the Olympics, or elite power lifters.

Significance of the Overlapping Lines Concept

What set of lines do you think most people have in mind when making decisions in youth sport about athletes' abilities, support for training, and whether youth sports should be mixed or separate by sex? The relationships between male and female performance and body characteristics in youth sport are almost always represented by the first three sets of lines. Yet our culture automatically thinks of gender as depicted in the D and E sets of lines, and policy decisions in youth sport are often made based on this thinking. Cultural competence includes understanding the overlap that typically occurs between girls and boys in youth sport. For skill instruction and competition before puberty, skill level may be a more useful way to group youth athletes than gender.

Average Gender Differences in Physical Characteristics and Motor Skills

Now that we've contemplated gender overlap, we can identify several average gender differences apparent in the physical characteristics and motor skills of females and males. These differences tend to start small and then increase through childhood and particularly after adolescence. With regard to strength, speed, and aerobic endurance, there are small differences between girls and boys before age 12 but considerable differences after this age, with males growing stronger and faster with more endurance capabilities. Females are more flexible and have better fine motor skills at all ages, but these differences are not large. Gender differences also are apparent in fundamental motor skills. Females are better than males at hopping, skipping, and leaping, while males are better at manipulative skills like throwing, catching, and kicking (Barnett, van Beurden, Morgan, Brooks, & Beard, 2010). Overarm throwing is a motor skill that has shown the greatest differences between genders, even at early ages (Hyde, 2005; Petranek & Barton, 2011).

REASONS FOR GENDER DIFFERENCES IN YOUTH SPORT

Average gender differences in sport and motor skills may be attributed to physical–biological differences, as well as the differential socialization of boys and girls in our society.

Physical and Biological Differences

Several physical characteristics of postpubescent males predispose them to outperform females in sports that require strength, power, and speed. Adult males tend to be taller with longer limbs. The breadth of their shoulders allows for more muscle on a larger shoulder girdle, the main contributor to postpubescent males' advantage in upper-body strength. Adult males have more overall muscle mass and less body fat than females, even in trained samples. Male athletes average 4% to 12% body fat compared to 12% to 23% in female athletes. Males develop larger skeletal muscles, as well as larger hearts and lungs and a greater number of red blood cells (which absorb oxygen for an

aerobic advantage). Without question, males and females differ on several physical characteristics that influence sport performance. But what about the gender differences that appear before puberty, when the physical differences between males and females are still very small?

Gender Stereotyping

The answer lies in how girls and boys in our culture learn about and internalize gendered beliefs, values, and practices. This is called **socialization**, a process in which we actively formulate ideas about who we are and how we're supposed to act (and not act). Males and females are socialized very differently in most cultures. As a result of this socialization, stereotypes are often formed. A **stereotype** is a popular belief about specific types of individuals in certain categories.

Gender stereotyping is a process in which children's biological sex determines the activities they engage in (and not engage in), as well as the manner in which they are treated in these activities. Sports are generally considered a masculine domain, and this stereotype results in boys' perceiving greater ability and attaching greater importance to sport than girls. This contributes to the gender differences observed in sport. Following are some specific examples of gender stereotyping.

1. **Females have not been as encouraged by parents to be physically active.** Parents have been shown to provide less encouragement for physical activity, offer fewer sport-related opportunities for their daughters than for their sons, and perceive their sons to have higher sport competence than their daughters (Fredricks & Eccles, 2005).

2. **Females are less apt to be taught and to engage in fundamental motor skills during sensitive periods.** In chapter 5, you learned that the sensitive period for learning fundamental motor skills is between the ages of 2 and 8 years in children. This

is the limited time in human development when the effects of learning experiences on the brain are particularly strong. Sensitive periods are the most fertile time to learn motor skills; and although skills may be acquired later, it is much more difficult, and typically athletes fail to reach the same levels of proficiency as those who began acquiring them during their sensitive period. On average, boys are superior to girls on most fundamental motor skills, particularly object control (throwing, catching, kicking) and body control (agility) skills.

When females fail to develop these critical fundamental skills during their early years, they are disadvantaged later when they wish to participate in sport. It may be a lack of opportunity or instruction or peer socialization that blocks girls from participation. An example of peer socialization is boys' derogatory remarks to girls about sport involvement. Here is a sample of comments made by boys about girls playing sports with them on the playground: "Girls are too weak," "They are girly-girls," "It's a man's game," and "They're too weak, fragile, short, and they might break a nail" (Oliver & Hamzeh, 2010). Just make some simple observations at your local pool, park, or playground, and we bet you'll notice differences in how children play and engage in fundamental motor skills. Boys' play tends to be more active and sport related, whereas girls' play often is more passive, physically restricted, and quiet.

3. **Gender-stereotypical toys have been emphasized throughout childhood and adolescence.** See the Water Break section for a discussion of this topic.

4. **Youth are often pressured into "gender-appropriate" sports.** If someone tells you that she has a child playing ice hockey and another doing figure skating, what assumption do you typically make about these kids? The gendered assumption would be that a boy plays ice hockey and a girl figure skates. Kids do gender-type sports as more or less appropriate (e.g., gymnastics for girls because they're flexible and it's a girls' sport, football for boys because it is rough with lots of contact) (Hannon, Soohoo, Reel, & Ratliffe, 2009).

5. **Female athletes are constantly sexualized by the media. Sexualization** occurs when people value a girl or woman primarily for her sexual appeal and view her as an object for sexual use. Male athletes are rarely depicted as sexual objects when they endorse a product or are on a magazine cover, while female athletes are most often shown in sexualized poses as opposed to a sport action photo. Sexualization of girls begins at puberty, which is a big reason their self-esteem drops during this period. Sexualization leads to depression, bodily shame, low self-esteem, and disordered eating in females. When high school and college females observed pictures of female athletes actively engaged in their sports, their feelings about their physical abilities increased and they were more motivated to be physically active (Daniels, 2009). When they viewed pictures of female athletes in sexualized poses, girls felt more negativity about their own physical appearance and body image. Media depictions of sexualized athletes directly counteract all the positive benefits that sport participation brings to young girls.

6. **Boys who are not physically skilled or good athletes experience ridicule and embarrassment, based on the rigid male stereotype that includes strength, muscularity, athleticism, and lack of empathy for other participants** (Tischler & McCaughtry, 2011). Boys who are good at sports are often popular among peers, with enhanced self-esteem and self-image and positive identity. The ridicule experienced by boys who don't fit the culturally prescribed gender role may cause them to struggle with self-esteem and social relationships. Boys who didn't meet the prescribed masculine athlete stereotype have explained

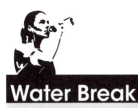

Water Break

Barbie and Easy-Bake Ovens

Children socially learn, as early as 18 months, which toys are appropriate for girls and which are appropriate for boys. Most kids' rooms are furnished with "gender-appropriate" colors and toys. Boys tend to have more sport equipment, construction sets, and superheroes—more active toys that elicit more gross motor activities. Girls are more likely to be given and choose dolls (e.g., Barbie), child-sized household items (e.g., Easy-Bake oven), and stuffed animals, which elicit quiet, more constrained play. One Barbie doll is sold every 3 seconds somewhere in the world. Having a son and a daughter, we were always dismayed when ordering a kid's meal at McDonald's and being asked "Is this for a boy or a girl?" Couldn't kids just choose a toy based on their interests?

Although both sexes receive strong gender-stereotypical messages about toys and activities, research shows that boys are much more narrowly gender stereotyped than girls (Wood, 2002). Girls can play with a variety of toys that are typical of both genders, but there seems to be an unyielding expectation that boys play only with "masculine" toys. In addition,

fathers were found to have more rigid gender-stereotypical views than mothers, particularly about toys purchased for their sons.

Although we still live in a gender-typed world, there are some movements toward more gender neutrality. Some have occurred due to backlash, as in the 1990s, when Barbie was programmed to say "Math class is tough" and "Party dresses are fun." Outrage over such damaging gender-stereotypical statements pressured Mattel into removing the programmed comments. In 2012, Mattel debuted Mega Bloks Barbie construction sets, and Hasbro developed a line of Nerf Rebelle crossbows for girls and a black- and blue-colored (more masculine) Easy-Bake oven for boys. Lego now has five different female mini-dolls, including Emma, who is shown in her karate uniform. What do or will your kids play with? And how might these toy choices influence them? It is our hope that children can choose toys (and aspirations) based on individual interests and abilities as opposed to being constrained by narrow gendered identities.

the negative effects (Tischler & McCaughtry, 2011): "Sometimes I am so nervous about the [sport] activities that I feel sick. One time I threw up because I was so nervous about doing this . . . and I'm not good at it. I did not want the other kids to see me" (p. 43). "People make fun of you . . . and if you screw up the other kids yell and scream at you and make fun of you" (p. 44).

Why Does Gender Stereotyping Occur With Kids?

Many parents explain their gender-stereotypical parenting practices as coming from a desire for their kids to fit in and be accepted in the culture. Yet, children and adolescents need to be educated about harmful gender stereotypes that have been limiting and destructive to both females and males in sport. The use of derogatory terms such as *tomboy, dyke,* and *fag* indicates that a big part of gender stereotyping is the result of **homophobia,** which is an irrational fear or intolerance of gay, lesbian, and bisexual people. However, toys that parents buy and activities they herd their children into are not going to make the difference in the child's sexual orientation. Finally, gender stereotyping preserves the dominant social position of males and subordinate position of females in sport, which many people in society would like to continue. We think there's room for girls in sport, boys in sport, and boys and girls together in sport, in all kinds of sports—and that our culture is enriched because of it.

Moving Beyond Gender Stereotypes

So how would you respond to the young male wrestler who refuses to wrestle against a female (described at the beginning of the chapter)? You could tell him that girls' wrestling is one of the fastest-growing high school sports in the United States and that it is also an Olympic sport for females. You could ask him to describe the feelings and thoughts that are making the situation difficult for him, and help him move from sexualizing his opponent based on her being female to viewing her simply as another competitor.

We hope that adult leaders will not ignore tired sexist comments such as "You throw like a girl"; "Boys will be boys"; and "Bros before hos." Such statements are unacceptable and damaging to everyone. When the 3rd-grade teachers at New Roads School in Santa Monica, California, heard their students say "You throw like a girl," they presented their class with a short documentary on Mo'ne Davis. Davis was the first female pitcher to earn a win and to pitch a shutout in the Little League World Series (2014), with a 70-mile-per-hour (113 kilometers per hour) fastball and a curve that froze batters in their cleats. In her team's 4-0 victory over

Nashville, she pitched six innings, struck out eight, and gave up two infield hits. She made the cover of *Sports Illustrated* and inspired young girls to go beyond rigid boundaries of gender-appropriate sports. Students from the school wrote Mo'ne about her impact, one saying, "Dear Mo'ne—I saw your video. I thought it was so cool because it gave me the feeling that I can do anything I put my mind to" (Chen, 2014, p. 152).

Invite competent females as coaches, and change the stereotypical assigning of menial duties to "team moms" to moms and dads (and change the name to "team manager"). Provide opportunities and expectations for girls to be active and part of any and all sports (and have them dress in comfortable clothes and sneakers so they can actively run and climb and jump to build fundamental motor skills). Provide support and counsel for young boys who don't fit the male athletic stereotype, and help them find outlets through which they can remain physically active.

RACE AND ETHNICITY IN YOUTH SPORT

As most of us are aware, racial and ethnic minorities face oppression and prejudice, even genocide, all around the world. Racial discrimination has a long history in sport (the story of the 1955 Cannon Street All-Star Little League in chapter 2 is a youth sport example of discrimination). **Race** refers to a category of people who share genetically transmitted characteristics; one such characteristic is skin color. However, race is confusing, because the characteristics associated with a particular race are in reality quite broad or fluid. African American athletes are also known as black athletes, but there are many shades of skin color across the group of people identified as African. Tiger Woods is only one-quarter African American, but he is widely identified as a black golfer.

Ethnicity refers to the cultural heritage of a particular group of people. Examples of ethnic groups include Americans, Asian Americans, Hispanics, and African Americans. Hispanics are the largest minority group in the United States; the term refers to people whose ethnic heritage may be traced to Spanish-speaking countries. Asian Americans are also a fast-growing minority group in the United States.

There is a tendency in society to try to explain racial differences, particularly between blacks and whites, based on biology. It's beyond the scope of this book to discuss this tendency at length, but sport sociologists indicate that oversimplified biological explanations for racial differences in sport performance are misleading. No one has tried to identify the inborn characteristics of Canadians that lead to their success in hockey or the biologically advantaged cardiorespiratory systems of Norwegians that enable them to be dominant cross-country skiers (Coakley, 2009). Everyone knows that hockey is emphasized in Canadian sport and that Norwegians learn to ski at about the same time they learn to walk. Yet, article after article has been written about the biological advantages of East Africans in distance running and of Jamaicans in sprinting.

Racial Stereotypes

Racial stereotypes are common in sport and are destructive in many ways. Historical black athlete stereotypes include them being perceived as "natural" athletes, endowed with speed and jumping abilities and less able to engage in complex strategies and decision making. Such stereotypes influence coaches and athletes in terms of what sports, events, and positions are viewed as "appropriate" based on one's race. I (first author) clearly remember when there were no black quarterbacks in the National Football League and very few black pitchers in Major League Baseball. Obviously, these were stereotypical, discriminatory practices based on decades of racism. But similar stereotypes persist in coaches' minds. All youth athletes should be evaluated and coached based on their performance skills, without any stereotypical preconceived notions about their race.

A phenomenon known as **stereotype threat** occurs when the knowledge of a negative stereotype about a group leads to lowered performance on a task. When black athletes were told that a golf putting test was a test of "sport intelligence," they performed more poorly than those who were told it was a test of "natural athletic ability" (Stone, Lynch, Sjomeling, & Darley, 1999). Thus, stereotypes influence our beliefs about our abilities to perform specific skills, based on racial or gender categories to which we belong.

Combating Negative Racial and Ethnic Stereotypes

Racial and ethnic differences on youth sport teams can teach kids two things: (1) that people of different races and ethnicities are more alike than different (similar to our overlapping lines concept with gender); and (2) that becoming aware of other subcultures is enriching and helps people understand and appreciate the world much better. In the scenario of the Muslim tennis team member mentioned in the chapter introduction, the team could learn about the Muslim females' practice of wearing hijabs and why modest clothing is an important ethnic tradition for this athlete. When a referee barred a soccer player from competing in a game for Overland High School in Colorado because she was wearing a hijab, all of her teammates decided to wear hijabs for the next game (Chiari, 2014). As a consequence of their showing their support for their teammate, the officials relented and all the team members were allowed to play while wearing hijabs.

Adult coaches and leaders could stretch their cultural competence by recognizing and supporting diverse holidays and celebrations, remembering that not everyone celebrates Christmas and Easter. Racist comments and slurs must be confronted immediately and deemed inappropriate, and even stereotypical comments could be viewed as providing teachable moments (discussed more in chapter 14) so kids can move forward in developing their own cultural competence. We strongly advocate that youth sport leaders address negative stereotypes explicitly by discussing them with young athletes. Guard against subtly communicating low expectations of athletes because of their race, ethnic background, or social class (Martens, 2012). Avoid preferential treatment and greater frequency and warmth of communication with athletes who have the same cultural background as you. And find opportunities for athletes to share their cultural heritage with team members to enhance young athletes' understanding of and appreciation for cultural diversity.

Water Break

Coach Vivian Stringer on Cultural Competence

We can all learn cultural competence from Vivian Stringer, coach of the Rutgers University women's basketball team. In 2007, after a successful season that ended in the National Collegiate Athletic Association National Championship game, national radio talk show host Don Imus derided the team members on the air by calling them "nappy-headed hos." In an emotional news conference jammed with spectators and reporters after the incident, Stringer and her players spoke eloquently and passionately about the inappropriateness of the remark and how it detracted from the team's joy in their success.

Coach Stringer remarked, "They worked hard in the classroom and accomplished so much and used their gifts and talents to bring smiles and pride within this state to so many people, and then we had to experience racist and sexist remarks that are deplorable, despicable, abominable, and unconscionable. It hurts me. Let me put a human face on this. These young ladies are valedictorians, future doctors, musical prodigies, and yes, even Girl Scouts. They are all young ladies of class." And to help us understand how racism and sexism harm society, Coach Stringer added, "It's not about the players as black or nappy-headed. It's about us as people. When there has been denied equality for one, there has been denied equality for all" (Strauss, 2007).

Although this situation did not occur in a youth sport context, it could be used as a teachable moment for coaches as well as young athletes to internalize a greater understanding of and commitment to cultural competence. Coach Stringer's eloquent response went a long way toward moving our society beyond the use of destructive, racist labels.

SEXUAL ORIENTATION AND YOUTH SPORT

If you went to the 2014 Winter Olympic Games in Sochi, Russia, and expressed in any way your practice or support of gay rights, you could have been thrown in jail as a criminal. Brian Burke, general manager of the Calgary Flames and U.S. men's hockey director of personnel, responded to the situation: "You don't have to be a gay man to care about this. You don't have to have a gay son or daughter to recognize an organized effort by a county to target and destroy a minority group. History has taught us that, left unchecked, this sort of bigotry will only escalate. The rest of the world cannot bear silent witness" (Burke, 2013). Burke's statement, published in *Sports Illustrated,* is a great example of cultural competence and a model for all of us to speak out against injustice.

Sexual orientation refers to an enduring pattern of emotional, romantic, or sexual attraction to females, males, or both sexes and is a significant part of identity development in youth. Sexual orientation is usually categorized into three groups: gay-lesbian (same-sex attraction), heterosexual or "straight" (opposite-sex attraction), and bisexual (both same- and opposite-sex attractions). Middle and high school youth who identify as gay, lesbian, or bisexual are more likely to be bullied and physically assaulted and are more than twice as likely to have attempted suicide compared to heterosexual youth (www.cdc.gov/lgbthealth/youth.htm).

American society has improved its cultural competence in supporting difference in sexual orientation (as have several other countries), but more needs to be done. For youth to thrive in their communities, they need to feel socially, emotionally, and physically safe and supported. Coaches and teachers have historically viewed the issue of sexual orientation as a subject to be avoided in sport and left up to families to work out in the privacy of their homes. But to avoid it is to tacitly approve of discrimination and prejudice. Homophobic slurs (e.g., fag, dyke), like gender and racial slurs, are destructive and without question should be addressed as a serious problem. Our kids told us about the statement "That's so gay" used by some adolescents to describe what they see as inappropriate or stupid behavior. When people use such a slur, they should be questioned: "What do you mean when you say 'That's so gay'? How do you think a gay or lesbian person feels when they hear that statement? Do you think it's right to say things that make fun of other people that are different from you?"

We understand that many people don't feel they have the cultural competence to lead a discussion or to counsel a young athlete about sexual orientation. That's okay. But what we do urge youth sport leaders to do is to identify local educators and mental health providers (e.g., school counselors and psychologists, counseling professionals in the community) as referral sources who can be on call for athletes, parents, and coaches. We encourage coaches to remain involved with athletes who have been referred to other professionals so that coaches are part of the support team (instead of just giving an athlete or parent a phone number to call).

Youth sport directors could add acceptance of and support for different sexual orientations to program mission statements. Youth sport coaches must immediately challenge any slurs or negative stereotypes on the part of youth athletes. Coaches and athletes could visit the You Can Play website (youcanplayproject.org), which has powerful video testimonials from many sport teams supporting inclusion of gays and lesbians in sport. The slogan "If you can play, you can play" means that everyone is welcome in sport; your ability to play is the only qualification. Its tag line reads, "Gay athletes. Straight allies. Teaming up for respect." High school programs can submit their own videos to appear on the website to show their

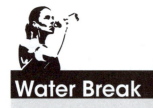

Water Break

Speaking Out for Being Out

Positive Coaching Alliance founder Jim Thompson offers this perspective on supporting sexuality differences in sport (www.positivecoach.org): "The Positive Coaching Alliance is about Better Athletes, Better People, and no one can become their best if they can't embrace who they are as a person. The very best athletes effectively put much of their energy toward accomplishing their goals. If one of your goals is to hide who you actually are, there is less productive energy available to put toward goals that can help yourself, your team and our world, which badly needs the creative energy of all people."

support for the eradication of homophobia in sport. Another educational website is AthleteAlly (www.athleteally.org), dedicated to educating and empowering allies in the sport world to stand up for gay rights.

DISABILITY AND YOUTH SPORT

Disabilities, or biomedical conditions that limit a person's ability to perform specific tasks, are discussed in chapter 1 as a potential barrier to youth sport participation. However, a common theme in federal disability laws and policies is that disability is a natural part of the human experience and in no way diminishes the right of individuals to live independently, enjoy self-determination, and enjoy full inclusion in society, including in youth sport. Sport is for everyone, so it's important for youth sport leaders to enhance their cultural competence in understanding disability.

Common Disability Groupings

Athletes with disabilities are often unable to participate in most sports without some accommodation, such as special equipment or rule modifications (e.g., using a wheelchair to compete in basketball or track and field). The Paralympic Games are the highest level of competition for athletes with disabilities and are held right after the Olympic Games in the same hosting cities. There are very specific groupings for sport competition for athletes with disabilities, with classifications differing based on types of sport (e.g., www.disabledsportsusa.org, www.paralympic.org). Some common disability groupings are shown here, divided into the broad categories of sensory, physical, and mental disabilities:

Sensory impairments

- Deafness: Hearing loss that makes it impossible to understand speech
- Blindness: Range of vision impairments

Physical disabilities

- Amputation: Elbow, wrist, knee, or ankle joint missing or no functional movement in one of these joints
- Cerebral palsy: Disorder of movement and posture caused by brain damage
- Spinal cord injuries: Complete or incomplete quadriplegia or paraplegia
- Les autres: Means "the others" in French; other conditions that limit movement

Mental disabilities

- Intellectual disabilities: Typically individuals with intelligence quotients of less than 70
- Learning disabilities: Developmental speech and language disorders, academic skill disorders (dyslexia), and motor coordination disorders
- Attention disabilities: For example, attention deficit hyperactivity disorder (ADHD)

Adapted from Martens 2012.

Where Should Disabled Youth Athletes Participate?

The bottom line is that children with disabilities have the same right to play as other children. Legally, the Americans with Disabilities Act requires organizations that offer sport programs to provide comparable opportunities to people with disabilities. Youth sport programs must make reasonable accommodations to allow athletes with disabilities to have access to sport programs. All individuals have the right to play on recreational sport teams and to try out for elite, competitive teams, but the law recognizes that not everyone has the right to play on elite sport teams (Martens, 2012). When it is unsafe or not appropriate for athletes with disabilities to compete on sport teams with able-bodied athletes, youth sport leaders can work with parents to identify opportunities for kids to learn skills and compete in sport programs specifically designed for young people with disabilities.

Obviously, some disabilities would preclude a child from participating in certain sports, but it is very typical for athletes with certain disabilities to participate on youth sport teams. Youth sport programs leaders may want to confer with parents, the athlete, the coach, and perhaps medical consultants about the safety and appropriateness of kids with disabilities participating in certain sports. Kevin Laue participated fully in youth basketball and earned an athletic scholarship to Manhattan College in 2009, even though he was born with a left arm that ended just below his elbow. Kevin's achievements led to the film *Long Shot: The Kevin Laue Story* (2012), and his story is included in *Opening the Gate: Stories & Activities About Athletes With Disabilities* (Floyd, 2013), a compilation of inspiring stories about athletes with disabilities that is written for children.

Recommendations for Youth Sport Leaders

We understand that you may not feel culturally competent in knowing about various types of disabilities and how to talk to and coach athletes with disabilities. However, the first obligation that all of us have is to seek to learn and understand more about the specific disabilities of athletes in our programs. We urge you not to avoid this responsibility but to embrace it and increase your cultural competence. There are many print (e.g., Davis, 2010; Winnick, 2011) and Internet resources to help you understand specific disabilities in relation to sport participation. Youth sport leaders don't need to have all the answers about how to adapt the situation for athletes with disabilities, but should welcome these athletes and their families by saying, "Welcome to our program—we'll do our best to figure out how to make it work for you" (Balyi, Way, & Higgs, 2013).

An important consideration is to use *people-first language.* Preferred language when one is discussing athletes with disabilities refers to the individual first and the disability second. It is culturally competent to say "a runner who is blind" or "a child who is autistic" as opposed to "blind runner" or "autistic child." The term *intellectual (or cognitive) disability* is preferred over *mental retardation,* and the word *retarded* is viewed as a hurtful, derogatory term that should not be used. Language is important in our attempt to eliminate generalizations, assumptions, and stereotypes. People-first

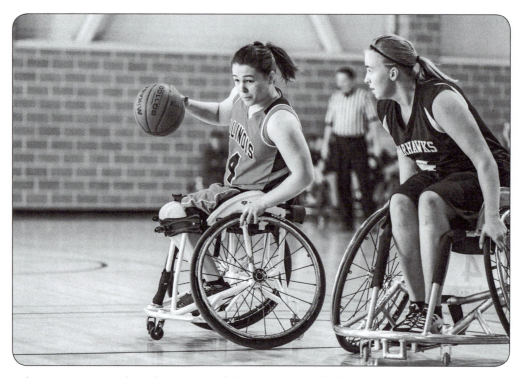

Youth sport programs must make reasonable accommodations to allow athletes with disabilities to have access to sport programs.

language expresses what a person has or does, not what a person is.

Seek out ways to modify your sport to accommodate athletes with disabilities. Parents and even the athletes themselves may have suggestions about how to adapt activities. Know your athletes with disabilities well; treat them as special—not for their disabilities, but just as you would treat each of your athletes as special (Martens, 2012). Allow them to experience risk, success, and failure without overprotecting them.

All of us in youth sport, and society, should say to a child, "How can I help you to be the best that you can be?" (Floyd, 2013). Children 10 to 12 years old with physical disabilities described their good days and bad days in physical education classes (Goodwin, 2009). Good days included companionship and support from classmates in doing physical activities ("They cheer me in the relays"), being able to physically participate ("It makes me feel strong"), liking the feeling of movement ("It's fun"), and acknowledgment by others of their

skill proficiency ("It's nice when they see me swimming on their level or ahead of them"). Bad days included feeling socially isolated or rejected or like an object of curiosity ("There's always one or two kids that are making fun of you"), having their competence questioned or assumed to be lacking ("You can't do this"), or having their active participation restricted ("My teacher won't let me do anything"). These insights helps us to reflect on ways we can structure youth sport to help athletes with disabilities be the best that they can be. Such sensitivity and cultural competence is an important part of developmentally appropriate practice in youth sport.

SEXUAL ABUSE IN YOUTH SPORT

Jerry Sandusky, American football coach and founder of a charity organization to help disadvantaged youth, was convicted in 2012 on 45 counts of sexual abuse of young boys. Former British Olympic swimming coach Paul Hickson was sent to prison in 1995 for rape and 15 other sexual offenses against young girls in his care. Renowned Canadian ice hockey coach Graham James was convicted in 1997 of sexually abusing a young athlete in his care over 350 times from the time the athlete was 14 years old. Sexual abuse of young athletes is a worldwide problem that occurs with startling frequency.

Sexual abuse refers to any sexual activity for which consent is not or cannot be given, which typically involves manipulation and entrapment of athletes (International Olympic Committee, 2008). Sexual abuse often begins with **sexual harassment**, which is sexualized verbal or nonverbal behavior that is unwanted or coercively imposed. Sexual abuse is a misuse of power and trust granted to an adult, with male coaches more often reported as abusers than females. Youth athletes are frequent targets because of their maturational vulnerability and their trust that coaches are important, caring adults committed to athletes' well-being.

Common warning signs of sexual abuse by coaches include giving individual players special gifts, spending extra time (by phone, e-mail, text, or in person) with athletes outside of official practices or games, and keeping secrets or telling players not to share their conversations or activities with parents (www.positivecoach.org). Risk situations include the locker room, away trips, coaches' cars or homes, and social events, particularly when alcohol is involved. Sexual abuse typically occurs as a process in which the abuser begins with seemingly innocuous behaviors such as giving rides home or offering special privileges and then progresses to sexual harassment (making explicit sexual remarks) and actual physical sexual abuse. Young athletes are often confused about what is happening to them, and abusive relationships with coaches continue based on athletes' guilt, embarrassment, and feelings of dependency on coaches (which these coaches strongly reinforce) (Brackenridge, Bishopp, Moussalli, & Tapp, 2008). Victims

of sexual abuse are at great risk for posttraumatic psychological distress.

This is a cultural problem for youth sport, and one that everyone must address in terms of recognition and commitment to change. Youth sport provides coaches with almost unquestioned authority over athletes, with loyalty and obedience to coaches considered the norm. Child sexual abuse is a result of overconformity to masculine socialization, with an emphasis on power and dominance over weaker individuals (Burke, 2001). Thus, the first place to protect children is at the organizational level.

All youth sport organizations should develop policies and procedures, including mandatory education of coaches, for the prevention of sexual harassment and abuse. A good idea is to view sexual abuse prevention as an ongoing initiative, with multiple messages provided to coaches, as opposed to a one-shot intervention in the form of a 20-minute presentation. The goal is to raise (and maintain) awareness of problematic cultural practices that do great harm to youth athletes. Some organizations require background checks of coaches as well, since abusive coaches can be fired from positions but not prosecuted, which simply allows them to move on to abuse athletes in other programs. The Positive Coaching Alliance (positivecoach.org) provides a Youth Sexual Abuse Prevention Policy & Procedures outline that can easily be adapted by youth sport programs.

Parents should also be educated (in a clinic setting or via a printed brochure) about sexual abuse, including how to identify warning signs, what to do when possible violations occur, and how to talk to their children about sexual abuse. Adolescent athletes should be educated firsthand about sexual harassment and abuse so they understand how these processes evolve from seemingly innocent, unintentional behavior that is in fact abusive. The objective is to raise everyone's awareness of the abhorrent practices of sexual harassment and abuse to safeguard the well-being of youth sport athletes.

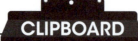

Protecting Youth Athletes From Sexual Abuse

A. What can you do as a youth sport leader?

1. Require that all coaches watch video(s) on protecting athletes from sexual abuse.

2. Have established policies and a publicized action plan for protecting kids and reporting suspected abuse.

3. Prohibit coaches from being alone with individual athletes (including in cars), except in emergencies. Individual instruction should occur in a public setting where a parent or other adult observes the training.

4. Conduct background checks of prospective coaches.

B. What can you do as a youth sport parent?

1. Ask your organization for its policy on protecting athletes from abuse.

2. A major key to child protection is "no secrets." Tell your child that any problems, favors, gifts, or touching should never be a secret.

3. Give children the language to use if someone is making them feel uncomfortable. Teach them to say "Please stop! This makes me feel uncomfortable."

4. Encourage kids to tell you any time when someone's behavior is making them feel unsafe or uncomfortable. Explain that you want them to tell you even if they're not sure, even if it's really uncomfortable to talk about, or even if someone might get upset.

5. If something makes you uncomfortable, address the coach calmly and respectfully. If you're still concerned, talk to the organizational leader or even a police officer.

6. Don't allow your child to practice alone with a coach. Make sure that the setting is public and that at least one other adult (or multiple teammates) is present.

Adapted, by permission, from Positive Coaching Alliance, 2014, *Youth sexual abuse prevention policy & procedures.* Available: http://devzone.positivecoach.org/resource/article/youth-sexual-abuse-prevention-policy-procedures.

WRAP-UP

There are many groups that deserve our sensitivity and commitment to cultural competence. Maybe as the youth coach of an athlete with a hearing impairment, you learn a few words you can say to her in sign language. Perhaps you include an athlete with a physical disability somewhere in your sport program so he can enjoy being part of a team (and remember not to make him a token but rather an important and valued member of the team). Don't worry if you don't feel culturally competent in all situations—none of us are. But what all of us can do is commit to enhancing our cultural competence by being self-reflective about our own biases and open and accepting about learning more about different subcultures and groups.

One word we hear a lot when teaching about difference is *natural.* An obstacle for many is their belief that certain characteristics are natural, which makes alternative practices "unnatural." We hear that males naturally like sport more and are better at it than females, and that heterosexuality is natural and being gay is unnatural. If this is what you believe, we advocate that you take some time to examine your beliefs about the naturalness of things, which ends up valuing and privileging some people over others. We urge you not to ignore what you perceive as unnatural, but rather to learn more to see if your opinions are indeed supported by evidence and fact. Your task is to evolve in your own personal quest for cultural competence, and we believe that youth sport and our society will benefit greatly from the work that we all do in this area.

LEARNING AIDS

Key Terms

cultural competence—Our ability to interact effectively with people of different cultures, subcultures, and backgrounds, as well as being aware of our own cultural identity and personal views about difference.

disability—Biomedical condition that limits a person's ability to perform specific tasks.

ethnicity—The cultural heritage of a particular group of people.

gender—The characteristics, behaviors, and activities that society considers appropriate for males and females, typically labeled as masculine and feminine.

gender stereotyping—A process in which children's biological sex determines the activities they engage in (and not engage in), as well as the manner in which they are treated in these activities.

homophobia—An irrational fear or intolerance of gay, lesbian, and bisexual people.

race—A category of people that share genetically transmitted characteristics.

sex—A biological characteristic based on a person's chromosomes, hormonal profiles, and internal and external reproductive organs.

sexual abuse—Any sexual activity for which consent is not or cannot be given, which typically involves manipulation and entrapment of athletes.

sexual harassment—Sexualized verbal or nonverbal behavior that is unwanted or coercively imposed.

sexualization—When people value a girl or woman primarily for her sexual appeal and view her as an object for sexual use.

sexual orientation—An enduring pattern of emotional, romantic, or sexual attraction to females, males, or both sexes.

socialization—A process in which we actively formulate ideas about who we are and how we're supposed to act (and not act) in a particular culture.

stereotype—A popular belief about specific types of individuals in certain categories.

stereotype threat—When the knowledge of a negative stereotype about a group leads to lowered performance on a task.

tokenism—A superficial action, similar to "going through the motions," to include members of different groups.

Summary Points

1. The five levels on the cultural competence continuum are competence, precompetence, blindness, incapacity, and destructiveness.

2. "Treating everyone the same" typically means assuming that everyone fits with the dominant cultural practices of the day.

3. Sex is biological and fixed, whereas gender is culturally constructed and fluid.

4. The overlapping lines concept shows that male and female youth sport athletes are more similar than different.

5. Average gender differences in sport and motor skills may be attributed to physical–biological differences as well as to the differential socialization of boys and girls in our society.

6. Racial stereotypes can lead young athletes to underperform on certain tasks.

7. Middle and high school athletes who are gay and lesbian are more likely to be bullied and physically assaulted, and are more than twice as likely to have attempted suicide compared to heterosexual youth.

8. Sexual abuse occurs when adult coaches misuse power to take advantage of youth athletes' maturational vulnerability and trust.

9. Youth sport leaders have an obligation to learn more about disabilities, such as how to adapt sport and use people-first language.

Study Questions

1. Identify and explain, using an example for each, the five levels of cultural competence.

2. Explain the difference between sex and gender, and provide two examples for each.

3. Explain what is important about the concept of overlapping lines, and provide examples of two sets of lines as well as characteristics that fit these sets of lines.

4. Identify several biological as well as social reasons for average gender differences in sport or motor skills.

5. Provide guidelines to combat negative stereotypes based on gender, race-ethnicity, and sexual orientation.

6. What is sexual abuse in youth sport, why does it occur, and how can we prevent it?

7. Identify several strategies that youth sport leaders can use to help athletes with disabilities have positive experiences in youth sport.

Reflective Learning Activities

1. Visit a local toy store or the toy section of a department store. Evaluate 20 different children's toys and how they are packaged. Create a toy log to use in note taking, and for each toy, enter (a) name of the toy, (b) type of toy (from the toy categories listed here), (c) the key word or phrase used by the manufacturer to market the toy (e.g., "for tough guys only"), and (d) whether girls or boys are pictured on the package, along with their approximate ages. Types of toy categories include these:

   a. CB: construction-building

   b. D: make-believe domestic (e.g., kitchen set, dolls)

   c. A: make-believe action (e.g., swords, action figures)

   d. SPA: sport–physical activity equipment

   e. E: educational-computer

Write up your conclusions after examining your toy data. You can include your own insights, but overall you want to figure out whether there was a tendency for either sex to be associated with certain types of toys and marketing of these toys. Discuss how you think the toy trends you found are part of the socialization process and whether you did find that toys are gender stereotyped. What implications might this have for children's aspirations, self-concept, physical skill development, and physical fitness?

Adapted, by permission, from K.M. Haywood and N. Getchell, 2001, *Learning activities for life span motor development,* 3rd ed. (Champaign, IL: Human Kinetics).

2. Rate your cultural competence (using the levels provided in table 13.1) regarding gender, race-ethnicity, sexual orientation, and disability in relation to sport. For each area, explain your cultural competence rating, why it is what it is, and share specific strategies that you will use to enhance your cultural competence in each area.

3. Identify or create three different activities you could do with a youth sport team to build their cultural competence. These activities could be about any of the topics discussed in the chapter.

Resource Guide

Protecting Youth Athletes from Sexual Abuse: Key Actions for Youth Sport Leaders (YouTube) (www.youtube.com/watch?v=kn-z6Y_KHac).

Protecting Youth Athletes from Sexual Abuse: Key Actions for Parents & Coaches (YouTube) (www.youtube.com/watch?v=xR5Sk-_w6Rw).

You Can Play Project (youcanplayproject.org).

www.disabledsportsusa.org.

www.paralympic.org.

chapter 14

COACHES AND YOUTH SPORT

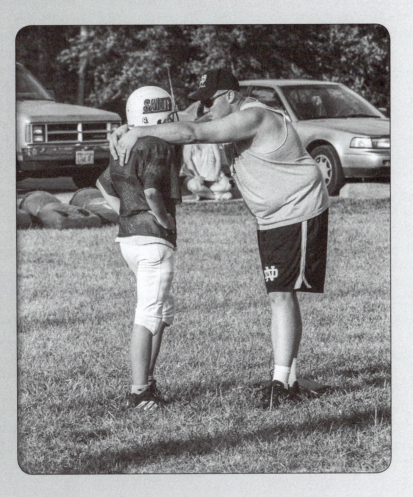

CHAPTER PREVIEW

In this chapter, you'll learn

» about youth sport coaching education programs,

» how to recruit and evaluate youth coaches,

» the skill set needed by youth coaches, and

» how coaches' expectations can influence children's learning and achievement.

Laid out before me was my life as a sports story, a narrative with each mile marker underscoring a coaching relationship. I saw . . . the kind of coaches who use players as tools to meet their personal needs for validation, status, and identity. They held their power over us to elicit the response they wanted. I obeyed these coaches out of necessity, but I never accepted their belief systems or bought into their programs. Coach first, team second, and players' growth and needs last, if at all, were their modus operandi (Ehrmann, 2011, p. 5).

This quote is by Joe Ehrmann, former professional American football player and author of the groundbreaking book *InSide-Out Coaching: How Sport Can Transform Lives* (2011). We'll talk more about *InSide-Out Coaching* later in the chapter, but this quote is about a common problem in youth sport coaching—placing coaches' needs or winning ahead of young athletes' developmental needs. In a nutshell, coaches make or break youth sport in terms of the quality of the sport experience for athletes. Reflect back on the various coaches in your personal sports story, and identify both positive and negative examples of coaches who influenced you as a person or athlete. Isn't it amazing that coaches influence athletes' experiences more than anything else? More than winning championships, more than training in fancy facilities—coaches are "it" when it comes to making the difference for kids in youth sport.

Coaches at the youth sport level have the special challenge of coaching children and adolescents. Coaching athletes during the most significant developmental years of their lives is far different from coaching college and adult athletes. Consider the following example of a coach failing to understand the cognitive maturational level of youth basketball players:

When I walked onto the court and said, "Set a pick," you just assume that these kids know what you're talking about. And they don't. It took me a while to figure out that, hey, you almost gotta go back to the basics. Like when I mean "zone," I say, "Protect the house," and that stuff. When I say, "Play big," I mean "put your hands in the air" (Wiersma & Sherman, 2005, p. 329).

As we've noted repeatedly, the emphasis in youth sport coaching must be on developmentally appropriate practice. All of the chapters in this book relate to effective coaching in youth sport as based on this principle. When asked what made their first youth sport coaches effective, expert athletes explained that it was their coaches' understanding of the needs of children more than their technical knowledge of the sport (Monsaas, 1985). Youth coaches need "people skills" and particularly "little people skills" to provide the interpersonal environment that works best for youth athletes.

Most coaching at the youth level is an incidental or occasional "temp" job, often done by parents, typically on a volunteer basis with no pay. Middle school, high school, and some club teams pay for coaches who often have more sport experience and technical knowledge, although these payments for coaching services are modest. Coaching as a full-time profession typically occurs only at the collegiate, professional, and elite (Olympic or national teams) levels. An exception to this in youth sport is the private club coaches of sports like tennis, gymnastics, figure skating, and golf; these coaches may train many athletes as part of a full-time position, typically at one facility or private sport academy.

COACHING EDUCATION AND CERTIFICATION

Youth sport coaching in the United States is largely unregulated, with the majority of youth sport coaches uncertified by any type of coaching education program. This is troubling because of the powerful influence that adult coaches have on youth athletes, as well as coaches' prominent role as supervisors of athletes' safety and well-being. If we require lifeguards at our local pools to be certified in swimming, lifesaving techniques, and basic first aid, why in the world do we allow uncertified coaches to coach our kids?

One answer to this question is tradition and the belief that if you've played a little sport, then you're qualified to coach children. Nothing could be further from the truth. We can ride bicycles, but that doesn't mean we know how to build one. Only in sport, it seems, do people believe that anyone can coach or buy into the erroneous idea that playing experience makes one a good coach.

The other answer to the question about why we allow uncertified coaches in youth sport is the need to search constantly for volunteer coaches to staff youth sport programs. We understand this dilemma and empathize with youth sport directors attempting to staff their programs with volunteer coaches. But we feel that it's time for a cultural shift in how we think about youth sport coaching. It must become part of our culture to require that anyone who coaches children complete at least a minimal educational program that certifies her to work with a specific age group. With the multiple educational programs available online, only a small amount of time and no travel are needed to gain important understanding about coaching kids in youth sport.

Canada's National Coaching Certification Program

The gold standard for coaching education programs is Canada's National Coaching Certification Program (NCCP). Begun in 1974, the NCCP is a collaborative program of the Canadian government, sport federations, and the Coaching Association of Canada. The NCCP is designed to meet the needs of all types of coaches, from the first-time youth sport coach to the head coach of an elite national team.

As shown in figure 14.1, the NCCP has three streams based on the type and needs of participants to be coached: Community Sport, Competition, and Instruction streams. Different contexts within each stream mean that coaches receive training to fit the unique needs of participants in a very specific context. For example, the Initiation context in the Community Sport stream focuses specifically on coaching very young children who are being introduced to a sport. Following developmentally appropriate practice, the focus is on fun, safety, and the development of fundamental motor and basic sport skills. The Competition stream is for competitive sport coaching, and the Instruction stream is for coaches who deliver lessons and skill development sessions to athletes but who do not coach in formal competitions.

The unifying core competencies (e.g., valuing, critical thinking) shown at the bottom of figure 14.1 are interwoven throughout the program. This is particularly noteworthy because it shows that the NCCP incorporates thoughtful self-awareness and personal development activities for coaches, as opposed to just providing rote managerial information. These core competencies lead into specific coaching outcomes that make up all the programs' content, representing outcomes that all coaches need to be able to achieve (e.g., making ethical decisions, planning practices, analyzing performance).

Who am I coaching? (based on participants' needs)

Community Sport stream

Initiation context
Usually very young children
Kids' first introduction to sport
Focus on fun, safety and development
of fundamental and basic skills

Ongoing context
Youth in recreational programs
Encourage continuing participation
for fun, fitness, skill development,
and social interaction

Competition stream

Introduction context
Children and adolescents taught basic
sport skills preparing them for mostly
local competition

Development context
Adolescents coached to refine basic
skills and develop more advanced
skills and tactics

High-performance context
Advanced skills and tactics
and preparation for national
and international competition

Instruction stream

Beginners context
Participants with no or little experience
taught basic sport skills

Intermediate performers context
Participants with some experience
refine skills and learn more
complex techniques

Advanced performers context
Experienced, proficient performers
continue to advanced development

What do coaches need to be able to do? (coaching outcomes)

| Make ethical decisions | Plan a practice | Manage a program | Design a sport program |
| Support athletes in training | Analyze performance | Support athletes in competition | Establish sport-specific outcomes to be achieved |

What core competencies do all coaches need?

Valuing   Interacting   Leading   Problem solving   Critical thinking

Figure 14.1 Canada's National Coaching Certification Program (NCCP).

Adapted from *Canada's National Coaching Certification Program.*

An NCCP certification database is kept online, and coaches may receive three types of certification (called accreditation). *In training* means that coaches have completed some of the required training for a context; *trained* means that coaches have completed all the required training for a context; and *certified* means that coaches have participated in a formal evaluation process and have demonstrated competence at a high enough level to be declared a certified coach. Any coaching education program that requires an evaluation to achieve certification is preferred in that it assesses the degree to which knowledge has been internalized by coaches. Emphasizing lifelong professional learning, the organization requires NCCP-certified coaches to participate in continuing professional development activities to maintain certification.

Other International Coaching Education Programs

New Zealand, Great Britain, and Australia are other English-speaking countries that have implemented national coaching education programs. Similar to Canada's NCCP, New Zealand's program focuses on training coaches for specific contexts based on the needs of participants. These coaching communities include foundation coaching (for first experiences of primary school children), development coaching (for later years of primary school and secondary school participants), performance coaching (for athletes with higher ability levels who seek to compete at district or regional competitions), and high-performance coaching (for elite national or international athletes). We love New Zealand's guiding statement for the program, which is that coaching should first and foremost be about the needs of the athletes being coached (Sport New Zealand, 2012a). As you already know, we agree that it's all about the kid.

Sports Coach UK has published "minimum standards for active coaches of children and young people," recommending types and levels of coaching education in the United Kingdom (www.sportscoachuk.org). Governing bodies of various sports work with Sports Coach UK to set educational requirements for coaches at various levels.

The Australian Sports Commission developed the National Coaching Accreditation Scheme (NCAS) as a progressive coach education program offering courses at various levels. The NCAS includes assessment of coaches in completing each component of the program, and also requires reaccreditation to ensure that coaches stay up-to-date in their learning. Overall, these examples of international coaching education programs are impressive, as they provide comprehensive youth sport coach education and certification specifically targeted to benefit kids at all levels of sport.

Coaching Education in the United States

Youth sport coaching education in the United States is more decentralized and entrepreneur oriented when compared to that in other countries. There is no national education–certification program but rather several programs sponsored by different agencies from which youth sport programs can choose. The website www. usacoaching.org provides information and resources for coaches in sport science and technical sport-specific content, but does not provide a specific education or certification program. The National Council for Accreditation of Coaching Education (NCACE) provides accreditation for coaching education programs, based on "national standards for sport coaches" (it costs $21 just to view the standards).

Several coaching education programs are available, most of which offer online training. Most middle schools and high schools in the United States require basic coaching certification in sport sciences, sport management, and first aid. (You can find the specific coach education requirement for your state at nfhslearn.com/statepricingregs.aspx.) Two programs are targeted for and recognized by middle and high school athletic departments as appropriate certification to coach at these levels: the National Federation of High School Associations (NFHS) and the Human Kinetics Coach Education.

Both programs offer a coaching fundamentals course and a sport first-aid course, as well as many other educational courses, including sport-specific courses. Both the NFHS and the Human Kinetics Coach Education programs are accredited by the NCACE, and both include online examinations required for certification by the programs. The NFHS offers coaches the distinction of becoming an Accredited Interscholastic Coach by completing four courses: coaching fundamentals, concussion in sport, first aid, and a sport-specific course. The Human Kinetics Coach Education also offers similar recognition for coaches who complete multiple courses.

For nonschool, community-oriented youth sports, the Human Kinetics Coach Education offers a Coaching Essentials certification program for coaching youth age 13 and under. The Human Kinetics Coach Education also offers many sport-specific courses (e.g., coaching youth tennis, coaching youth softball). The National Youth Sports Coaches Association (NYSCA) has offered coaching certification clinics since 1981, which can now be done online. The NYSCA program is required by some community youth sport programs, although it involves only a 3-hour clinic or online experience compared to the more comprehensive coaching certification programs. The Positive Coaching Alliance (PCA; positivecoach.org) provides three online courses for coaches that are very specific to the PCA educational philosophy (e.g.,

Thompson, 2003, 2010b). The PCA programs are excellent and very applied, focusing on the philosophy and psychology of coaching.

Individual sport organizations have implemented their own coaching education–certification requirements, often incorporating some of the programs just discussed. For example, USA Track & Field requires the NFHS Fundamentals of Coaching for coaches, and then offers three levels of certification, one of which is a youth specialization program. The United States Tennis Association (USTA) offers multiple developmentally appropriate online courses for youth coaches (www.usta.com). The American Youth Soccer Organization requires coaches to complete its online training program called Safe Haven, as well as age-specific training based on the level of athletes.

Summary of Coaching Education and Certification

Overall, progress has been made in the education and certification of youth coaches. Although the United States does not have a standardized national certification program as do other countries, several quality programs are available for youth sport programs to adopt. The advent of online coaching education–certification programs has made it easier and more practical for coaches to receive quality training. We are heartened that interscholastic coaches are required to become certified, and we envision that this requirement will become automatic at the community youth sport level as well.

In table 14.1, we've identified what we view as eight topics that should be included in youth sport coaching education programs. Minimally, we feel that coaches must learn about and become aware of the philosophy and objectives of their youth sport programs. In addition, a minimal requirement should be to learn about teaching sport-specific skills and tactics, as well as safety, injury prevention, and basic first aid. Beyond this minimal education, we feel that coaches also need to learn about physical conditioning; motivation and communication; and the developmental aspects of growth, maturation, and readiness. And finally, a complete coaching education program should also include the topics of organization and management as well as subcultural understanding.

An important development in coaching education has been the creation of specific educational streams for different types of coaching situations (e.g., community recreation vs. high school coaching), as opposed to the older model of progressive levels of coaching education without any specific contextualization. This is a terrific idea, as the content areas (such as shown in table 14.1) can then be contextualized and made practical for specific types of coaches. We urge you to lead the cultural change in attitude

Table 14.1   Topic Areas for Youth Sport Coaching Education Programs

Minimal	Needed	Complete
Philosophy and objectives	Philosophy and objectives	Philosophy and objectives
Teaching sport skills and tactics	Teaching sport skills and tactics	Teaching sport skills and tactics
Safety, injury prevention, and basic first aid	Safety, injury prevention, and basic first aid	Safety, injury prevention, and basic first aid
	Physical training	Physical training
	Motivation and communication	Motivation and communication
	Growth, maturation, and readiness	Growth, maturation, and readiness
		Organization and management
		Cultural competence

that is needed so that coaches view education–certification programs as a professional responsibility and an important opportunity to learn and improve.

RECRUITING YOUTH SPORT COACHES

The quality of a youth sport program depends on the coach. With this in mind, youth sport directors should make the recruitment of coaches a systematic year-round effort. Through designing and publicizing the need for coaches in different sports and ages across the year, people in the community have time to consider their interest in coaching and even to prepare for their coaching roles by completing a coaching education course or sport-specific coach training program.

Strategies to recruit coaches might include local newspaper articles, posters, and flyers; personal presentations at local civic clubs or college coaching classes; blast e-mails to former and prospective coaches in the community; and a website that explains and invites people to get involved in coaching youth sport. Sample job descriptions for coaching may be found on the Internet as well as in print sport management guides (e.g., Martens, 2001). Creating a coaching intern partnership with a nearby university is an excellent way to recruit coaches. Both the undergraduate and graduate coaching students at our university partner with local recreational and interscholastic programs to serve as intern coaches.

Both interscholastic and community youth sport programs should consider creating the position of director of coaching for the program. We realize that many programs are financially strapped, which would make it difficult to hire an additional person. But perhaps this could become the main division of labor for someone on staff, which places an emphasis on selecting, preparing, and evaluating coaches. There are also retired coaches in communities who may be interested in such a position. Overall, the idea is to make the program's commitment to quality coaching systematic and ongoing.

EVALUATING YOUTH SPORT COACHES

The adage "What gets measured gets done" applies to supervising and evaluating coaches. Again, youth sport program directors tell us that they are stretched too thin to have the time to do this. But there may be creative ways to engage in coach supervision, similar to our ideas about finding people in the community who could help in this endeavor. Retired teachers and coaches might be interested in observing coaches and providing feedback.

Overall, the intent of evaluation is to provide coaches with useful feedback, from which they can learn and get better at coaching. The purpose is not to find fault or look for weaknesses and mistakes. The best case would be to observe and provide feedback to all coaches, and this can be done in an informal and relaxed manner so as not to threaten or stress novice coaches. A sample coaching appraisal form (adapted from Martens, 2001) is provided in appendix L. Most of us get a bit nervous about being evaluated, so it's most effective to describe this process to coaches as an opportunity to get recognized for their commitment to kids and to learn through feedback provided by another person (preferably a master coach, to heighten the credibility of the feedback). The feedback should be pertinent and honest but should be provided in a positive and helpful manner. The specific comments should always close with thanks to the coach for his time and effort on behalf of the organization. Coaches should have the opportunity to share their thoughts about the evaluation with the program director as well.

Another way to use a coaching appraisal form is to ask coaches to complete it about themselves at the end of the season. They could summarize at the bottom of the form

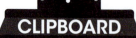

CLIPBOARD

Self-Evaluation Questions for Youth Sport Coaches

1. Do my athletes come to practice excited and motivated to play?

2. Have my athletes and my team shown improvement? *All* my athletes?

3. Is my team working together as a unit? Are they interacting well with each other?

4. Do I come to practice and competitions each time showing enthusiasm and belief in my athletes?

5. Are athletes generally enjoying their sport experience? Am I?

6. Do I interpersonally connect with every athlete on the team in a positive way each practice?

7. Am I meeting the developmental needs of my athletes through appropriate teaching, training, and communication?

Based on Dicicco and Hacker 2002.

with areas to improve. Coaches could also assess their own performance by answering questions featured in the Clipboard sidebar. These questions would be useful for coaches to read and consider periodically to remind them of their role in youth sport.

The most meaningful evaluation should come from the athletes who have been coached. Appendix M provides a sample end-of-the-year evaluation form for athletes to provide feedback to their coaches. Not only is it athletes' right to evaluate their coaches; such evaluation also provides a unique perspective for coaches to consider. Youth sport directors should decide on the appropriate way to administer these evaluation forms to athletes, preferably by a program director, student intern, or even a volunteer parent. Emphasize to the athletes that their responses are anonymous (explain that this means no one will know who said what) and that they should be honest and thoughtful in providing feedback to their coaches.

BUILDING THE YOUTH SPORT COACH'S SKILL SET

Like all positions we take on in life (e.g., parent, tennis player, mayor), coaching requires a unique skill set to be successful.

A **skill set** is a combination of abilities that enable us to succeed in certain positions. We think there are three primary skill sets needed by youth sport coaches: technical, managerial, and personal. All of these skills can be developed and improved—and should be.

Technical Skills

Technical skills are coaches' abilities to teach skills and tactics in training, as well as knowing how to use tactics when coaching in competition. Volunteer coaches often experience initial difficulties in teaching sport-specific skills appropriately to children. Coaches have asked for help to teach kids to use proper progressions and develop a collection of basic drills for use in practice (Wiersma & Sherman, 2005).

Should coaches worry if they are not highly skilled or able to perform the skills of the sport they are coaching? Is it true that having played the sport makes one a better coach? It may help, at least, in gaining initial credibility with athletes. Adolescent athletes have expressed the desire for coaches who are effective teachers and can perform the skills of the sport (Martin, Dale, & Jackson, 2001), and playing and coaching experience enabled volunteer coaches to be more confident (Feltz, Hepler, Roman,

& Paiement, 2009). However, coaches can use assistant coaches who possess higher levels of skill and can demonstrate skills more easily.

There is no correlation between how effective a coach is and how skilled she is or was at the sport. What is most important is that coaches engage in developmentally appropriate skill development, and that does not automatically transfer from having played the sport. We have observed coaches who were outstanding athletes but ineffective in planning learning progressions and teaching children the skills of the sport. Likewise, we have observed coaches who were not outstanding athletes in their sport but who had the ability to structure the learning environment so that kids developed skills and got better. There is a wealth of sport-specific instructional books and online courses (e.g., www.HumanKineticsCoachEducation Center.com) that coaches can use to enhance their technical skills. Those without coaching experience could begin as interns, or even as assistant coaches with a more experienced head coach, to improve their technical skills.

Managerial Skills

Managerial skills are needed for planning, for organization of programs, and for administration responsibilities (the dreaded paperwork). Managerial skills enable coaches to develop a systematic approach to their coaching through planning, implementing, and evaluating. Coaches may have great technical skills, but without effective management skills to conduct an efficient program, technical knowledge is wasted.

A common and useful practice is to use a division of labor strategy and invite assistant coaches or parents to manage certain tasks. Drafting eligibility forms, purchasing postgame snacks, setting up equipment, and ordering uniform and gear are examples of managerial tasks that can be shared by others to free up the head coach to focus on teaching and coaching duties. The NFHS

Fundamentals of Coaching certification program includes a unit on the coach as manager, and the Coaching Principles course in the Human Kinetics Coach Education certification program includes units on managing teams, relationships, and risk.

Managing risk means that coaches fulfill their legal duties; failure to do so is termed **negligence.** Negligence may occur because of an inappropriate act (requiring full-pads football practice on an extremely hot and humid day without adequate hydration of athletes) or failure to act (not teaching appropriate football tackling technique). The answer to all four of the following questions must be yes in order for coaches to be found negligent:

1. Did the coach have a legal duty to the injured party?
2. Did the coach fail to fulfill this duty?
3. Was there injury to the athlete to whom the coach owed the legal duty?
4. Did the coach's failure to fulfill the duty cause the injury?

Youth coaches have 10 legal duties that they should understand in the unique context of their sport. These duties have been developed by courts of law; they change over time and may vary from state to state. However, those listed are the most prominent duties expected of youth coaches (Martens, 2012).

The best way for coaches to manage their risk is to ensure that they explicitly fulfill each of these duties as would be expected of adults coaching in their specific sports These duties are presented in various chapters of this book—for example, protecting athletes from sexual harassment and abuse (chapter 13) and evaluating athletes for injury, warning of inherent risks, and providing appropriate emergency assistance (chapter 12). The Volunteer Protection Act (known as the Good Samaritan law) provides volunteer coaches in nonprofit organizations with immunity against frivolous lawsuits. However, coaches are still liable in the case of gross negligence. Completing a coaching education program with a risk management or sport law segment is recommended for all youth coaches. And risk management education-certification should be mandatory for program leaders or supervisors of coaches.

Personal Skills

Personal skills needed by coaches may be divided into intrapersonal and interpersonal. We believe this skill set is the most critical one in coaching youth athletes because it focuses on coaches' personal competence in building relationships with their athletes.

Intrapersonal Skills

Intrapersonal skills involve coaches' abilities to be self-aware and emotionally competent, and to fit with the philosophy and objectives of youth sport. Intrapersonal skills are typically overlooked as a requisite for coaching success, but a wealth of sport psychology and business literature emphasizes that these skills are critical for people (like coaches) who work closely with others (e.g., Collins, 2001; Covey, 2013; Vealey, 2005).

Being personally authentic involves being who we are and being honest about ourselves when communicating with others. Authenticity develops trust, respect, and credibility with athletes. Emotional competence is about how well we manage our feelings when relating to others, and it enables coaches to respond openly and rationally without becoming defensive. These intrapersonal skills enable coaches to be more effective in their interpersonal connections with others, particularly their athletes. An example of how intrapersonal skill leads to interpersonal skill and coaching success is the InSideOut coaching approach described in the Water Break section.

Interpersonal Skills

Interpersonal skills are coaches' abilities to build relationships and communicate with others, such as in providing instruction and feedback to athletes as well as responding to parents and officials. (Some guidelines to help coaches effectively interact with youth sport parents are provided in chapter 15.) The majority of research and practical guidelines on youth sport coaching effectiveness focus on the interpersonal skills of coaches; thus, the remainder of the chapter deals with this important topic.

YOUTH SPORT COACHES' META-SKILL: COMMUNICATION

Communication is youth sport coaches' meta-skill, meaning it is a higher-order skill that allows coaches to effectively engage in all other skills (managing, teaching, leading). Research examining youth sport coaches' interpersonal (communication) skills has generally focused on four areas: coach effectiveness training, controlling versus autonomy-supportive coaching, transformative leadership, and coach expectancy theory.

Coach Effectiveness Training

The Coach Effectiveness Training (CET) program was begun at the University of Washington in the late 1970s to provide an ongoing, systematic approach to the study of coaches' interpersonal skills.

Development of the Coaching Behavior Assessment System

The CET investigators first developed a system that identified interpersonal behaviors commonly exhibited by youth sport

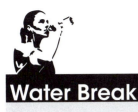

Water Break

InSideOut Coaching

In his acclaimed book *InSideOut Coaching* (2011), Joe Ehrmann emphasizes that the intrapersonal skills of coaches form the foundation for their coaching effectiveness. InSideOut coaching means that coaches have to start with honest self-reflection and self-understanding (inside) before they are able to transform the lives of their athletes (outside). In Ehrmann's opinion (supported by research on parenting), coaches cannot teach athletes critical life skills until they learn these skills themselves.

This intrapersonal work requires coaches to reflect on their positive and negative sport and life experiences, particularly understanding unfulfilled needs and considering how these unmet needs now drive them as coaches and adults. An InSideOut coach does the reflective work to answer four questions: Why do I coach? Why do I coach the way I do? What does it feel like to be coached by me? How do I define success?

Ehrmann developed his InSideOut coaching movement because of his distaste for how young boys were socialized in sport to be stereotypically "manly" (lacking empathy and emotional connections with others). Here's Ehrmann's

answer to why he coaches: "I coach to help boys become men of empathy and integrity who will lead, be responsible, and change the world for good" (p. 110). Without an InSideOut approach, he feels that coaches are too often serving themselves at the expense of their athletes' needs.

Ehrmann's program offers many examples of "Outside Lessons" for athletes and coaches. Examples include "Moments of Greatness," in which athletes are asked to describe something they or a teammate did that week to positively affect another person; brief lessons at the start of each practice; and discussions about dating abuse and gender violence. An InSideOut code of conduct for coaches goes beyond normal coaching platitudes to include such guidelines as "Don't be afraid to apologize! We all make mistakes."

We wholeheartedly endorse InSideOut coaching as a fresh, athlete-centered approach to coaching young athletes. The easy-to-read book *Season of Change* (2012), by Walter Sparks, is the story of how one coach and his staff implemented InSideOut coaching with their youth football team; this is another helpful resource for youth coaches who want to be more InSideOut in their coaching.

coaches (Smith, Smoll, & Hunt, 1977). This system was called the **Coaching Behavior Assessment System (CBAS,** pronounced *SEE-bass*). Researchers were trained to identify these specific coach interpersonal behaviors; then they went out and observed

coaches and coded their behaviors onto a recording sheet to assess how often they engaged in different types of interpersonal behaviors. I (first author) spent time in graduate school hanging out around Little League baseball coaches and coding their behavior onto the CBAS forms. It was a great education.

How Coach Behaviors Relate to Athlete Outcomes

The most positive outcomes occurred when children played for coaches who engaged in high levels of reinforcement for good performance and effort and who responded to mistakes with encouragement and technical instruction (Smith & Smoll, 2007). Children liked these coaches more and had more fun when playing. In contrast, the more punishment oriented the coaches' behavior, the less the athletes liked the coach and the sport experience. These findings were particularly strong for youth athletes with low self-esteem, indicating how influential coaches' interpersonal behavior is to kids who lack self-esteem. Notably, the team's win–loss record was unrelated to how well the athletes liked their coaches and how much they wanted to play for these coaches in the future.

Results of the CET Program With Coaches

The investigators then developed the CET program, a training program for coaches that taught youth coaches to increase reinforcement, instruction, and encouragement and to decrease their use of punishment and nonreinforcement. The CET program also emphasized and taught coaches how to develop a mastery-oriented climate that put athlete and skill development ahead of winning. When trained coaches were compared to untrained coaches (Smith & Smoll, 2007), the results were impressive.

CET-trained coaches

- increased their use of reinforcement, encouragement, and instruction (and decreased their use of punishment) and
- were better liked by athletes and rated as better teachers by athletes.

Youth athletes who played for CET-trained coaches

- enjoyed sport more and experienced less anxiety,
- significantly increased their self-esteem from the previous year, and
- had a lower dropout rate (5%) from sport as compared to athletes who played for untrained coaches (26%).

Overall, CET demonstrated that working with youth sport coaches to enhance their interpersonal behaviors had very positive effects on athletes who played for these coaches. These findings have been replicated by others using the CET model (Coatsworth & Conroy, 2006) and extended to develop the Mastery Approach to Coaching (MAC) program. The MAC program showed decreased anxiety in athletes over the course of the season (as compared to athletes with non-trained coaches, whose anxiety increased) (Smith, Smoll, & Cumming, 2007).

Coaches' interpersonal behaviors have also been examined in relation to specific situations that occur in sport, with the intent of identifying each coach's unique **behavioral signature** (Smith, Shoda, Cumming, & Smoll, 2009). Certain coaches' instructional behaviors declined and punitive behaviors increased when their teams were losing. As you might expect, coaches who became more punitive in losing situations were less liked by athletes. Observing behavioral signatures seems to be the "acid test" of coaches' interpersonal skills in identifying their true interpersonal tendencies in response to emotion-provoking situations in sport, such as losing.

Controlling Versus Autonomy-Supportive Coach Behavior

Controlling versus autonomy-supportive behavior by coaches is another research area related to the effects of coaches' interpersonal behavior on athletes. This is usually studied in relation to motivation, which is why we discuss it in chapter 6 of this book. As defined in that chapter, **autonomy-supportive coaching** means that youth sport coaches listen to and attempt to understand their athletes, provide them with opportunities for input and choices, and minimize demanding or controlling behaviors. Youth athletes who perceive that their coaches are autonomy supportive feel more competent and connected to teammates and also experience less burnout and greater well-being (Adie, Duda, & Ntoumanis, 2012; Coatsworth & Conroy, 2009).

Strategies for becoming more autonomy supportive, as well as the interpersonal skill of disciplining athletes, are discussed in chapter 6. The traditional autocratic style of coaching, using intimidation and threat, is automatically adopted by many youth sport coaches because this is what they believe coaches should use. Consider the following example of a youth sport coach (found to be ineffective in his coaching) using excessive controlling interpersonal behavior:

> *Somebody cursed and I asked them who did it. At first they wouldn't tell me, so I made them run. So they ran, got back to the baseline, and I said, "Now tell me who did it." They still wouldn't tell me—I made them run again. So finally when we got back this time they said, "Well, Mike did it." So I made them run again 'cause it's like, you don't snitch on your teammates (Flett, Gould, Griffes, & Lauer, 2013, p. 331).*

Such controlling behavior is ineffective and inappropriate in youth sport. Coaches may need help in recognizing their inappropriate behaviors driven by a need for excessive control (some intrapersonal skill is required to figure out why they need excessive control). Following are some checklist items[9] that coaches can use for self-reflection

---

[9] These items were taken from the Controlling Coach Behaviors Scale (Bartholomew, Ntoumanis, & Thogersen-Ntoumani, 2010) and do not represent the entire scale.

regarding their tendency to engage in controlling behaviors:

- Do I pay less attention to an athlete who has displeased me?
- Do I threaten to punish my athletes to keep them in line during training?
- Do I only use rewards and praise to make athletes train harder?
- Do I expect my athletes' entire lives to center on their sport participation?
- Do I embarrass athletes in front of others if they don't do what I want them to do?
- Am I less supportive of my athletes when they are not training or competing well?

Transformative Leadership

A third area of study that focuses on interpersonal effectiveness in youth sport coaching is **transformative leadership.** This style of leadership emphasizes the relationship between coach and athlete, with the coach helping to shape athletes' beliefs and attitudes. Joe Ehrmann's (2011) InSideOut coaching is a perfect example of transformative leadership. Transformative coaches engage in the four I's (Bass, 1985): **I**nspirational motivation, **I**nfluence through modeling the right behaviors, **I**ndividualized attention to athletes, and **I**ntellectual stimulation (encouraging athletes to be creative and learn on their own). Research in youth sport has shown that transformative coach behavior enhances adolescent athletes' confidence, motivation, enjoyment, and effort (Arthur, Woodman, Ong, Hardy, & Ntoumanis, 2011; Price & Weiss, 2013).

Coach Expectancy Theory

Have you ever had a coach who believed in you so much that it increased your belief in yourself and made your performance soar? Or conversely, have you ever underperformed

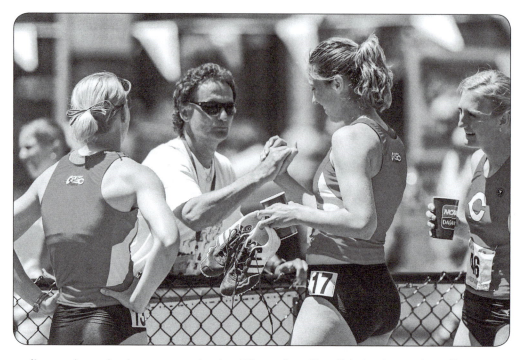

Coaches often unknowingly communicate differently with athletes based on the expectations that they have for these athletes.

because you had a coach who didn't value your abilities and made you feel less confident? This psychological influence of coaches on athletes is based on **coach expectancy theory,** which proposes that the expectations that coaches form about the abilities of individual athletes have the potential to determine the level of achievement each athlete ultimately reaches (Horn, Lox, & Labrador, 2015). This is also called self-fulfilling prophecy, as the coaches' expectations create a process in which these expectations (or prophecies) come true for athletes.

The Four-Step Coach Expectancy Process

Four steps explain how coach expectancy creates a self-fulfilling prophecy (as shown in figure 14.2). (1) The coach forms an expectation for each athlete in terms of level of ability and predicted performance. (2) Often without the coach's realizing it, this expectation influences his interactions with the athlete. (3) The interpersonal behavior

of the coach toward the athlete influences her perceived competence, motivation, and overall ability to learn. (4) The athlete's subsequent behavior and performance conform to the coach's original expectation. What a powerful process! Let's go over each step, so you can better understand the vast potential that youth sport coaches have to influence their athletes.

Step 1: Coaches Develop Expectations About Athletes

It's typical for coaches to make judgments about the abilities of athletes, but the important thing is to make these judgments in a certain way using certain kinds of information. The information sources coaches use to assess athletes fall into three categories: personal, psychological, and performance characteristics (Horn et al., 2015). Personal characteristics include gender, race, body size and shape, physical attractiveness, style of dress, and family background. Psychological characteristics have to do with coaches' perceptions of things like athletes' coachability,

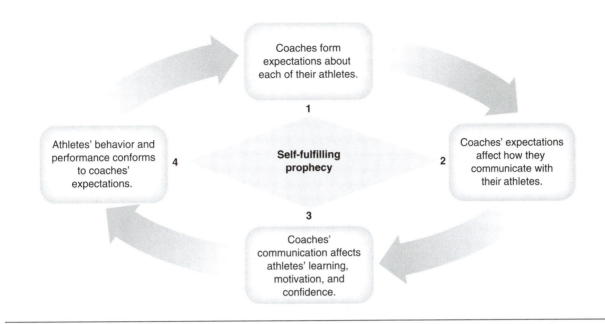

Figure 14.2 How coaches' expectations may create self-fulfilling prophecies for athletes.

mental toughness, and emotional maturity. Performance characteristics include performance of athletes observed in training and competition, individual statistics or performance charts, and past performance accomplishments.

Which sources do you think are better for coaches to use in evaluating youth athletes? Obviously, personal characteristics are a poor choice, as they often represent stereotypes. Late-maturing boys could be labeled as low-ability athletes when in reality they're just behind in maturation and physical skill development. Stereotypical coach expectancies also might include viewing female athletes as less skilled because they're girls, or African American athletes as naturally gifted and less hardworking than white athletes. Youth athletes who display Mohawk haircuts, tattoos, and alternative-type clothing are often stereotyped in negative ways.

Psychological characteristics are an important part of what an athlete brings to a youth sport situation. However, coaches should remember that their perceptions of these characteristics are just perceptions and could actually be inaccurate. Performance characteristics represent the best source of information about the abilities of young athletes. However, the ways in which performance are assessed is crucial. To obtain the most accurate assessment of athletes, coaches need to engage in multiple, performance-based assessments of athletes' abilities across time. Coaches' initial assessments of athletes' abilities may be inaccurate, so they should continuously reevaluate athletes' performance to give every athlete the chance to demonstrate performance improvement.

Step 2: Coaches' Expectations Influence Their Communication With Athletes Multiple studies have supported that coaches often communicate differently with athletes based on the expectations they have for the athletes (Horn et al., 2015). Coaches tend to spend more time and show more interpersonal warmth with high-expectancy athletes as compared to low-expectancy athletes. Low-expectancy athletes often spend more time on nonskill-related activities (shagging balls, waiting in line) and are held to lower standards of performance than high-expectancy athletes. For example, a low-expectancy volleyball player might receive praise for simply hitting a spike inbounds, whereas a high-expectancy athlete may get immediate feedback from the coach on how to more accurately find the hole in the defense with his spike. This additional corrective or prescriptive feedback that high-expectancy athletes receive provides them with a powerful learning advantage. Giving low-expectancy athletes unearned praise for mediocre performance is another negative coach expectancy behavior that only sends these athletes the message that they're not very good and that coaches don't expect a lot from them.

Step 3: Coaches' Communication With Athletes Affects Their Confidence, Motivation, and Ability to Learn

Young athletes who consistently get less effective instruction and attention from coaches will not show the same degree of skill improvement as their high-expectancy teammates. Research has shown that different types of communication from coaches can influence athletes' self-esteem, self-confidence, motivation, anxiety, and decisions to continue in sport (Horn et al., 2015).

Step 4: Athletes' Behavior and Performance Conform to Coaches' Expectations

This final step confirms to coaches that their judgments, or expectations of their athletes, were accurate. Not all athletes are susceptible to the coach expectancy effect. However, young children (9 years and younger) are particularly influenced by the feedback and evaluation of significant adults, including coaches. Thus, children in sport may be particularly susceptible to the expectations and communication of coaches about their abilities as athletes. Because childhood is such an important time for motor skill development, youth sport coaches should be extremely mindful and take thoughtful steps to avoid sending negative expectancy messages to kids.

Strategies for Coaches

Not all coaches fall into the coach expectancy trap, although we all are susceptible to it simply because we are human. Youth sport coaches should remain mindful that their expectations and impressions are very powerful influences on their communication with young athletes. Here are three strategies for coaches to use to avoid the negative coach expectancy trap:

1. Maintain high expectations for all athletes based on their unique skill levels. Everyone can learn and improve her individual skills. A mastery focus on skill development and improvement is helpful.

2. Coaches should keep their expectations for athletes flexible and open to constant change by creating a "clean slate" each day of training and competition to accurately assess athletes' developing abilities. Kids are constantly maturing and developing, and they often surprise us with performance improvements as a simple result of development.

3. Coaches should focus on the interpersonal coaching skill of providing specific, information-loaded instruction and feedback to all athletes. They should avoid general evaluative comments that don't allow young athletes to understand what and why they did well in the game that day. "Your defense was great today—you fronted the post the entire time and really boxed out well" beats the more general "Good job today." This lets each athlete know that a coach paid specific attention to his performance and contributions to the team that day.

WRAP-UP

When we ask college students in our classes to identify their heroes, coaches are often prominently mentioned. It's amazing to hear students' stories about the coaching heroes that made such a difference in their lives. Youth sport needs more "hero coaches" who believe it's all about the kid, as opposed to "zero coaches" who focus on their own selfish needs.

What does it take to be a hero coach? Does it require the heroism displayed by Frank Hall, who in 2012 was a football coach at Chardon (Ohio) High School when a shooter opened fire on students in the school cafeteria? Coach Hall chased the shooter from the school and then gently comforted the fatally wounded students in their last moments. Filled with grief, Coach Hall stated that he was no hero for his actions that horrific day. However, his athletes called him a hero for his coaching style; he practiced the InSideOut coaching philosophy of teaching his players how to be better men, not just football players.

All youth sport coaches can be heroes simply by understanding and meeting young athletes' needs to learn skills, enjoy what they're doing, and develop confidence and relationship skills. All youth sport coaches should reflect on their powerful influence on kids; they should be thoughtful and take great care to use this power and influence in developmentally appropriate ways.

LEARNING AIDS

Key Terms

autonomy-supportive coaching—A behavioral style in which coaches listen to and attempt to understand their athletes, provide them with opportunities for input and choices, and minimize demanding or controlling behaviors.

behavioral signature—Coaches' typical interpersonal tendencies in response to emotion-provoking situations in sport, such as losing.

coach expectancy theory—Theory proposing that the expectations coaches form about the abilities of individual athletes have the potential to determine the level of achievement each athlete ultimately reaches.

Coaching Behavior Assessment System (CBAS)—A categorization system that identifies interpersonal behaviors commonly exhibited by youth sport coaches.

interpersonal skills—Coaches' abilities to build relationships and communicate with others.

intrapersonal skills—Coaches' abilities to be self-aware and emotionally competent and to fit with the philosophy and objectives of youth sport.

managerial skills—Coaches' abilities to plan and organize programs and fulfill all administrative responsibilities.

negligence—Failure of coaches to fulfill their legal duties due to an inappropriate act or failure to act.

skill set—A combination of abilities that enable people to succeed in certain positions.

technical skills—Coaches' abilities to teach skills and tactics in training, as well as knowledge of how to use tactics when coaching in competition.

transformative leadership—A style of leadership that emphasizes the relationship between coach and athlete, with the coach helping to shape athletes' beliefs and attitudes.

Summary Points

1. Coaches influence the youth sport experience for young athletes more than any other factor.

2. The majority of nonschool youth sport coaches are volunteers, without formal coaching certification.

3. Canada, Australia, New Zealand, and Great Britain all have nationally sponsored coaching education–certification programs; coaching certification is more decentralized and entrepreneur oriented in the United States.

4. Most middle and high schools in the United States require basic coach education-certification, with most using the NFHS Fundamentals of Coaching program or the Human Kinetics Coach Education Coaching Principles course.

5. Recruiting and evaluating youth sport coaches should be a systematic year-round process, using multiple resources within communities such as college students and retired coaches and teachers.

6. The three primary skill sets needed by youth sport coaches are technical, managerial, and personal.

7. Coaches must fulfill their legal duties to avoid negligence and manage their risk of lawsuits.

8. Athletes who played for coaches trained in the Coach Effectiveness Training (CET) program enjoyed sport more, experienced less anxiety, increased their self-esteem, and had a lower dropout rate from sport as compared to athletes who played for untrained coaches.

9. Coaches who use autonomy-supportive coaching styles and engage in transformative leadership positively influence youth athletes' confidence, motivation, enjoyment, and effort.

10. The coach expectancy theory states that the expectations coaches form about the abilities of their athletes have the potential to determine the level of achievement athletes ultimately reach.

11. To avoid negative coach expectancy effects, youth coaches should use multiple performance assessments, provide specific and informative feedback to all athletes, and keep their expectations for athletes flexible and open to constant change.

Study Questions

1. Why is there resistance to requiring coach certification in youth sport?

2. Describe the contextualized coaching education–certification programs sponsored by the Canadian and New Zealand governments, and explain the advantages of these types of programs.

3. How is youth sport coaching education in the United States different from that in other countries?

4. What are some strategies youth directors can use in recruiting and evaluating youth sport coaches?

5. What are the three primary skill sets needed by youth coaches? Explain the importance of each, as well as how coaches can develop these skills.

6. What is negligence, how is it determined in a court of law, and how can coaches manage their risk of charges of negligence?

7. What were the findings of the research on Coach Effectiveness Training, and why are these findings important?

8. Describe the four-step process outlined in coach expectancy theory.

9. What are the best sources of information for coaches to use in evaluating athletes' abilities? Why are these sources preferred over others?

10. Explain three case examples of how coaches may behave differently toward high-expectancy versus low-expectancy athletes in practice or competition.

Reflective Learning Activities

1. Identify a youth sport coach you can interview. Prepare an interview guide with questions you will ask the coach about his or her development of the skill set needed and used in his or her coaching. (It may or may not be one of the skill sets explained in this book.) Interview the coach to understand how he or she developed these skills, what he or she feels are the skills needed to coach youth sport, and his or her thoughts about and experiences with coaching education programs.

2. Using the CBAS, observe a coach in one training session, and code his or her behaviors using the CBAS categories. Write up a summary of this coach's communication pattern based on the results of your observation.

3. Complete a CBAS evaluation of a coach as described in question 2; but beforehand, ask the coach to rank from top to bottom the ability of all the athletes on the team. Split the athletes into high-expectancy and low-expectancy groups based on the coach's rankings. Conduct your CBAS assessment by coding the coaches' responses to individual athletes to see if there are any differences in the types of communication provided to the different expectancy groups. (Note: You will have to become familiar with and learn the names of each of the athletes to be able to code coach behaviors in relation to each.)

4. Assign a percentage to each of the specific CBAS categories for how much of coaches' communication to athletes should be included in that category. All your assigned category percentages should add up to 100%. The idea is for you to consider the ideal amount of each type of interpersonal communication within coaches' overall communication to athletes.

Resource Guide

Martens, R. (2012). *Successful coaching* (4th ed.). Champaign, IL: Human Kinetics.

Thompson, J. (2008). *Positive coaching in a nutshell.* Portola Valley, CA: Balance Sports.

Thompson, J. (2010). *The power of double-goal coaching.* Portola Valley, CA: Balance Sports.

Multiple sport-specific coaching books and online certification programs (www.Human KineticsCoachEducationCenter.com).

Sport-specific coaching courses and Fundamentals of Coaching national certification program, National Federation of State High School Associations (www.nfhslearn. com).

chapter 15

PARENTS AND YOUTH SPORT

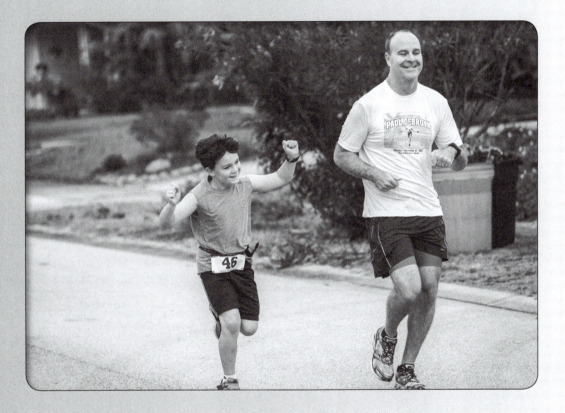

CHAPTER PREVIEW

In this chapter, you'll learn

- » types of parenting styles,
- » the three M's that represent youth sport parent roles,
- » about optimal parental push in youth sport, and
- » guidelines for better youth sport parenting.

Dear Daddy,

Thank you for cheering me on at soccer games and not yelling at me and telling me what to do. I know that some parents from other teams do that and some of our parents too. But I know that I have to make my own decisions when I play and most of the time it's distracting when people tell me what to do. I think you're setting a good example for all the other parents and plus me. When I grow up I will try to do everything you taught me. Even though I might make mistakes.

Love,

Stasianne Marie Mallin

A 9-year-old soccer player wrote this letter to her father, Kevin, who, as a former student of ours, shared it with us. What useful insights we can gain from Stasianne's words! Cheering works, but yelling and coaching from the stands doesn't. She reminds us that young athletes have to play the game themselves and make their own decisions as well as mistakes. She explains that when parents overstep their boundaries, kids are distracted from playing and learning the game on their own. A gift that Kevin gave his daughter was the permission to make mistakes and accept them as part of life and learning. His parenting approach served as a strong model for her, and as she suggests, for other parents as well.

Because young athletes are minors and dependent children, parents are a major part of youth sport. In fact, youth sport would cease to exist without the cooperation, support, and leadership of parents. Extreme examples of negative youth sport parenting earn a lot of media attention, but the majority of parents contribute positively to the success of youth sport and the well-being of young athletes. Parents are critical in helping children effectively navigate the world of youth sport. Equally important, yet often overlooked, are parents' abilities to effectively navigate the world of youth sport for themselves. Parents' own past experiences affect how they view sport and how they respond to their children's participating in youth sport. Therefore, the objective of this chapter is to explain how parents influence their children's participation in youth sport and are influenced by it.

FOUNDATIONS OF THE PARENT–CHILD RELATIONSHIP

Let's start off with some basic aspects of the parent–child relationship to provide a foundation for understanding youth sport parenting.

Attachment

The deep emotional bond that connects parents to children is called **attachment** (Bowlby, 1988). Attachment results in parents responding sensitively and appropriately to their children's needs, with parents becoming a secure base for their children. Attachments typically form with those who respond most accurately to children's needs, not with those they spend the most time with. The critical period for attachments is from birth to 5 years, with irreversible developmental consequences occurring for children who do not have this secure base.

Understanding attachment helps explain some of the irrational parent behavior in youth sport. The emotional bond that parents have with their children often short-circuits their rational sense and ability to reason when they feel their children are mistreated, hurt, or distraught. We certainly can remember times when we reacted emotionally at our children's youth sport events, only to realize later that our emotional displays were inappropriate. Parents feel deeply about their kids and even feel what their kids are feeling, which clearly influences their behavior as youth sport parents.

When parents perceived that their child was treated poorly compared to other children, or when their child was not given the same opportunities as teammates, they were more likely to act inappropriately at youth sport events (Wiersma & Fifer, 2008). Parents admitted that observing their kids in the competitive environment often changed them from rational, good-natured adults to people who acted in emotionally explosive ways that they later regretted. Their behavior appeared to be influenced by their parental attachment and an instinct to protect their child from harm or unfair treatment (Wiersma & Fifer, 2008). Attachment also leads parents to more positive vicarious experiences, as in when they feel great joy in observing their children's enjoyment, improvement, development, and success in youth sport (Wiersma & Fifer, 2008).

Evolution of Parent–Child Relationships

Another factor that influences youth sport parents is the idealized cultural norm regarding what it means to be a good parent. Parent–child relationships have evolved over time, with many changes in what is viewed as socially acceptable. Children were exploited in the labor market through the 1800s, until child labor laws finally protected them (mostly poor children) from oppressive jobs. Also during this time, religious beliefs led parents to use sternness and whippings to "shape" children to obey their parents. Noted clergyman John Wesley admonished, "Break their wills that you may save their souls."

It wasn't until the last quarter of the 20th century that children came to be viewed as more than parental property and instead as human beings with rights who required special protection and treatment (Rutherford, 2009). Widespread use of contraception and family planning in the 1970s led to smaller family sizes so that children came to be planned for and viewed as "golden" (Tofler & DiGeronimo, 2000). These golden children enjoyed greater economic privilege even if their parents had to sacrifice their own needs to achieve it. Quite often, children came to be seen as collateral for parental investments of money, time, and attention. This often led to children's sacrificing their own goals to those of their parents, which certainly can and does occur in youth sport.

The style of "hothouse parenting" (Marano, 2008) that arose in the United States in the 1980s (and continues today) is mentioned in chapter 2 as having a strong influence on youth sport. This parenting style focuses on preparing children to be special, as opposed to the earlier parenting practice of protecting kids' childhood years to ensure them normal childhoods (Farrey, 2008). The hothouse parenting ideal has led to the frenzy of overscheduled, tightly controlled, highly specialized, financially draining activities to push children to achieve, as often occurs in youth sport.

We raise this point to increase your awareness of cultural changes in parenting ideals so that you won't uncritically accept the current norm for parent–child relationships in our society. Ideas about child-rearing and the rights and needs of children have been and will continue to be culturally and historically shaped. It's important that we continue to consider the effectiveness of current child-rearing practices, keeping in mind both the optimal development of children and the well-being of all family members, including parents.

Parenting Styles

Think about your parents and consider the ways in which they interacted with you.

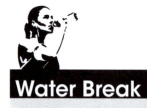

Water Break

Youth Sport Parenting as Business?

Professional golfer Sean O'Hair endured a childhood as a business project for his father, Marc, the intent being to turn Sean into a golf superstar. From an early age, Sean was forced into a military-like regimen of training and endured punishments for less than desirable performances, such as being forced to run certain distances for making bogeys or finishing over par at tournaments. In a hurry to cash in on his investment, Mr. O'Hair directed Sean to turn pro in 1999, at age 17, after his junior year in high school. At that time, Mr. O'Hair forced Sean to sign a contract requiring him to pay his father 10% of all professional earnings for life. Mr. O'Hair states, "I know how to make a profit . . . it's material, labor, and overhead. [Sean's] pretty good labor. I told [Sean], I can't blow this kind of money without a return. When you make it, there has to be a payback someday" (Elling, 2005). Looking back, Sean said, "We have never had a father–son relationship. It has always been the investor and the investment" (Elling, 2005).

In 2005, Mr. O'Hair, who claims he spent $2 million on his son's career, released Sean from their contract. Mr. O'Hair stated for the media, "Even though Sean must sooner or later assume responsibilities for his own actions, I will bail him out of another one of his problems by releasing him from liability concerning the contract" (Cybergolf, 2014). Sean's attorney stated that the contract would likely not hold up in court since Sean was less than 18 years old when he signed it.

Now happily married with a young daughter, Sean has moved on and has enjoyed relative success on the Professional Golfers' Association tour. Sean also sounds like a successful father in stating, "There's a fine line [between] being supportive and being overbearing. I want the best for my daughter. But you have to know when to let them make their own mistakes, and let them learn on their own." Mr. O'Hair, however, retains a different view, stating, "I feel like a damn fool. I thought I would get every penny back" (Elling, 2005).

What did they do (or not do) that influenced your development the most? What made them effective or ineffective as parents? Your description of your parents probably situates them in one of several categories of parenting styles. **Parenting style** is the overall manner in which parents interact with their children, based on parents' attitudes and values about what the relationship should be between parent and child (Darling & Steinberg, 1993).

Most simplistically, parenting styles are based on levels of responsiveness and demandingness[10] (Baumrind, 1989) (see figure 15.1). Responsiveness is the extent to which parents support children's autonomy and respond to their needs. Demandingness is the extent to which parents set limits and expect adherence to rules and mature behavior. As shown in figure 15.1, four parenting styles emerge from different combinations of responsiveness and demandingness.

[10] Many different types of parenting styles have been identified (see Horn and Horn [2007] for a review). The styles presented in this book are the most widely used in discussions of parenting effectiveness.

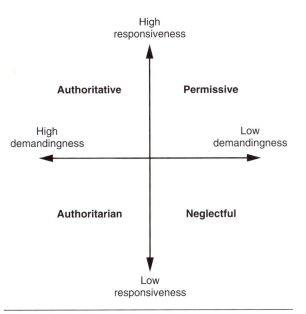

High
responsiveness

Authoritative   Permissive

High   Low
demandingness   demandingness

Authoritarian   Neglectful

Low
responsiveness

Figure 15.1 Parenting styles as combinations of responsiveness and demandingness.

Adapted from Baumrind 1989.

The **authoritative parenting style** is high in both responsiveness and demandingness. It involves setting high standards and limits, showing respect for and reasoning with kids, and being nurturing and responsive to their emotional needs. An authoritative parent might say things like "I encourage my child to talk about his feelings" and "I provide my child with reasons for the expectations I have for him." Parents with an **authoritarian parenting style** are demanding but less responsive. They emphasize obedience without explanation or any attempt to reason with children. Those with a **permissive parenting style** are high in responsiveness but less demanding. They are reluctant to impose rules and standards and thus provide little structure, preferring to let their children regulate themselves. Those with a **neglectful parenting style** are neither demanding nor responsive—they're disengaged and unsupportive.

Hmmm . . . so what style did your parents fit into? Which parenting style would you prefer? Authoritative parenting leads to more positive outcomes for children and adolescents in terms of life satisfaction, academic competence, higher self-esteem, and lower rates of risky health behaviors (Horn & Horn, 2007). Authoritative parenting predicted greater athlete satisfaction, compliance with rules, team cohesion, and motivation in youth ice hockey (Juntumaa, Keskivaara, & Punamaki, 2005); it also has been associated with healthy (as compared to unhealthy) perfectionism in youth soccer players (Sapieja, Dunn, & Holt, 2011). Authoritative, or autonomy-supportive, parenting is identified as an important component of youth sport parenting expertise (Harwood & Knight, 2015).

Overall, understanding attachment, idealized cultural norms for parenting, and parenting styles helps explain a lot of parent behavior in youth sport. Parents act based on their deep emotional connections with their children, because they are trying to be culturally prescribed "good" parents, and based on the parental style that they value and believe in. Keeping these foundations of the parent–child relationship in mind enables us to better understand both positive and negative parenting behavior in youth sport.

THREE ROLES OF YOUTH SPORT PARENTS

Parenting is a challenge. A favorite ornament on our family Christmas tree each year is inscribed with the words "Motherhood is not for wimps." To be culturally competent, we'll amend that to "Parenthood is not for wimps." Parenting requires a broad skill set (Fredricks & Eccles, 2004; Harwood & Knight, 2015), most of which we learn on the job. To help categorize this skill set, we propose that youth sport parents have to fulfill three important roles[11]: manager, model, and meaning maker (see figure 15.2). You can think of these as the three M's of youth sport parenting.

[11] Fredricks and Eccles (2004) frame parents' roles as interpreters of experience, providers of experience, and role models. Harwood and Knight (2015) discuss a range of competencies required of youth sport parents, which they categorize as intrapersonal, interpersonal, and organizational. We chose to simplify these authors' categories into the three roles of youth sport parents presented in this book, which we call the three M's of youth sport parenting, for practical clarity.

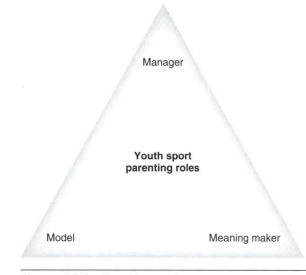

Figure 15.2 The three M's representing youth sport parenting roles.

Manager

Boy, do parents need management skills if they have children involved in youth sport! Serving as parental managers for youth sport participants includes providing financial support, coordinating travel and ride schedules, sacrificing personal time for young athletes' training and competition, volunteering to coach or manage youth sport teams, and aiding in team activities such as fund-raising and end-of-season banquets. Parents who have multiple children participating in youth sport can attest to the challenge of juggling extensive parental management responsibilities.

These responsibilities have grown due to the increasing professionalization of youth sport, with youth athletes commonly training longer hours and traveling more extensively. When Olympic and professional basketball star Maya Moore was 12, her mother moved them to Atlanta so Moore could play and travel with a high-level Amateur Athletic Union (AAU) basketball team, the Georgia Metros (with whom she won four national championships in four years). Eugene Heyward, father of professional

baseball star Jason Heyward, arranged his job and life around the youth baseball schedule of his son. Jason Heyward states, "They had a plan, my parents. I appreciate that they did everything they could to get me in front of all the right people. But my dad said, 'Without you saying you wanted it, it wouldn't have happened.' Every year he asked, 'Do you still want to play baseball?'" (Verducci, 2010, p. 64).

An important managerial role of parents is to introduce children to a variety of sport and physical activity experiences. As you learned in chapters 5 and 10, childhood is a time of sampling, during which kids try out many different activities to find those that suit them best. Parents are instrumental in providing opportunities for kids to sample a wide variety of sport activities, particularly before adolescence, when fundamental motor skill development is needed.

Attempting to fulfill the parent manager role in youth sport is often difficult and has led to strained spousal relations, constricted social opportunities for parents, sibling resentment, and parental job conflicts (Harwood & Knight, 2009). Many parents have admitted that the monetary expenses of modern youth sport are a burden, and that juggling kids' training and competition schedules and constant transportation needs along with other tasks (family meals, homework) is very difficult. However, despite these demands and the strain on family time, most parents stated that the benefits of youth sport for their children made it all worthwhile (Wiersma & Fifer, 2008).

Model

The second important role for youth sport parents is to serve as **models** for their children, which means they set standards or provide examples for imitation or comparison. Parents' modeling of physical activity and sport participation, moral behavior and life skills (e.g., respecting coaches and officials, effectively managing emotions), work ethic, and participation in gendered activities has been shown to influence kids' perceptions and behavior (Wiersma & Fifer, 2008). Although active parents tend to have active children, parents' own participation in sport or physical activity is not as influential on kids as parental support, encouragement, feedback, and overall valuation of sport or physical activity (Horn & Horn, 2007). Parents' beliefs in the value and usefulness of sport participation have been related to children's feelings of sport competence, the value they place on sport participation, and their actual levels of participation (Clark, 2008; Fredricks & Eccles, 2005).

So it's helpful for kids to have parents who are active in sport or physical activity, which provides opportunities for children to learn from and play with their parents. However, if parents don't have the skills or time to engage in sport, they still can be positive models for youth athletes by demonstrating the value that they see in their child's sport participation. Parents don't necessarily need to be good athletes—they just need to be encouraging and supportive parents!

Some children of former elite athletes have admitted feeling pressure to become high-performing athletes like their parents, even though their parents did not overtly pressure them to pursue elite status (Fraser-Thomas, Cote, & Deakin, 2008b). I (first author) consulted with a college hockey player whose father had been a well-known National Hockey League star. The college player expressed appreciation for the opportunities he had gained from his father, but admitted that "it sucked" as a youth athlete trying to live up to expectations of being as good as his father. Parents and coaches may consider counseling children with elite athlete parents to help them enjoy their accomplishments and participation apart from any comparison with their accomplished parents.

Meaning Maker

The third M representing an important youth sport parent role is meaning maker. Youth athletes need constant guidance in understanding and thinking about their sport participation, as in "How should I feel about competing in front of others today?" "What if I mess up?" "How did I do?" "Am I any good?" "Which sport is right for me?" "Why do I play?" "Does it matter if I lose?" "How should I act when I win?" "What if other kids are better than me?" The ways in which parents guide young athletes in answering these questions strongly influence kids' enjoyment, motivation to continue in sport, self-esteem, and feelings of competence (Fredricks & Eccles, 2004) (see some meaning-making examples in table 15.1).

Parents' emotional support and encouragement is a critical aspect of parents' meaning-maker role. It has been linked to the quality of the sport experience, continuing motivation, enjoyment, and self-esteem in youth athletes (e.g., Lauer, Gould, Roman, & Pierce, 2010a, 2010b). Parents' emotional support acts as a buffer in helping children cope with performance failures and competitive stress (Cote, 1999). Tennis champion Chris Evert speaks of the emotional support provided by her father: "His was the voice I wanted to hear after a tough loss—he always found a way to soothe me and point out the positives" (Evert, 2010). Relating back to the secure base that children feel from attachment with parents, perhaps the most important emotional provision parents can give to their children is unconditional love and acceptance. This means that the secure base is solid, without any conditions about performing well, winning, or living up to parents' expectations and standards.

Other types of meaning that parents can provide to young athletes include productive attributions for their performances, permission to make mistakes, praise for effort and mastery (not outcomes), and

Table 15.1 Parenting Meaning-Making Examples

Situation	Sample parental response
Athlete is anxious and worried about important competition.	"Most all athletes feel nervous before big competitions. It means your body is getting ready to play, which is a good thing. Have fun today and work hard—that's what's important."
Athlete loses or performs poorly, and you're in the car riding home.	Don't assume that a discussion is necessary. Kids often get over losses more quickly than adults. You can ask, "How'd you feel about the game today?" If the child expresses negative feelings, you can say, "I know you're disappointed, but you're the kind of person who won't let this keep you down. You can rebound from this." Add "I'm sure you and your coach can find a good strategy to get better."
Athlete makes mistake and looks at you in the stands.	Take care to control your nonverbal responses, as kids easily read your posture and facial expressions. Avoid nonverbal signals that it's the end of the world and that you're upset. Smile and give an encouraging signal to signify that it's okay and to brush it off and move on.
Athlete has a hero moment and the team wins.	As with not overreacting to losing, don't overreact to winning. Praise effort and training that enabled the hero moment to happen. Be careful with "I'm so proud of you"; rather, show pride in controllable things like preparation and dedication that paid off.

Adapted from Thompson 2009.

autonomy-supportive behaviors (all discussed in chapter 6). Tiger Woods' father Earl implemented a unique way to support and develop Tiger's autonomy and responsibility as a junior golfer. Once they arrived at a tournament, they would reverse roles, and Tiger would check them in and out of the hotel and plan the schedule, including when to get up, when to eat, and when to leave for the course. After the tournament, they would reverse roles again (Callahan, 2006).

Youth sport parents have admitted that performing effectively in this meaning-maker role is challenging. Parents understand the importance of helping their children interpret competitive experiences—for example, in the car ride home after competition—but they have struggled in knowing what to say and how to help their kids process things in a productive way (Wiersma & Fifer, 2008). Parents have also struggled in helping children maintain their commitment to practice and competition when they perceived that they were not as good as the other kids on the team (Wiersma & Fifer, 2008). These concerns of parents are understandable, as we've struggled with knowing what to say to our children with regard to devastating losses, lack of playing time, or decreased motivation to continue in the sport. Research with youth sport parents showed that over time, they gained needed perspective and maturity in their meaning-maker roles (particularly after they had had experience with older siblings) (Wiersma & Fifer, 2008).

The meaning that parents help athletes derive from their sport participation also helps them to perform better. Talking with children to help them understand and accept nervousness as a normal part of competing is helpful; focusing on lessons learned after losing helps them understand the nature of competition. Parents help children internalize expectations for achievement striving, such as high standards, effort and focus, and commitment to their sport training (Pomerantz, Grolnick, & Price, 2005). By providing honest, pertinent feedback in response to children's performance attempts, parents help children form accurate perceptions of their competence to enhance their motivation and persistence in pursuing challenging goals in sport.

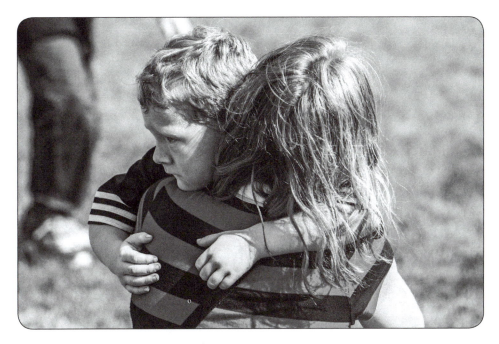

Emotional support from parents has been linked to the quality of the sport experience, continuing motivation, enjoyment, and self-esteem in youth athletes.

Water Break

Making Meaning by Providing Choice

Chris Evert, winner of 18 Grand Slam singles titles, explains how her father enabled her to make her own decisions about the importance of tennis in her life. "He never once got mad when I lost a match; he never yelled or put pressure on me to excel. As long as I tried my best, my dad was satisfied. He wasn't driven to nurture a Grand Slam champion or fulfill his own career dreams. In the eighth grade, I was competing in tournaments and doing quite well. At the same time, I wanted to feel like just another one of the girls at school. So I tried out and made the cheerleading squad. It would have been a significant time commitment that interfered with tennis. My dad told me I had a decision to make. He wasn't going to give me his full support and spend all his free time with me on the court if what I wanted was to become a cheerleader. I thought about it, and in the end it was a fairly obvious choice to make. Still, that was a defining moment for me, because I realized I would have to make sacrifices in order to reach my potential. And I have always respected my dad for allowing me to come to that conclusion on my own" (Evert, 2010).

WANTED: POSITIVE PARENT BEHAVIORS IN YOUTH SPORT

Most youth sport parents are helpful and supportive. Observational research has shown that around two-thirds of parent behaviors at youth sport competitions are positive and appropriate, with one-third assessed as negative or inappropriate (Bowker et al., 2009). Youth sport coaches have assessed 70% of parents they work with as "golden," with the rest ranging from "temperamental" to "raging maniacs" (Gould, Lauer, Rolo, James, & Pennisi, 2008).

What Kids Want

As the letter at the beginning of the chapter indicates, kids are quite perceptive about parenting behaviors that help and hurt them. The bottom line: Kids want support, but not pressure, and certainly not a spectacle! Specifically, kids prefer parents to show respect and support and use positive body language, as well as commenting on effort and attitude rather than performance (Knight, Boden, & Holt, 2010; Omli & Wiese-Bjornstal, 2011). Youth athletes don't want parents to be overly loud or to embarrass them, attempt to coach from the sidelines, or make negative comments. In the view of a 9-year-old athlete, parents "should just be quiet, and if you do a good thing, then clap" (Omli & Wiese-Bjornstal, 2011, p. 708).

Youth athletes have identified preferred parental behaviors for certain times (Knight, Neely, & Holt, 2011). Before competition, kids appreciated parents' helping them physically prepare in terms of getting ready and eating well. Most athletes preferred not to talk about performance issues and concerns before competition. During competition, athletes liked parents to encourage the entire team, focus on effort rather than outcome, control their emotions and not draw attention to themselves or their children, and avoid coaching and arguing with officials. After competition, youth athletes preferred feedback that was positively phrased but also honest and contingent on their performance. Athletes also appreciated when their parents gave them time to process negative emotions before asking them to talk about things.

Parental Behavior Backfires

It's helpful to know what kids want from their parents. However, it is often the case that well-meaning parents pressure youth athletes without even realizing it. We call these "backfires" because the positive intent of parents often turns into something negative.

"I'm Proud of You"

A common thing that parents say to kids after a great performance is "I'm so proud of you." This seems like a supportive comment, but it has the potential to create a lot of pressure for kids. It turns children's accomplishments into something they've done to elicit parental pride instead of something they should be proud of themselves. Parents are typically trying to encourage their children and instill in them a sense of pride in their accomplishments. However, "I'm proud of you" is often seen as a judgment or a controlling statement that may create pressure or expectations that they continue to achieve to gain the reward of parental pride and approval (Elmore, 2014; Pickhardt, 2009). African American activist Charleszetta Waddles stated, "You can't give people pride, but you can provide the kind of understanding that makes people look to their inner strengths and find their own sense of pride" (AZ Quotes, 2015).

Consider this example of how these words can affect kids' sense of competence and self-worth (adapted from Schafer, 2010).

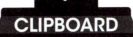

Interpersonal Tips for Empowering Conversations Between Parents and Youth Athletes

Following are some guidelines for parents to consider when engaging their daughters and sons in conversations about youth sport. Parents often rush to the "giving advice" phase of a conversation. Think about these strategies for demonstrating support and willingness to listen and consider the needs of kids.

1. Stay on your child's "side of the fence." Remind yourself that you want to support your child in this conversation and to let her know that you are on her side. The goal of the parent should not be to always give advice on how to be a better athlete. The child should feel a parent's unconditional support, not pressure or an obligation to perform in a certain way.

2. Maintain an attitude of "tell me more" to make the parental role more that of a listener and less that of a lecturer. Prompts like "I really want to hear how you feel about it," "Go on," and "Can you tell me more about that?" hopefully will lead to the child's doing most of the talking and the parent's doing most of the listening.

3. Be a patient, attentive, open, nonjudgmental, often silent listener. Listening is one of the most critical skills for parenting. Even if you know how the game went or exactly what your child needs to do to improve, ask her what she thinks and listen patiently. Ask open-ended questions that tend to allow the young athlete to express herself more fully, such as "What did you think about the game today?" or "What did you learn that can help you in the future?" Put effort into listening—make eye contact, nod your head, say things like "Uh-huh," and "I see," be comfortable with silence, and keep your body posture open. Giving advice or solving problems is not listening.

4. Let the young athlete lead into the conversation when he is ready to talk about things. Avoid the formal "Come sit on the couch" grilling that most kids don't want. You can spark conversation just by spending time together and doing activities such as preparing a meal, raking leaves, or playing a card game.

Over time, when kids have learned that their parents will listen to them without judging or advising, they will be more apt to seek out discussions and trust that their parents will listen and support them.

Adapted from Thompson 2003.

Fourteen-year-old Emma says to her mom, "Mom, I'm so glad you don't say 'I'm proud of you.'" Mom replies, "Really? Why is that?" Emma explains, "You know how I just made the starting lineup for soccer? I just told my friend Natalie and she smiled and said, 'I'm so proud of you' and it felt awful. It made me feel like I have to start for her to think I'm any good. That she doesn't think I'm a good athlete unless I start. She doesn't understand that I worked just as hard when I wasn't a starter." Mom replies, "But I was excited too when you told me about being in the lineup. Do you feel like I'm judging you as well?" Emma answers "No, Mom, what you said was totally different. You said you were excited for me and happy that I got what I was going for. I loved hearing that support and belief in me."

So what should parents say? A better choice is to say "You should be really proud of yourself." Other alternatives are "Good for you!" or "I'm so happy for you." It's also helpful when parents focus on the attributes and behaviors that children personally control, such as hard work, effort, and sportsmanship (as opposed to performance outcomes). An example is "You should be so proud that you worked so hard to accomplish this." When college athletes were asked what their parents said that made them feel great, they identified the powerful phrase "I love to watch you play" (Elmore, 2014). We've used this one a lot with our kids, including variations such as "It was so fun for me to watch you swim today." The idea is to avoid judgment and pressure to achieve and just focus on your love of watching your kids participate and strive to achieve.

"You Should Win This"

A second well-meaning yet pressure-inducing comment (before competition) is "You should win this." Parents often view this as an expression of confidence in a young athlete, but it puts the monkey of high expectations right on the athlete's back. Even with adult athletes, focusing on outcomes before competition is not a good mental strategy (Gould, 2015). Words like *should, must,* and *have to* make a statement unrealistic and convey an unreasonable demand, which in turn creates pressure and anxiety for young athletes (Ellis & Dryden, 1987). Parents should help youth athletes focus on the excitement of competition, the process of playing, and the feeling that they're prepared. In fact, distraction and doing other things before competition is preferred over parental lectures, analyses, and outcome-focused pep talks.

Unintentional Nonverbal Communication

Parents are much better at controlling their verbal communication during youth sport events as compared to their nonverbal responses. I (first author) have had to work very hard on this, as my daughter can always read my thoughts and feelings just by looking at me in the stands during her volleyball matches. Kids look to their parents and even misread them sometimes, as a youth tennis player explains: "Sometimes Dad has a really serious face and you're not sure what it means, so it's something really distracting because you're thinking about what he's thinking" (Knight & Holt, 2014, p. 161). Parents should attempt to manage their nonverbal responses to their children's performances by showing physical signs of encouragement and positive support.

Meeting Developmental Needs in Parenting

Successful parents are sensitive to the changing needs of developing children. Parental roles change in youth sport as athletes move through different levels. During the sampling years of entry into sport until about age 12, parents' roles include introducing children to different activities, focusing on fun and skill development, and providing a lot of support, encouragement, and guidance (Cote, 1999).

The specializing years between 13 and 15 often require greater financial and emotional support based on competitive demands, with athletes taking more personal responsibility for their own training and self-management. Coaches become more central in athletes' lives, with parents' roles becoming more secondary and behind-the-scenes supportive. This is a time for appropriate letting go for parents, avoiding making too many decisions and doing too many things for athletes, which breeds overdependence on parents (Lauer et al., 2010a). During the elite or late teenage years, parents' involvement typically becomes less direct, entailing encouragement and support. Athletes have stated that too much directiveness on the part of parents at this advanced sport level creates feelings of pressure and distraction (Lauer et al., 2010a).

Although parents' degree of involvement shifts over time, certain parenting characteristics are viewed as important across all stages of youth sport. The parental secure base for emotional support should be unwavering and constant. Key values should continue to be emphasized, such as hard work and sportsmanship. Appropriate parent behaviors, such as emotional control and appropriate reactions to mistakes and losses, remain important in assisting young athletes with the pressure of competition (Lauer et al., 2010a, 2010b).

UNDERSTANDING PARENT TRAPS

The emotional investment and attachment between parents and children can lead to what we call parent traps. These traps occur when parents' investment in youth sport becomes so great that the main point—"What is best for my child?"—is forgotten.

How Much Should Parents Push?

A question many parents wrestle with is "How much should I push my child?" We've emphasized that being supportive of athletes' autonomy is an important parenting practice, and youth athletes have indicated that parents who engage in excessive direction create pressure and detract from athletes' sport enjoyment. Excessive pressure from parents to perform is a parent trap that has been linked to lower self-esteem, anxiety, burnout, and avoidance of the activities that parents are pushing as "good for you" (Fraser-Thomas, Cote, & Deakin, 2008a; Gould et al., 2008).

Yet, there is evidence that some push from parents is needed. An athlete explains:

There were times I didn't want to practice and it wasn't like, "Too bad, you're practicing" (from my parents' perspective). It was like, "[Son], you want to do well at this. Do you want to do that?" [I would say,] "Yeah, I do." [My parents would respond,] "Well, then I think you should practice." And I would say, "Okay, fine" (Lauer et al., 2010b, p. 490).

Parents can be critical with regard to teaching young athletes by saying things such as "If you're going to do it, do it right" and "Follow through on your commitments." As parents, we insisted that our daughter try out for volleyball as a 6th grader even though she was uncertain about doing so. We felt that she needed that push from us to try it. She loved it and went on to enjoy high school and club volleyball.

Parents should strive for **optimal push**, or directive behaviors that challenge children to strive for achievement, while supporting their autonomy and avoiding excessive pressure. Research with youth swimming families showed that parents' level of push (how much they directed their children and emphasized achieving performance goals) was related in a curvilinear manner to children's enthusiasm (a combination of effort, competitiveness, and enjoyment) (Power & Woolger, 1994). This result showed that too little push, as well as too much push, was not as effective as moderate levels of parental push in enabling kids to achieve in sport. Similarly, a study with youth athletes from a variety of sports showed that greater amounts of parental directive behavior, coupled with praise for effort and emotional support, were associated with greater success for kids in sport (Wuerth, Lee, & Alfermann, 2004).

As discussed in chapter 11, parental pressure created only anxiety in youth swimmers when the parents focused on outcomes, such as winning or beating opponents (O'Rourke, Smith, Smoll, & Cumming, 2011). Parents who engaged intensely with their children to encourage effort, learning from mistakes, and focus on self-improvement were viewed as directing their children in an adaptive manner, which enabled their kids to concentrate on controllable goals. This is another example of optimal push by parents.

Although putting excessive pressure for achievement on kids without emotional support is to be avoided, so is being under-involved and failing to provide enough push in the form of encouragement, active engagement, and directive behaviors that youth athletes need in order to strive and thrive in sport (Hellstedt, 1987). Shanyn, a local club swim coach, explained her experience with loving and supportive yet underinvolved parents as part of an assignment in our class:

> I wish I had felt more push from my parents. Growing up, they directed my siblings and I to participate in sports to keep us active and to have fun. They never had dreams for us to grow up and be Olympians or anything, which was totally fine because all pressure was off. However, when I was 11, I decided not to swim year-round and try club volleyball. I really wish my parents would have helped me weigh that decision more and directed me back to club swimming after I found I didn't like volleyball.

> On entering high school, I began to realize that I was a fairly decent swimmer, and based on my success, I began to develop dreams of swimming in college. I had never had those dreams before because my parents never acted like it was possible. As I began to win and drop time, I felt that my parents didn't realize my potential or understand the talent I felt I had. I wish they had pushed me to pursue opportunities to test my abilities and become faster.

> My senior year in high school, I made the decision to join a club swim team to work to qualify for Nationals. I did

> qualify, but they didn't seem proud or excited for me. They seemed annoyed about having to travel to Texas and sit through hours of swimming for my one race. This hurt my feelings because I had worked very hard to drop enough time to qualify. When I told my mom I wanted to be recruited to swim in college, she said "Don't get your hopes up." Because of this, I never truly believed that swimming in college was an option for me. Girls that I swam with and against who had similar or slower times than me went on to swim at [various colleges]. I feel like if my parents had pushed me more to try and maximize my talent and self-belief, I could have been a collegiate swimmer instead of a swammer.

Optimal push seems to occur when parents use the right amounts of push and pressure while also listening and demonstrating unconditional emotional support for their children. Parental push without emotional and autonomy support is an all-take, no-give parent trap. Conversely, not enough push by parents may hinder young athletes' abilities to pursue their goals in sport. Additional research is needed to help us better understand the most advantageous recipe of parent behaviors in relation to optimal push in youth sport.

From ABP to ABPD

A second parent trap occurs when parents cross the line from normal, supportive parenting to abnormal, distorted parenting. Due to emotional attachment, parents strongly identify with their children. They derive pleasure from their children's achievements, called **achievement by proxy (ABP)** (Tofler & DiGeronimo, 2000). In a healthy by proxy experience (ABP), parents vicariously experience their children's success and failure, but at the same time, they realize that children are separate individuals with their own unique needs and goals. A teenage Tiger Woods described his highly involved father in ABP terms: "My dad doesn't live through me, which is what some parents do" (Callahan, 2006).

The parent trap happens when ABP turns into **achievement by proxy distortion (ABPD)**. Achievement by proxy distortion is a psychological state in which parents' need for social recognition or financial benefits through the accomplishments of their children takes priority over the needs and goals of the children (Tofler & DiGeronimo, 2000). This need for parental gain in ABPD can be conscious or unconscious, and it pushes parents to risk their children's physical and emotional health. Achievement by proxy distortion often begins when parents start making sacrifices of excessive time and money, move to more favorable training locales, or send children to specialized training academies. Because of these sacrifices, athletes are expected to reciprocate with their own sacrifices as repayment to parents.

An elite gymnast recalls her mother's response to her weight gain and desire to discontinue elite participation: "No! You won't. You're going back to the gym on Monday. I won't let you eat! I'll lock the cabinets! You're not going to throw this away after all the time and money we've spent" (Sey, 2008, pp. 258-259). The young athlete becomes objectified, a product to be improved rather than a person with needs and feelings. This emotional abuse may lead to physical abuse when parents completely lose the ability to differentiate their own needs and goals from those of their children. Olympic gymnast Dominique Moceanu recalls her father striking her in the face because she had eaten some candy, strictly forbidden in the weight-controlled world of elite gymnastics (Moceanu, 2012). At age 17, Moceanu filed for the right to be declared a legal adult because of the abuse she endured from her father.

A figure-skating parent explains the ABPD trap:

I got hooked the first time I saw Tess on the medal stand. What you don't realize is how it pulls you in. I kept coming back for more. There were always better competitions to enter, tougher opponents to face. After a while I stopped listening to Tess. I wanted her to win, but for me, I think. I needed it. The last few years were pretty bad. Tess wanted out a long time before I realized that it had to be that way. I just hope I didn't waste her childhood (Murphy, 1999, p. 84).

Parents of elite young athletes who discontinued sport participation have described themselves as lost and admitted struggling psychologically for years after their children's retirement (Lally & Kerr, 2008).

Youth sport parents need to be aware of the ABPD trap. They should continuously monitor their motives for and feelings about their child's sport participation. Parents should find it useful to complete the 100-Points Exercise (Thompson, 2009) provided in appendix A, rating a number of objectives for youth sport programs based on how important they think each one is for their child. Parents should keep their 100-Points list in a prominent place to remind them of their parenting priorities, which hopefully are developmentally appropriate and ABP-like. Another exercise is to develop a family sports mission statement by addressing the following questions (Ginsburg, Durant, & Baltzell, 2006, p. 11):

- When my child is 21, what kind of person do I want her or him to be, and how will youth sport help us, as parents, get our child there?
- What are the three most important lessons that I want my child to learn through involvement in youth sport?

By working on self-awareness in order to understand ourselves better, we can lessen our tendency to unwittingly pressure our kids to meet our needs as parents. As much as possible, parents should put their own desires aside and focus on the needs and goals of their children.

Should Parents Coach Their Own Kids?

A potential parent trap arises when adults serve as coaches of their own children in youth sport. Volunteer parent-coaches are plentiful in youth sport, and the motivation to coach one's own child (and do it appropriately) is a big reason for parents to volunteer their time. An informal survey carried out over the past 25 years in our classrooms indicates that the majority of athletes who were coached by their parents had positive experiences. Male youth athletes have identified many positive aspects of playing for their fathers, including additional technical instruction, optimal push and motivation, involvement in decision making, and their fathers' unique understanding of their abilities and strengths (Weiss & Fretwell, 2005). Being kids, they also noted that playing for their dads meant they were never late for practice, and that "[they] always get the trophy and [they] get to keep it at [their] house" (p. 291).

Of course there are also negative aspects of having a parent as a coach, such as pressure and expectations and being held to higher standards than other athletes on the team. The aim of the latter is often to avoid perceptions of favoritism. As one young athlete said, "If I do something good and then the other person does the same thing, he'll say good job to them but not to me . . . he doesn't want to say something that would seem like he was being nice to me" (Weiss & Fretwell, 2005, p. 293). A particular problem is the dual role of parent-coaches. Unlike adults or older athletes, young children are less able to distinguish between criticism from Mom and criticism from the coach. For the child, criticism is always from Mom (Murphy, 1999).

Parent-coaches should attempt to manage their dual roles and clearly return to being Mom or Dad once practice and competition are over. A junior tennis player explains,

"My biggest problem was there was no separation between the role of the father and the coach. So we wouldn't talk about anything but tennis . . . he didn't leave any room for like personal feelings" (Gould, Tuffy, Udry, & Loehr, 1997, p. 265). A father-coach offers useful advice for separating parent and coach roles: "When the game is over, you're the parent, and you've got to make a fairly quick transition . . . now you have to treat your child supportively, and whether he played well or poorly, you're there not to deal with his soccer skills or his mastery of the game. You're now there to deal with him emotionally in terms of how does he feel about how he played" (Weiss & Fretwell, 2005, p. 299).

We believe that parents can competently serve as coaches of their own children, and we suggest that parents talk to their children about the dual-role situation. Parent-coaches can create some guidelines and expectations for their kids, such as how parent-coaches should be addressed at team events and the parent-coach's intent to be a coach at games and a parent once the game is over. Ask kids how they feel about being coached by you, the parent, and discuss their concerns when making the decision whether to coach or not. Some school programs and club sports have established a rule that parents cannot coach their own children. This may be a good idea in some cases, but at the grassroots youth sport level, volunteer parent-coaches are still the norm. In our community, we have observed the vast majority of volunteer parent-coaches doing a great job of providing a positive experience for youth athletes, including their own children.

Sibling Issues

At 14-year-old gymnast Chris Sey's first national competitive meet, the announcer introduced him this way: "Up on vault, Chris Sey, whose sister Jennifer Sey, the new national champion, is in the audience. Jennifer, could you stand up, please" (Sey, 2008, p. 245). In her book, Jennifer Sey talks about how devastating this incident was for her brother. Siblings of highly successful youth athletes often feel marginalized due to the attention and resources provided to the star athlete in the family (Blazo, Carson, Czech, & Dees, 2014; Cote, 1999; Harwood & Knight, 2009). It is difficult when the more talented child works on her sport expertise with extra training while siblings are asked to pick up the slack in everyday household chores (Tofler & DiGeronimo, 2000). Siblings begin to feel, often with hidden resentment, that they are less important to the family. A young athlete explains:

> It's not like I was jealous of his achievements, just some of the opportunities maybe . . . I mean, my dad supported me, sure but . . . my dad seemed to make him a priority, tenniswise, more than me . . . I felt like he was just focused on helping [older sibling] with tennis rather than trying to help me with whatever sport I choose other than tennis (Blazo et al., 2014, p. 44).

Parents should attempt to do what they can to create a more family-centered atmosphere, as opposed to an athlete-centered atmosphere in which everything revolves around the most talented child. Parents should show sincere interest in all children's activities and allot time to spend with all children. Children need to get the message that parents love them for who they are, not for what they do. Parents can find ways to make a big deal out of activities and accomplishments of all children. Families can discuss how to create an equitable distribution of household responsibilities. When children are involved in the scheduling and distribution of responsibilities, they typically harbor less resentment toward a sibling who spends more time on sport training (Tofler & DiGeronimo, 2000).

Parents can attempt to avoid the sibling resentment parent trap by making a focused effort to emotionally connect and support each child in the family. And in many families, siblings serve as positive models and emotional supporters to help their brothers and sisters out in their youth sport participation (Fraser-Thomas et al., 2008b).

PARENT EDUCATION IN YOUTH SPORT

Many youth sport parent education programs have been developed to provide practical information to parents about children and youth sport. The free Positive Sport Parenting course is available online at nfhslearn.com. The Human Kinetics Coach Education (HumanKineticsCoachEducationCenter.com) offers the SportParent Course, which youth sport administrators can deliver to parents in their communities. The Human Kinetics Coach Education provides all the materials and the detailed SportParent Facilitator Manual with key points that administrators or coaches can follow. The National Alliance for Youth Sports offers an online course for parents as part of its educational mission (www.nays.org/parents). The Parent Mental Trainer (PMT) program

Personal Plug-In

What Parent Traps or Backfires Have You Experienced?

You've read several examples of how well-meaning behaviors on the part of parents can backfire or serve as parent traps. Have you experienced any of these, either as a son or daughter or as a parent? Are there other parent traps or backfires that you have experienced? How did these experiences influence your sport participation and your self-perceptions?

is offered online as a resource provided by Mental Training, Inc., and the Institute for the Study of Youth Sports at Michigan State University. Other parent education programs are available from specific youth sport associations (e.g., US Youth Soccer). Short, practical, positive sport parenting books are also available (e.g., Thompson, 2009, 2010a).

At the very least, we advocate that youth sport administrators or coaches (or both) conduct a brief parent orientation meeting before the competitive season. The objectives and focus of the program could be clarified, and details about schedule, travel, length of practice, and team rules and guidelines could be presented. We've seen this done in very informal ways by coaches, who appeal to parents to make the experience all about the kid. It's useful if the tone of the meeting communicates a sense of partnership between coaches and parents and questions from parents are invited and openly discussed. An alternative to a meeting is a parent information sheet or newsletter that is offered a few times across the season. Youth sport organizations may consider partnering with university programs to use student interns to create and distribute parent information guides and newsletters.

Strategies for Coaches in Interacting With Youth Sport Parents

1. Make parents allies of your program. Involve parents and families in social activities and even hold a parent–athlete competition (either parents playing against the athletes or parents teaming up with their kids in a competition). Ask parents for help (e.g., fund-raising, staffing the snack bar, providing rides, line judging in volleyball) and express your appreciation for their leadership and service.

2. Provide information, preferably in a parent orientation meeting, about your coaching philosophy, objectives, guidelines, and rules. Provide time for parents to ask questions.

3. Make it a point to talk to and connect with all parents, and be positive about their kids.

4. Require athletes to talk to you first (before their parents) about playing time or playing positions.

5. Establish a rule that you will not talk to parents about playing time, positions, or strategies on competition days. Parents must set up a meeting with the coach at another time to discuss such issues.

6. Be aware of parental "manager" duties. As discussed previously, many parents struggle to manage the time, travel, and transportation requirements that are part of youth sport. Try to make all this as easy as possible for parents, and thank parents for fulfilling this role.

7. These are some suggestions for when parents challenge or raise issues with you as the coach (adapted from Haefner, 2015):

   a. Listen calmly with your professional face on.

   b. Don't interrupt or get emotional.

   c. When given time, explain your point of view slowly and clearly. Focus on their child and don't compare their child to other players.

   d. No matter what, don't lose your cool. Use a calm voice at a normal conversational level. Be a professional!

   e. Thank parents for voicing their concerns and let them know that you've heard them and will consider their viewpoints.

Suggestions for Being a Better Youth Sport Parent

1. Support and accept the decisions made by the coach, even if you disagree. Thank the coach repeatedly for his time and energy.

2. Ask coaches how you can help.

3. Honor the game (Thompson, 2010b) by not disrespecting or talking negatively about any official, opponent, athlete, or coach.

4. Remember, your role as a parent is different from the coach's role. Your role is not to instruct, offer strategy, or provide feedback during competitions and practices. Your role is to be a parent and support your child and the team.

5. Work to recognize your reactive tendencies, and plan and rehearse strategies to use to keep your composure (refocusing, taking a walk, re-establishing perspective [this is a U-9 soccer game, not the World Cup]) (Wiersma & Fifer, 2008).

6. Manage the three relationships of a youth sport parent (Thompson, 2003). Your primary relationship is with your child, as a supportive and emotionally tuned-in parent attempting to provide optimal push. Your second relationship is with your child's coach. Be supportive and positive, allowing the coach to do her job. The final relationship parents need to manage is with themselves. Remember that it's all about the kid and not about your goals and desires for your child. We admit that it's hard to juggle these three relationships, particularly the third one. Simply being aware of the importance of these three relationships is a start to being a terrific youth sport parent.

WRAP-UP

Much of youth sport parenting advice focuses on meeting the needs of young athletes. The idealized parenting culture of today fuels the perception that being a good youth sport parent means running ragged to enable children to meet their overscheduled youth sport commitments. You hear a great parenting tip every time you begin an airline trip. The advice to parents: If the airplane loses cabin pressure, put on your own oxygen mask before attending to your children.

We don't know of many parents who would automatically follow this advice. Our instinct as parents is to attend to our children's needs ahead of our own. However, research clearly shows that children are negatively affected by their parents' stress. A national stress survey found that 86% of children were negatively affected by their parents' stress (Novotny, 2012). Youth sport parents need to renew their focus on their own oxygen masks, for their personal well-being and for the well-being of their children. Parents are much less able to engage in good parenting if they don't prioritize their own oxygen masks. We understand and admire the acceptable sacrifices that parents, often gladly, make for their children. But we think that the culture of youth sport will be enhanced if parents thoughtfully consider their needs and the overall needs of their families, to avoid risky sacrifices and mentally unhealthy practices that are hidden parent traps in youth sport today.

LEARNING AIDS

Key Terms

achievement by proxy (ABP)—When parents vicariously experience their children's success and failure yet at the same time realize that children are separate individuals with their own unique needs and goals.

achievement by proxy distortion (ABPD)—A psychological state in which parents' need for social recognition or financial benefits through the accomplishments of their children takes priority over the needs and goals of the children.

attachment—The deep emotional bond that connects parents to children, resulting in parents' responding sensitively to children's needs and becoming a secure base for their children.

authoritarian parenting style—Style that is demanding but less responsive to emotional needs; emphasizes obedience without explanation or any attempt to reason with children.

authoritative parenting style—Style that is high in both responsiveness and demandingness; involves setting high standards and limits, showing respect for and reasoning with kids, and being nurturing and responsive to their emotional needs.

models—The ways in which parents set standards or provide examples for imitation or comparison.

neglectful parenting style—Style that is neither demanding nor responsive; disengaged and unsupportive.

optimal push—Directive behaviors that challenge children to strive for achievement while supporting their autonomy and avoiding excessive pressure.

parenting style—The overall manner in which parents interact with children, based on parents' attitudes and values about what the relationship between parent and child should be.

permissive parenting style—Style that is high in responsiveness but less demanding; parent is reluctant to impose rules and standards and thus provides little structure, preferring to let children regulate themselves.

Summary Points

1. Attachment results in parents' responding sensitively and appropriately to their children's needs, with parents becoming a secure base for their children.

2. The hothouse parenting style focuses on preparing children to be special, as opposed to earlier parenting practices of protecting kids' childhood years to ensure a normal childhood.

3. Parenting styles differ based on levels of responsiveness and demandingness and include authoritative, authoritarian, and permissive styles.

4. The three M's representing youth sport parenting roles are manager, model, and meaning maker.

5. Active parents tend to have active children, but parents' encouragement and support for sport or physical activity are most influential on children's sport participation.

6. Youth athletes desire parental support but prefer parents not to give coaching advice or make negative comments.

7. Parental roles change in youth sport as athletes move through different levels of sport.

8. Optimal push occurs when parents use the right amounts of push and pressure while also listening and demonstrating unconditional emotional support for their children.

9. Achievement by proxy distortion occurs when parents' desire for social recognition or financial benefits through the accomplishments of their children take priority over the needs and goals of the children.

10. Parents can attempt to avoid the sibling resentment parent trap by making a focused effort to emotionally connect with and support each child in the family.

Study Questions

1. Explain why parent–child attachment relates to parental behaviors in youth sport.

2. What is the idealized cultural norm for parenting in today's society? How and why has that changed? Can you predict how it might change in the future?

3. Explain the three parenting styles, using the continuums of responsiveness and demandingness. Although one style is recommended for youth sport parents, could any of the other styles be useful in certain circumstances in youth sport?

4. Describe the three M's representing parents' roles in youth sport. Provide examples for each M.

5. Describe the research findings on what kids want with regard to parental behaviors in youth sport.

6. How should parents' roles change as their children move through the youth sport system?

7. Explain the concept of optimal push, and provide guidelines for parents to achieve it.

8. How and why does ABP turn into ABPD? Provide some examples for each.

Reflective Learning Activities

1. Design an interview guide with questions for a youth sport parent. The guide should focus on a specific area or multiple areas in which you are interested regarding parents and youth sport (e.g., parenting style, coaching one's own child, any other aspects of youth sport parenting that may or may not have been discussed in this chapter). Interview two youth sport parents, and include anonymous demographic information to set up the case description. Write up an analysis of your interview results, how your results fit with chapter ideas, and what you learned from these parents.

2. Do the interview assignment as described in question 1, but plan and conduct your interview with two youth athletes about their perceptions of and preferences for various parenting styles and behaviors related to their sport participation and overall development. You must get parental permission to interview minor children, and you should provide a copy of your interview questions to the parent.

3. Create an educational guide or newsletter for parents in a specific youth sport situation (e.g., 9- and 10-year-old softball players). Make sure that your guide or newsletter provides parents some education beyond the typical schedule and team rules and guidelines. Include information presented in a colorful way that affords parents insights about youth sport parenting beyond aspects they may have already considered.

Resource Guide

Thompson, J. (2009). *Positive sports parenting.* Portola Valley, CA: Balance Sports.

Thompson, J. (2010). *The high school sport parent.* Portola Valley, CA: Balance Sports.

Human Kinetics Coach Education SportParent Course (HumanKineticsCoach EducationCenter.com).

Engaging Effectively With Parents, NFHS free online course (nfhslearn.com).

Parent Mental Trainer (PMT) (www.parentmentaltrainer.com). PMT is an online certification course for parents designed by leaders in youth sport research. It helps parents engage in their child's youth sport experience in the most beneficial way for themselves, the athlete, and the coach. The online course covers how parents should act on the sidelines, how to support the athletes in a positive manner, and how to control emotions while watching a child participate in the sport.

The Role of the Parent in Sports, NFHS free online course (nfhslearn.com).

chapter 16

MORAL AND LIFE SKILLS DEVELOPMENT IN YOUTH SPORT

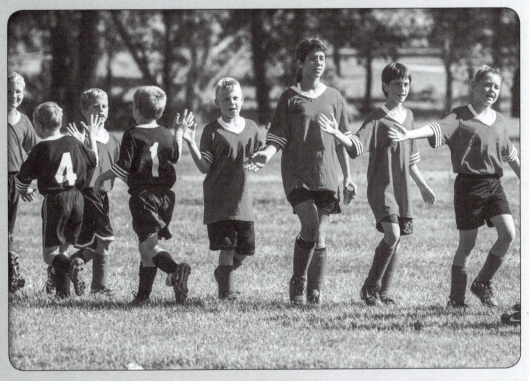

CHAPTER PREVIEW

In this chapter, you'll learn

» that sport doesn't automatically build character;

» how moral behavior and life skills are caught, taught, and bought; and

» practical strategies to enhance moral behavior and life skills in youth sport participants.

A common belief about youth sport is that children, when they participate in it, learn important life skills that enable them to become successful adults in our society. That is, many people believe that sport builds character. Do you believe this, and why or why not? This question was posed to you in the Youth Sport IQ Test in the introduction to this book.

If you believe that sport does not build character, you're probably thinking of the cheating, disrespect toward opponents and officials, and violent behavior that occur in sport. You may recall Utah soccer referee Ricardo Portillo, who died in 2013 after being punched in the face by a 17-year-old player after calling a foul on him and issuing him a yellow card. If you believe that sport does build character, you have observed sport teams in which adult leaders taught athletes to respect opponents, control emotions, and play fairly. You can cite positive examples, such as the humility and emotional maturity displayed by Major League Baseball pitcher Armando Galarraga in supporting umpire Jim Joyce, who admittedly blew the call that cost Galarraga a perfect game in 2010 (Verducci, 2010), or the impressive display of character in sport described in the Water Break.

The fact that there are many negative examples of bad behavior, as well as many uplifting examples like the Oak Harbor and Marysville-Pilchuck football teams' inspirational acts, emphasizes the key point of this chapter. Character, life skills, and moral actions are not automatically developed in youth simply through their participation in sport. Rather, these positive outcomes occur when knowledgeable adults structure

Water Break

A Display of Character

The high school football teams of Marysville-Pilchuck and Oak Harbor (Washington) were set to play for the league championship on the night of October 24, 2014. However, on the morning of the game, a troubled teenager killed four students and himself with a gun in the Marysville-Pilchuck cafeteria. In response to the devastating news, the Oak Harbor team forfeited the game to give the league title to Marysville-Pilchuck. Oak Harbor players and Coach Jay Turner attended a remembrance vigil in Marysville that night and offered their condolences to the Marysville-Pilchuck players. "I can't put into words what it meant to our guys," said the Marysville-Pilchuck coach, Brandon Carson. "This just goes beyond the game, and shows us what athletics can do" ("True Champions," 2014).

But what is even more amazing is how sportsmanship can pay forward by inspiring others to show moral integrity and compassion. Five days later, Marysville-Pilchuck players surprised the Oak Harbor team at practice (Oak Harbor had qualified for the playoffs, even though they had forfeited their league title) and presented them with the league championship trophy. Marysville-Pilchuck senior Corbin Ferry, explaining that all players were on board with relinquishing the championship trophy, said, "It's nothing compared to what they did for us."

developmentally appropriate activities, model and reinforce appropriate behaviors, and take the time to discuss moral issues so that youth sport participants develop reasoning skills and reach higher levels of moral development. Participation in sport can help athletes develop character, or important life skills, but only if the program is structured and delivered in ways that emphasize social and moral development.

UNDERSTANDING TERMS RELATED TO MORAL BEHAVIOR IN SPORT

A clear understanding about how sport participation affects athletes' character is impossible unless we clarify the vague term *character*. This term evolved from mid-19th-century Britain, where elite schools promoted sport participation as a means to develop important virtues for boys, such as leadership, honesty, self-control, courage, and persistence. Similarly, the concept of Muscular Christianity (the idea that sport participation leads to spiritual character) espoused by American Protestants grew into the YMCA competitive sport programs in the late 19th century in the United States. Thus, the term **character** refers to a group of positive moral or ethical qualities that are revered by a society. The problem is that the term is used loosely and inconsistently, making it impossible for researchers to answer the question whether sport builds character. To move beyond a vague idea of character, in this chapter we'll focus on more specific and contemporary terms such as *life skills, sportsmanship, moral behavior, aggression,* and *aggressiveness*.

Life Skills

Life skills include moral values as well as other skills that enable us to succeed in the culture in which we live (Danish, Nellen, & Owens, 1996). Life skills typically include physical competence (learning how to play a sport and be physically active), social competence (cooperation, effective empathy and communication, respect for others; often called **prosocial behaviors** because they benefit others), cognitive competence (decision making, academic skills), emotional competence (managing emotions, taking personal responsibility for one's behavior), and behavioral competence (pursuing personal goals, developing problem-solving strategies, productively contributing to one's community).

Youth sport parents believe that important life skills can be developed through sport participation, including learning how to win and lose, developing sportsmanship, working with teammates, following directions and communicating effectively, staying focused, and maintaining perspective when things don't go one's way (Wiersma & Fifer, 2008). As one parent stated, "Things will not be peachy their whole life, so they get to learn how to deal with that and they also learn to deal with people who might be jerks" (Wiersma & Fifer, 2008, p. 515).

So, like character, life skills include a number of qualities, but life skill development is even broader in that it focuses on human skills that allow individuals to function as effective citizens within society. These skills include, but are not limited to, moral and ethical behavior. We think the emphasis on learning life skills is an important objective for youth sport because it goes beyond the outdated idea, often referred to in a tongue-in-cheek way, of building character in sport. As discussed in chapter 3, an important objective of youth sport is to develop and enhance the physical, social, cognitive, emotional, and behavioral life skills of children and youth. Read the Water Break section for an example of how life skills may be taught in sport, and note particularly how the program is structured to extend the transferability of these skills beyond sport into other life contexts.

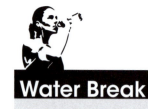

Water Break

The First Tee Life Skills Education Program

The First Tee (www.thefirsttee.org) is dedicated to building life skills in youth through the game of golf and focuses on nine core values: honesty, integrity, sportsmanship, respect, confidence, responsibility, perseverance, courtesy, and judgment. In the First Tee program, lessons for life are taught through a variety of golf-related activities designed with the primary goal of having fun. Participants learn about themselves as they move through the certification levels of Par (interpersonal communication and self-management), Birdie (goal setting), Eagle (resistance skills, conflict resolution), and Ace (advanced personal life planning). For example, youth participants learn how to be a STAR (Stop, Think, Anticipate, Respond) when faced with frustration or anger; practice the 4Rs (Replay, Relax, Ready, Redo) to respond effectively to mistakes; and internalize the mantra Be Patient, Be Positive, and Ask for Help. First Tee coaches are trained to use specific coaching strategies so that the learning process is activity based (doing vs. telling), mastery driven (emphasizing personal skill development), personally empowering (active decision making), and focused on continuous, lifelong learning. First Tee programs are offered in community as well as school physical education settings.

Independent research has confirmed that 73% of participants reported higher confidence in their ability to do well academically; 82% felt confident in their social skills with peers; 57% credited The First Tee for helping them develop their meeting-and-greeting skills; and all participants agreed that they had transferred the skills learned in the program to their school achievements (Weiss, Stuntz, Bhalla, Bolter, & Price, 2013; "Impact Report," n.d.).

Sportsmanship

Most often **sportsmanship** is defined as acting in ways that promote fairness and mutual respect in competition, even when these actions allow strategic gain by the opponent. Examples of good sportsmanship include calling lines fairly in tennis matches and shaking hands and respecting opponents even when you're angry about losing.

If you want to know what sportsmanship is, just ask youth sport participants. As shown in table 16.1, young athletes have a good idea of how to play fair and be a good sport. Entzion (1991) asked 6th graders to describe how to play fair, and their top 10 answers as shown on the left side of table 16.1 certainly are rules to live by. Over a thousand Canadian athletes age 10 to 18 defined sportsmanship in terms of five main factors, shown on the right side of table 16.1 (Vallerand, Deshaies, Cuerrier, Briere, & Pelletier, 1996). Both of these studies indicate that, on their own, youth athletes understand that sportsmanship involves a commitment to hard work; respect for teammates, opponents, and officials; emotional control; and cooperation with others. They are aware of the negative behaviors that occur in sport and understand that good sports avoid acting in these ways.

Table 16.1 How Youth Athletes Define Sportsmanship or Moral Behavior in Sport

1. Don't hurt anybody.	1. Showing up, working hard, and trying to improve all the time
2. Take turns.	2. Respect for rules and officials (even when you don't agree)
3. Don't yell at teammates when they make mistakes.	3. Respect for social conventions (shaking hands, being a good loser, recognizing good performance of opponents)
4. Don't cheat.	
5. Don't cry every time when you don't win.	4. Respect and concern for opponent (lending equipment, not taking advantage of injured opponents)
6. Don't make excuses when you lose.	
7. *Try* for first place.	5. Avoiding poor attitudes about sport (losing temper, selfish play, avoiding a win-at-all-costs approach)
8. Don't tell people they're no good.	
9. Don't brag.	
10. Don't kick anyone in the stomach.	

Adapted from Entzion 1991; Vallerand et al. 1996.

Moral Behavior

Although moral behavior is similar to sportsmanship, there is an important difference. Sportsmanship is about doing the right thing, whereas **moral behavior** is doing the right thing for the right reason (Shields & Bredemeier, 2007). People act morally because they have thought through what is fair and what is compassionate, and they act based on underlying moral values. An athlete can show respect for an official because he hopes to gain favor from the official during competition, or he can show respect because he believes it's the right thing to do. Doing something because you believe it's the right thing to do is moral behavior. Moral behavior results from an underlying reasoning process about why one should act in a certain way. In the movie *The Legend of Bagger Vance,* a golfer calls a penalty on himself for inadvertently moving his ball during play, even though no one saw it happen. The young boy serving as his caddy begs him to not call the penalty because, as he says, "No one will ever know" that the ball moved. The golfer replies, *"I'll* know." This powerful example demonstrates to the boy that cheating to win and disrespecting the game would make for a hollow and meaningless victory. As we'll discuss, the underlying moral reasoning levels of athletes are very predictive of their behavior in sport; thus, an important objective of youth sport is to offer life lessons so that children can develop mature moral values that will help them reason through the many moral conflicts inherent in sport and life.

Understanding Violence, Aggression, and Aggressiveness

The most extreme negative examples of lack of sportsmanship and moral behavior in youth sport are violent physical assaults on officials, coaches, and opponents, which have resulted in hospitalization and even death. A Pennsylvania youth baseball coach was convicted in 2006 for corruption of minors and criminal solicitation to commit assault by paying one of his players $25 to bean an 8-year-old autistic teammate to keep him out of the game and improve the team's chances of winning. The increasingly professionalized win-at-any-cost mentality and exorbitant financial and social rewards for winning have led to the acceptance of violence and hurting others as "part of the game."

The field of psychology uses the term **aggression** to mean violating the rights of another person with the intent to harm, for example to inflict pain or injury. It is similar to **violence,** which is rough or injurious physical force, although aggression may also be verbal. However, **aggressiveness** in sport is popularly thought of as competing in a forceful manner with great intensity of effort. Young athletes may confuse these terms when their coaches exhort them to "be aggressive out there." It is important to clarify the difference between aggression or violence and what we popularly call aggressive play for young athletes, so they understand that playing hard with great intensity is the goal and that attempting to hurt others is unacceptable in sport.

HOW SPORTSMANSHIP AND MORAL BEHAVIOR ARE LEARNED

How do children learn acceptable social and moral behavior? How do they learn to be good, as well as bad, sports? It's important to understand how and why children learn social behavior if we hope to develop and enhance life skills, sportsmanship, and moral behavior in youth sport participants. As you'll learn in this section, the social values that lead to moral behavior in young athletes have to be caught, taught, and bought.

Modeling

The 2008-2009 National Hockey League (NHL) preview article in *Sports Illustrated* was titled "Why Good Teams Fight" and included nine color photographs of professional male hockey players pummeling opponents with their fists (Farber, 2008). Certain players were identified as "fighting specialists" and featured prominently in the article as important to team success. What do you think youth hockey players learn from articles like this and from observing professional hockey? The message is clear—physically assaulting an opponent is an accepted and valued practice in adult hockey. This is called **modeling,** or observational learning, whereby children imitate the actions of significant adults (famous athletes, coaches, parents). Modeling is a form of **social learning** (Bandura, 1977), a major theory in psychology proposing that children become aware of and learn culturally valued behaviors or social norms as they develop into adults. They observe what is acceptable and valued in their culture and then internalize these behaviors as appropriate. In a word, appropriate behavior patterns are *caught* through constant observations and interactions with significant adults.

The effects of modeling on aggression were demonstrated in the famous Bobo doll experiment in which 3- to 6-year-old children watched an adult interact with a 5-foot-tall (152 centimeters) inflated doll (Bandura, Ross, & Ross, 1961). In the aggression condition, the adult struck the doll in the head with a toy mallet while repeating "Sock him in the face." In the nonaggression condition, the adult passively played with other toys and ignored the doll. The

---

Personal Plug-In

Your Life Lessons in Sport

How were you taught sportsmanship as a young athlete? What were the messages you received, and where did these messages come from? And did your view and practice of sportsmanship change as you moved through the youth sport system? How so?

children were then observed in a free-play situation, and those who had observed the adult striking the doll exhibited more physical and verbal aggression than those children who had observed the adult playing passively.

Emulating adult sport models has been documented in many youth sports. High school hockey players who selected role models that they perceived as more violent received more serious penalties (fighting, slashing, high sticking) than did players who chose role models perceived as less violent in their play (Smith, 1974). Sixty percent of 12- to 21-year-old hockey players said they learned how to aggress against an opponent (spearing, elbowing, tripping, slashing, high sticking) from watching professional hockey on television at least once a week. An example of what was learned was "[g]iving [an opponent] a shot in the face as he's coming up to you. The ref can't see the butt-ends [of the stick]" (Smith, 1982, p. 298). Similar results were obtained in a study of the effects of role models on youth football players (Mugno & Feltz, 1985). Ninety-four percent of the sample of middle school and high school players watched adult football and reported learning multiple forms of aggression against opponents (spearing, face masking, clipping, grabbing face masks). And 82% of those players admitted that they used one of these forms of aggression in their own games. Youth athletes ages 9 to 15 years across multiple sports admitted that they engaged in poor sportsmanship behaviors as a result of the ways in which coaches, parents, and spectators acted at their games (Shields, LaVoi, Bredemeier, & Power, 2007).

But the good news is that children can also catch positive values of sportsmanship and moral behavior. When asked to define, name, and identify characteristics of a hero, 11- to 16-year-olds ranked sport figures second after their parents and cited

helping behaviors, caring traits, courage, and trustworthiness as heroic qualities (White & O'Brien, 1999). Although former professional basketball player and noted brawler Charles Barkley famously stated, "I'm no role model," the fact remains that children and youth emulate the behavior of parents, coaches, and adult sport figures. An emerging practice is the development of codes of ethics for professional sport athletes, as well as youth sport coaches and parents, to emphasize the importance of modeling sportsmanship to young athletes.

We strongly encourage youth sport programs to develop codes for appropriate behavior on the part of parents and coaches, as well as athletes. In particular, we encourage you to develop a catchy, appealing theme that captures the spirit of sportsmanship and fair play without sounding preachy. A great example of this is "honoring the game" (Thompson, 2010b), which means that the game would not be possible unless we respected opponents, officials, and the rules of competition. So, you might present the concept of honoring the game to parents and coaches and ask them to model this. They, as well as participating athletes, could then sign a pledge that spelled out the various ways each group should behave to honor the game. A sample pledge for soccer is provided in the Clipboard (modified from "Sports: When Winning," Canadian Centres for Teaching Peace); you can revise this example to use in your specific sport, adding and modifying items as you wish. We also suggest that you create a signature and date line at the bottom, with the signature representing each person's pledge to comply with the code.

Reinforcement

Along with moral values being caught by youth athletes through effective models, these values are also *taught* through **reinforcement**

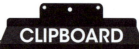

Honor the Game!

For Parents:

1. I will not force my child to participate in soccer.

2. I will remember that my child plays soccer for his or her enjoyment, not mine.

3. I will encourage my child to play by the rules and to resolve conflict without resorting to hostility and violence.

4. I will teach my child that doing one's best is as important as winning, so my child will never feel defeated by the outcome of a game.

5. I will make my child feel like a winner every time by offering praise for competing fairly and trying hard.

6. I will never ridicule or yell at my child or other children for making a mistake or losing a game.

7. I will remember that children learn best by example, and I will applaud good plays and performances by both my child's team and their opponents.

8. I will never question the official's judgment or honesty in public.

9. I will show respect and appreciation for the volunteer coaches who give their time to coach my child.

For Coaches:

1. I will be reasonable when scheduling games and practices, remembering that young athletes have other interests and obligations.

2. I will teach my athletes to play fairly and to respect the rules, officials, and opponents.

3. I will ensure that all athletes get instruction, feedback, and practice time in an equitable manner.

4. I will not ridicule or yell at my athletes for making mistakes or performing badly.

5. I will design practices so that athletes have fun, learn skills, and learn about the game of soccer.

6. I will make sure that equipment and facilities are safe and match athletes' ages and abilities.

7. I will set a good example by controlling my emotions, maintaining a calm, professional demeanor, and staying positive, even when I don't agree with the officials.

8. I will work in cooperation with officials and parents to honor the game.

For Athletes:

1. I will play soccer because I want to, not just because others or coaches want me to.

2. I will play by the rules to honor the game.

3. I will show respect for my opponents.

4. I will control my temper—fighting or "mouthing off" can spoil the activity for everyone.

5. I will do my best to be a team player by encouraging teammates and not yelling at them or getting upset if they don't play as I would like.

6. I will remember that coaches and officials are there to help me. I will accept their decisions and show them respect.

7. I will applaud all good plays and performances—those of my team and of my opponents.

8. I will remember that winning isn't everything—that having fun, improving skills, making friends, and doing my best are also important.

or the use of rewards and punishment. Like modeling, reinforcement is part of social learning about how one should act. Both good and bad moral behavior are positively reinforced in children through rewards such as praise and approval. In some situations, athletes get praise for calling penalties on themselves or shaking hands with an opponent after a physical collision. However, in other situations, athletes are encouraged to commit acts of aggression and are praised for doing so in the name of winning. In a famous scene from the movie *The Karate Kid*, a young athlete is instructed by his coach to "sweep the leg" of his opponent, or purposely injure his opponent's unstable knee to gain the advantage and win.

Influence of Coaches, Parents, and Teammates

Sport and team **norms**, or accepted and expected standards of behavior, have a strong influence on youth athletes' sportsmanship and aggression. Norms vary within teams and sports, and youth athletes quickly learn acceptable and valued normative behaviors for the given sport (e.g., conceding putts in golf match play). For example, athletes in heavy contact sports like ice hockey and American football have stronger tendencies to exhibit aggression and poor sportsmanship than athletes in lower-contact sports, indicating that the norms within contact sports support aggression as acceptable behavior (Bredemeier, Weiss, Shields, & Cooper, 1986; Shields et al., 2007).

Coaches and fathers encourage aggression in youth hockey, including fighting and other illegal acts, because they say it symbolizes strong character and helps teams win (Smith, 1982). Fathers' approval of illegal acts of aggression has been statistically linked to the number of fights their sons are in over a season's play. Similarly, over 40% of middle school football players admitted that teammates, coaches, and fathers influenced them to engage in illegal acts of aggression

on the field (Mugno & Feltz, 1985). Youth basketball players' tendencies to commit acts of aggression were strongly influenced by their perceptions that their coach would request this behavior and that their teammates would also commit acts of aggression (Stephens, 2001). Team norms supporting and encouraging aggression also predicted self-reported aggression in youth soccer players (Guivernau & Duda, 2002) and elite youth athletes (Long, Pantaléon, Bruant, & d'Arripe-Longueville, 2006). Ethnographic studies in sport (in which the researcher becomes part of the team and spends extended time over a season with the athletes and coaches) have described coaches'

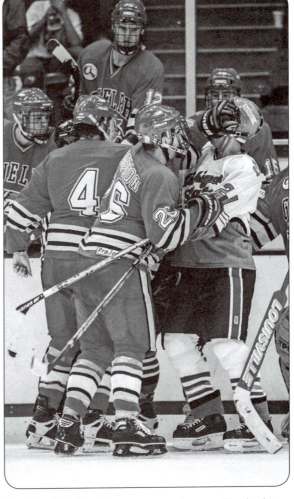

Youth athletes learn unsportsmanlike behaviors from norms established in that sport by coaches, parents, teammates, and the media.

teachings on sportsmanship as rhetorical lip service (Fine, 1987) or as hypocritically putting athletes in the "sticky situation" of weighing the contradictory goals of winning against sportsmanship (May, 2001). In a study by Fine (1987), Little League baseball players knew that coaches would occasionally instruct them to be good sports, but never in situations in which winning would be jeopardized.

But norms can work both ways. When coaches create an atmosphere in their teams in which individual improvement and personal mastery of skills (mastery climate) are emphasized over measuring oneself against teammates and beating others to feel competent (ego climate), athletes show higher levels of sportsmanship and prosocial behaviors and lower levels of aggression (e.g., Kavussanu, 2006; Ommundsen, Roberts, Lemyre, & Treasure, 2003). Moreover, the same finding holds for the positive influence of parents and peers on the sportsmanship of children. When children aged 8 to 10 and 13 to 15 years perceived a supportive mastery climate, they demonstrated greater respect for opponents, rules, and officials (d'Arripe-Longueville, Pantaléon, & Smith, 2006). Clearly, the ways in which adults structure youth sport programs have a direct impact on the moral behavior and values learned by children.

Influence of Media and Fans

One of the greatest challenges in enhancing moral behavior in youth sport is the glorification by the media and spectators of outrageous acts that demonstrate poor sportsmanship. On an ESPN *Outside the Lines* feature, former professional basketball player Joe Dumars, known for his outstanding sportsmanship, blamed the upsurge of unsportsmanlike conduct in the National Basketball Association on the media. Dumars spoke about how athletes know what it takes to lead off the television news show *SportsCenter,* saying that athletes quickly realize that the more outrageous their behavior, the more attention they receive.

Why hand the ball to an official in the end zone after scoring a touchdown as opposed to pretending to moon the crowd, autograph the ball with a Sharpie pen stuck in your sock, or run to midfield and spike the ball on the opponent's logo? All of these examples actually occurred in professional football and surely got the attention of youth athletes when they led off the sport news of the evening.

An article titled "2-4-6-Hate" describes inappropriate and destructive taunting orchestrated by high school fans against opposing athletes (Owens, 2006). Acceptable fun such as calling the hockey goalie a sieve or yelling during an opponent's free throw attempt has escalated to intolerant and inappropriate chants including racial epithets or stereotypes, homophobic heckling, and jeers about social class differences. Middle and high school administrators should review the honor the game code with student fans before contests and (a) define standards for what is acceptable and unacceptable, (b) communicate those standards, and (c) have a mechanism in place to enforce those standards (Owens, 2006).

Moral Reasoning

We've discussed how sportsmanship and moral behavior are caught by and taught to young athletes through modeling and reinforcement, respectively. However, productive social and moral values are not fully caught and taught until they are *bought.* True moral behavior requires individuals to "buy in"— that is, to act for the right reasons based on underlying moral values. So even though the modeling and reinforcement of moral values are important, without buy-in by the athlete, or the development of a mature and moral reasoning process, individuals will lack the internalized moral compass needed to reason through moral dilemmas throughout their lives. For example, athletes can grudgingly sign a pledge to honor the game because it is a participation requirement, or they can respectfully sign it because they believe that honoring the game is the right thing to do to preserve

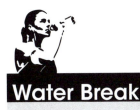

Water Break

The Myth of Useful Aggression

A widely held yet untrue belief is that a sudden eruption of aggression (e.g., fighting in hockey) is useful for "blowing off steam," or getting rid of inner frustration. The popular argument is that without fighting in hockey to release tension, players would resort to more vicious and dangerous assault with their sticks. This is known as the catharsis effect, in which releasing pent-up frustration through aggression serves to make one feel better and reduces the need to aggress more violently. However, the catharsis idea is a myth and has never been substantiated by research. Aggression is not cathartic and does not lead to a reduction in the desire to aggress. Instead, tempers flare and the behavior is socially rewarded by coaches and by fans. Michael Smith, who has extensively studied the culture of youth ice hockey, calls the idea of violence and fighting as catharsis "hockey's most durable folk theory" (1982, p. 294). He disputes that violence is an inevitable by-product of the game, because it doesn't occur across all teams and levels of play.

Let's be clear about why hockey players fight. The general manager of a NHL team stated, "I guarantee you, without the requisite level of hitting and fighting, we'd have empty buildings" (Farber, 2008, p. 62). Fighting is a learned behavior highly valued and rewarded in the culture. If professional hockey decides that its entertainment value is predicated on displaying violence and aggression on the ice, then leaders in the sport should simply acknowledge the fact. But spare us the senseless and baseless argument that fighting and aggression is a valuable release. As Smith (1982) argues, the real determinants of hockey violence are (a) the social organization of the hockey culture; (b) the ways in which the media portrays the professional game; and (c) the reinforcement players receive from parents, coaches, and teammates for aggression. To curb the growing violence in youth sport, adult leaders must be knowledgeable about such myths so as to educate parents, coaches, and athletes about why violence and aggression occur.

---

sport for everyone's benefit. These different reasons for signing the pledge represent different levels of moral reasoning, and these different levels of reasoning will ultimately influence how athletes behave in sport.

Developing Moral Reasoning Skills

Moral reasoning is the process people use in deciding what is the right thing to do. Typically, children go through developmental changes in their abilities to reason morally, and with age and appropriate learning and experience, they reach higher levels of moral reasoning. This process is called **moral development.** As children develop cognitive maturity, the basis for making choices moves from concrete, me-oriented ways of reasoning to a more abstract understanding of the world and a commitment to justice for all people. Figure 16.1 illustrates five levels of moral development to help you

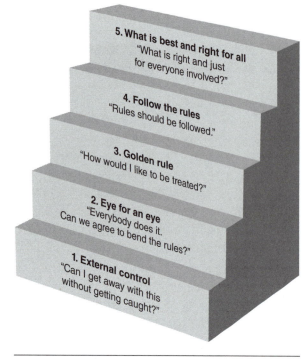

Figure 16.1   Levels of moral reasoning moving from self-interest to concern for others.

Based on Kohlberg 1984.

understand how people reason differently and how this may influence behavior in youth sport.

The moral reasoning staircase shown in figure 16.1 is modified from Kohlberg's (1984) famous categorization of how children mature developmentally in moving to higher levels of moral decision making. Individuals at levels 1 (external control) and 2 (eye for an eye) are characterized by self-interest. At level 1, individuals engage in moral behavior or do the right thing simply to avoid punishment. If they know they can get away with cheating and not get caught, they'll do it. Individuals at level 2 believe that everyone cheats or breaks rules a bit, so why not do it? They also may attempt to compromise with others to bend the rules, but self-interest is clearly still their focus. Two golfers in match play might agree to play winter rules, an illegal moving of the ball in the fairway to improve one's lie. At

this level, they see nothing wrong with the decision—"We're both doing it, so what's wrong with that?"

Individuals at level 3 begin to become aware of the feelings of others, but they do so to be "a good person" and expect others to treat them the same way (the golden rule: treating others as you wish to be treated). At level 4 (follow the rules), individuals are able to understand how rules and behaviors affect society or communities, and they make decisions to support the system in place. The highest level of moral reasoning is level 5, in which people reason about what is best and right for everyone involved even if it goes against the current system. Civil rights legend Rosa Parks demonstrated level 5 moral reasoning when she was arrested in 1963 for refusing to give up her seat to a white person on a city bus in Birmingham, Alabama. Ms. Parks followed her moral compass to demonstrate her belief that she, as an African American, had every right to sit on a bus, despite the racist Jim Crow laws of that city. Her act was a catalyst for the civil rights movement in the United States that moved the country to adopting more just laws to protect the rights of all citizens.

In a perfect world, all individuals would progressively move to level 5 as they achieve adulthood and engage in decision making and moral behavior that is in the best interest of their community. However, it's not a perfect world. Not everyone reaches level 5, and we don't always rise to the highest level of moral decision making that we are cognitively capable of (think of a particularly selfish coworker or family member here).

Moral Reasoning in Athletes

Unfortunately, competitive sport seems to be a particularly barren landscape within which to observe high levels of moral reasoning. Consider the following research findings (see

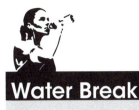

Water Break

Learning by Example

In October 2010, a Manchester High School (Connecticut) wide receiver lost his team's coded play card just before halftime, when it came off his armband. The play card was found and ended up in the hands of the opposing coach, D.J. Hernandez, of Southington High School. During the second half of the game, Manchester coach Marco Pizzoferrato noticed Hernandez looking down at his clipboard each time the Manchester quarterback began calling signals. Southington went to win the game 28-14, although the game had been tied at halftime. Caught in the act, Coach Hernandez was suspended for one game. He made the following statement: "I have had the opportunity to reflect on this entire situation, and I understand by using the card I did not set a good example for the young men that I coach" (Roberts, 2010, p. 102).

What would you have done if the opposing team's plays were given to you? This is a classic moral dilemma, with many possible responses. It is not our intent to denigrate Coach Hernandez, who realized in hindsight that his actions sent the wrong message to his young athletes about playing fairly. Rather, our intent in presenting this case example of a moral dilemma is to raise coaches' awareness of the many decisions that they face about what is right and fair to do in the heat of competition. What example are we setting for youth athletes in today's anything-to-win culture?

---

summaries by Shields & Bredemeier, 2007; Weiss, Smith, & Stunz, 2008; Wolverton, 2006):

- Athletes had significantly lower moral reasoning skills than nonathletes.
- Team sport athletes had lower moral reasoning skills than individual-sport athletes.
- The higher the level of contact in a sport, the lower the moral reasoning for both boys and girls.
- Male athletes had lower moral reasoning abilities than female athletes, but both had dropped in the past two decades.
- The lower the moral reasoning level, the more it was perceived as okay to engage in behaviors that might result in injuries to opponents.

- Athletes with less mature reasoning were rated by coaches as more likely to injure other athletes.

Reasons for Lower Moral Reasoning in Athletes

Are athletes bad or selfish people? What's going on in the sport world to explain this questionable morality of athletes? Several reasons may be offered. First, athletes tend to adopt **game reasoning** in making moral judgments in sport (see Shields & Bredemeier, 2007). Game reasoning is a form of bracketed morality in which lower levels of moral decision making are deemed appropriate in the context of sport, where winning takes precedence over other values. Game reasoning is supported by research showing that athletes use lower levels of moral reasoning in sport as compared to other life contexts (Bredemeier & Shields, 1986). The idea is that you can be nice off the court, but different rules apply once the ball is tipped.

Second, it may be that young athletes confuse aggression with aggressive play that is reinforced by well-meaning adults who fail to realize that children don't understand the

difference. Third, the model in professional sport of viewing opponents as obstacles to overcome rather than honorable participants in a contest of skill has trickled down to youth sports. In addition, the social and financial rewards in certain high-status sports have led to dubious practices not only in universities but also in middle and high schools, where athletes are entitled beyond other students,

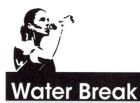

Water Break

Jack and Tiger on Learning Sportsmanship

Let's compare two of the greatest golfers of all time to see how they learned to be good sports, which helped them succeed as competitors in their careers. Jack Nicklaus recalls how his father reinforced the importance of sportsmanship to him: "Dad taught me that losing provides lasting lessons. I remember being 11 years old and playing with him. I had an eight-iron to the green, hit it into the sand, and I heaved the club darn near into the same bunker. Dad just said, 'OK, go pick up your club, we're going into the clubhouse. That's the last time I'll see you do that or you'll never go to the golf course again.' I had to learn how to behave as a young golfer, how to control my emotions and not let poor shots or other players affect me. My concentration and tight rein over my emotions [taught] me to perform under pressure and wall off distractions" (as cited in Ginsburg, Durant, & Baltzell, 2006, p. 176).

When Tiger Woods, still a preschooler, banged his club on the ground, his father, Earl, would ask him, "Who's responsible for that bad shot? That crow that made noise during your backswing? Your lie? The bag somebody dropped? Whose

responsibility was that?" "Mine," Tiger would reply. Then, each time Tiger banged his club he would say, "Daddy, I'm trying very hard [not to do it]." Mr. Woods would say, "I know you're trying, just keep trying. And as you grow and mature, you can turn this into an asset." Tiger would give his father progress reports. "Daddy, I wanted to bang my club today but I said no, I'm going to hit the next ball real solid." Mr. Woods explains that Tiger learned to play effectively while angry "all because we allowed him the space and then made him take responsibility for his actions. These are the kind of things we covered on life, through golf" (McCormick & Begley, 1996, p. 55).

Jack Nicklaus' father used firm reinforcement by allowing him to play golf only if he controlled his emotions and demonstrated proper behavior. A bit differently, Tiger Woods' father used more of a moral reasoning approach with his son to help him accept personal responsibility and make the choice to properly manage emotions. Obviously, both approaches worked, considering the combined success of these two golfing legends.

are not encouraged to think for themselves, and do not have to face the consequences of acting irresponsibly (Wolverton, 2006).

Addressing Moral Development in Youth Sport

The sobering report card of athletes' moral reasoning skills suggests that adult leaders in youth sport should more directly address moral development in children. First, it is important to understand that children must undergo a hierarchical transition through the levels and that, developmentally, young children are not able to reason at the higher levels. If I were working with 5-year-old soccer players, I would work toward level 3 to get them thinking about playing fair because everyone likes to be treated fairly. I might ask a child who makes fun of an unskilled teammate, "How do you think that makes Megan feel when you say that?" "What if that was you, and someone said those words to you—how would you feel?" Honoring the game at this age would be about being cooperative, fair, and supportive of teammates.

Second, we have to remember that moral development requires buy-in by athletes, which means that adults must go beyond modeling and reinforcement to help athletes reason and consider new ways of thinking about right and wrong in sport. Youth sport leaders can use the many **moral dilemmas** that arise in sport as teachable moments to discuss right actions with youth athletes. Moral dilemmas arise every day. These are some questions about moral dilemmas that you might get from your athletes: "If you cheat but win, isn't that okay?" "Why do all kids have to play in competition if some are better than others?" "If other people cheat, why shouldn't I?" "Why should I respect an official who makes a bad call and costs my team the victory?" "Why should I work hard in practice when I'm already better than the other kids?" "Why should I shake my opponent's hand when he was mean to me during the game?"

The point is not to answer these questions for children, but rather to engage them in a dialogue to help them think through the moral outcomes that stem from different alternatives. Our job as adults is to help them walk up the moral reasoning stairs shown in figure 16.1, to develop higher-level reasoning skills that will guide them not only in sport but also with the tough moral decisions they will face in life.

ENHANCING SPORTSMANSHIP, MORAL DEVELOPMENT, AND LIFE SKILLS IN YOUTH ATHLETES

As we've seen, moral behavior, sportsmanship, and life skills have to be caught, taught, and bought by young athletes, who need effective models, approval for positive behaviors, clear consequential penalties for negative behaviors, and life lessons learned through dialogue and a progressive understanding of what it means to play fair and be a moral person. In this section, we offer suggestions to foster the development of moral and life skills.

Sample Intervention Programs

Do moral and life skill development strategies work? Can children learn sportsmanship, enhance their moral reasoning skills, and transfer these skills to other life pursuits? The answer is yes, and this section provides some examples.

Intervention Programs in School Settings

An outstanding school-based model of a moral and life skill development intervention for children is Don Hellison's (2011) Teaching Personal and Social Responsibility (TPSR) through physical activity. As shown in figure 16.2, Hellison uses a moral reasoning hierarchy to get students thinking about how they can move from irresponsible behavior (level 0) to becoming a responsible, caring, self-directed individual (level 4). These levels are posted throughout the gym and discussed regularly in lesson plans that include counseling time, awareness talks, and group meetings so students can express opinions, as well as reflection time in which students evaluate how personally and socially responsible they were that day. As one youngster put it, "The levels were good. They let you know if you were acting like a fool or whatever" (Hellison, 2011, p. 33).

Research shows improvement in life skills and moral behavior, including their

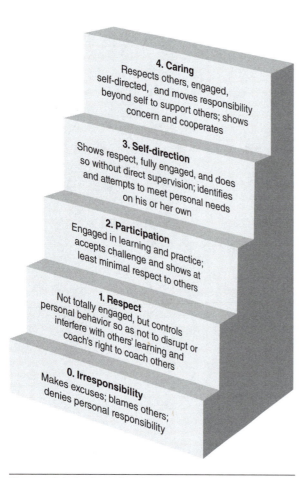

Figure 16.2 Levels of responsibility in Hellison's Teaching Personal and Social Responsibility program.

Adapted from Hellison 2011.

transfer into other life settings, with use of Hellison's TPSR approach (e.g., Martinek & Hellison, 2009). Perhaps the best evaluation examples are comments from kids in the program: "When someone messes up, I don't get mad now. I just tell them they can do better" (Hellison, 2011, p. 93) and "What I disliked about this program is that we should have had it a long time ago" (Hellison, 2011, p. 153).

National Intervention Programs

Earlier in the chapter, we presented the First Tee program as a national intervention program designed to enhance life skills in children through the game of golf (www.thefirsttee.org). Another example is Play It Smart, a national educational program targeted at high school football players from economically disadvantaged environments, where family and community support are often lacking (www.playitsmart.org). Life skills development is one of six measures of success in the program, along with improved scores on standardized tests, increased graduation rates, community service, and increased family involvement. The program has expanded from four schools in 1998 to 160 high schools, with more than 10,000 athletes participating. An outcome study showed that Play It Smart participants significantly improved on all measures of success (Petitpas, Van Raalte, Cornelius, & Presbrey, 2004).

The Playing Tough and Clean Hockey Program was developed to teach youth hockey players ages 12 and older to play within the rules and enhance their ability to respond positively to negative emotions (Lauer & Paiement, 2004). The Girls on the Run/Girls on Track program was developed as a life skills program for young girls to enhance self-esteem, to discourage them from participating in risky behaviors, and to foster a healthy lifestyle through running. The program has been shown to improve self-esteem, perceived competence, and interpersonal skills in participants (Sifers & Shea, 2013; Waldron, 2007).

CLIPBOARD

Taking the Direct Approach to Building Life Skills and Values in Youth Athletes

What can coaches do to directly work on life skill and moral development in youth athletes? A high school ice hockey program that was successful in life skill and moral development with players incorporated several strategies (Camire, Trudel, & Bernard, 2013). All players had handbooks, with the philosophy of the program on the first page. The philosophy of "focusing on the whole person" and using "ice hockey as a means to humanize the person" were emphasized from the beginning. A retreat was conducted with team bonding, communication, and values clarification exercises. Players kept journals in which they discussed personal events related to hockey or life, which the coaches collected and read weekly. Across the season, six player–parent–coach meetings were held that focused on the development of each player as a person and athlete. Players also participated in developmental activities such as goal setting and performed volunteer community service work.

Another specific strategy is the Captain's Leadership Development Program offered by the Institute for the Study of Youth Sports at Michigan State University (Gould & Voelker, 2010). Working with the Michigan High School Athletic Association, the program teaches leadership skills to high school students selected as potential candidates for captainship of their teams. The program involves participation at a clinic, after which all the athletes complete the self-study guidebook *Becoming an Effective Team Captain: Student-Athlete Guide*. Content includes captains' roles and responsibilities, key leadership principles, effective communication, understanding motivation, team building and cohesion, and how to handle tough team situations and common problems.

What is significant about both of these programs is that they involved active planning and implementation of specific strategies to build leadership and life skills in young athletes. We cannot assume that athletes designated as team captains understand how to provide leadership, nor can we assume that life skills are automatically developed through team membership. Research shows that coaches who directly address life skills development with their athletes strongly influence athletes' abilities to regulate emotions, engage in prosocial behavior, and link effectively with the community (Gould & Carson, 2010).

Practical Strategies for Moral and Life Skills Development in Youth Sport

Research has shown that moral and life skills can be caught by, taught to, and bought into by youth. So what can school and community youth sport leaders and coaches do to infuse moral and life skill development into their programs? The answer is to start small and consider simple and innovative ways to build social and moral skills along with the physical skills of the sport. We offer some tips in this section for how to do that, and we encourage you to think creatively about how you can teach important life lessons to children through sport.

1. As an adult leader, think about and prepare for the type of model you want to be for your youth athletes. Talk the moral talk by continuously reminding athletes of productive ways to think and act. Examples might be "There are no shortcuts to anywhere worth going"; "We never do anything to embarrass ourselves, our team, or our program [school]"; and "We call people by

their names, we don't call them names." In addition, walk the moral walk. Thoughtfully prepare for and model appropriate ways to manage frustration and anger, respond to setbacks, lose with dignity, and accept unfair decisions by officials.

2. Invite well-known athletes in your area (high school, collegiate, or professional) to talk to your team. These talks should be brief (10-15 minutes) and should be followed by an opportunity for athletes to ask questions. Role models who talk about how they overcame obstacles or how they made bad choices and experienced strong life lessons as a consequence might be especially powerful. Talk briefly with the speaker beforehand to make sure you're on the same page with regard to the lesson.

3. Clearly, emphatically, unemotionally, and repeatedly apply rules for acceptable behavior. Reward sportsmanship and penalize aggression, cheating, and disrespect. Use logical consequences in your reinforcement of athletes' behavior to emphasize their personal responsibility for the outcome. For example, explain to a disappointed athlete that she was not elected captain because she cuts corners by not working hard in practice, and her teammates don't respect her work ethic. When you remove a player from a game for losing his temper, remind him that he chose to behave that way and brought the consequence upon himself. Don't ever rescue athletes from the negative consequences of their behavior—for example, by revoking rules for a star player.

4. Sponsor a virtue on your team for a season or a few weeks within a season; you or your athletes choose a moral quality that you would like to highlight within the team (e.g., perseverance, responsibility, self-control, consideration, respect). Athletes could bring quotes or examples to practice each day, and you could post these on a bulletin board specifically designed to promote this social or moral virtue. You could also direct a team-building activity in which

the sponsored virtue is tested and then discussed among athletes.

5. Develop a theme for sportsmanship in your program, similar to the honoring the game (Thompson, 2010b) example provided earlier in the chapter. Examples might be Together Everyone Achieves More (TEAM); Winning With Honor; or Play Hard, Play Fair, Have Fun. Talk about your theme throughout the season, reminding athletes of ways in which they can and do live it each day.

6. Using your theme, create a pledge to specify desired and acceptable behaviors (see the example provided earlier in the chapter for coaches, parents, and athletes) and ask everyone to sign it.

7. If you're a school administrator, develop a sportsmanship plan to post on the school website that clearly defines acceptable and inappropriate behavior for all involved, including band members, spirit sections, cheerleaders, and spectators.

8. Give unannounced sportsmanship awards to athletes on your team for positive sport behaviors that they demonstrate. Encourage your athletes to notice these behaviors and honor their teammates as well. Select small, even silly, awards to give, and vary them each time. The point is to recognize and honor the behavior, not to give a big award.

9. Recognize and cultivate teachable moral moments as they arise in training and competition. If possible, group athletes to discuss what happened. If an athlete calls a teammate a name or makes fun of her, stop practice and lead a discussion. Make a point of not showing anger or directly punishing the athlete, but rather begin a dialogue by asking questions such as "What do you think happens to people when others call them names?" "Sarah, how did that make you feel?" "Amanda, how would feel if you were in her place?" "What happens in sport to make us act like that?"

10. In addition to teachable moments, consider planned moral dialogues that you can lead with your athletes. Occasionally, for 5 minutes at the end of practice, lead a discussion about such moral issues as inequity in sport, how to respond to rough play, what it means to be aggressive and what it doesn't, and why we have to cooperate to compete. For this to be effective, you must ask provocative questions to draw your athletes out to state their opinions. In the Miami University youth hockey school, all participants attend the Good Sports program, in which they discuss preplanned moral dilemmas scripted as hockey case studies. Examples of these deal with equal playing time, problem parents, trash talking, performance enhancers, and being a leader. The youth athletes work in small groups with coaches and write out their responses to the situations, then present them in front of the large group with discussion to follow.

11. Discuss sport incidents involving children, both positive and negative. For example, use the story of the Marysville-Pilchuck and Oak Harbor high school football teams described at the beginning of the chapter. Set it up as a moral dilemma by describing the circumstances, and then ask the athletes what they think should have happened in this situation. After some discussion, you can tell them how the story actually ended. Lead a discussion about how and why the acts of both teams honored the game and why that's important in sport. But also discuss negative occurrences like the use of illegal performance-enhancing drugs by athletes. The Positive Coaching Alliance (ww.positivecoach.org) encourages adults never to let poor sportsmanship examples in the media go undiscussed with youth athletes. If you don't discuss the immoral actions of children's sport heroes, they may be confused or interpret your silence as unspoken approval of the behavior. Speak out about what's going on in the world of sports, and in particular ask young athletes

how they view the issue. Instead of preaching, remember to ask open-ended questions about what they think.

12. Designate various athletes on your team as weekly assistant coaches. Give them responsibility and provide an opportunity for them to demonstrate leadership. They can come early and help set up practice, talk over and provide feedback about practice sessions, choose and lead certain drills, and perhaps present some team-building ideas or quotes for the day based on the team sportsmanship theme or sponsored virtue.

13. Simplify Hellison's (2011) levels of moral responsibility (see figure 16.2) and use this language within your team each day. For example, you could use the terms Rookie, Teammate, and Leader as three levels of social responsibility shown within the team. Rookies represent individuals at Hellison's level 0, who are disruptive and disrespectful to others. Teammates are engaged in practice and competition and show acceptable respect for others. Leaders distinguish themselves by demonstrating support and concern for others as well as taking personal responsibility to work hard to improve their skills beyond what is expected within the team. You can explain the terms to your athletes and begin to use them to reinforce behavior: "Who did you notice being a Leader today in practice and why?" or "Josh just cut in line—what kind of player does that?" The team learns to reply, "Rookie!" which hopefully helps Josh understand the problem with his behavior.

14. Although youth sport takes place within a competitive environment (as discussed in chapter 3), youth sport leaders can use cooperative games and activities to help kids learn life skills such as cooperation, teamwork, acceptance, communication, conflict resolution, and inclusion (Luvmour, 2007; Orlick, 2006). Such activities focus kids on the fun and process of playing, as opposed to outcomes. Many examples of developmentally

appropriate cooperative games and sport activities are available online.

WRAP-UP

Sometimes people ask why learning life lessons is such a point of emphasis in youth sport. Can't we just teach physical skills? Actually, the answer is no, for two reasons. First, striving to develop skills in any achievement area (e.g., music lessons, school) always involves social and moral learning as well. Children must learn to cooperate with others, respect rules, communicate effectively, respond appropriately to disappointment, persist through obstacles, and control emotions in pursuing most goals in life. Second, sport is a particularly fertile context within which to teach moral and life lessons because competition inherently involves a public striving to achieve goals while one's opponent is simultaneously striving to block one's goals. In addition, many children desperately want to achieve in sport because of its significance in our society. This adds up to a rich boiling pot of moral dilemmas, behavioral alternatives, and possible consequences.

Some have advocated de-emphasizing competition for youth in favor of cooperative games. Although these games should be part of youth development, we disagree that they should take the place of competitive youth sport. The competitive nature of sport constantly tests the character of young athletes; and through these tests, moral behavior, sportsmanship, and productive life skills can be learned and enhanced. However, it is up to adult leaders of youth sport to design and conduct appropriate moral tests for children and to prepare youth athletes to pass these tests. As adult youth sport leaders, it is our direct responsibility to enhance moral and life skill development in children, which is critical for the betterment of society.

LEARNING AIDS

Key Terms

aggression—Violating the rights of other individuals with the intent to harm them, for example, to inflict pain or injury.

aggressiveness—Refers to competing in a forceful manner with great intensity of effort.

character—A group of positive moral or ethical qualities that are revered in society.

game reasoning—A form of bracketed morality in which lower levels of moral decision making are deemed appropriate in the context of sport, in which winning takes precedence over other values.

life skills—Physical, social, cognitive, emotional, and behavioral skills that allow individuals to succeed in and effectively contribute to the culture in which they live.

modeling—A form of observational learning whereby children imitate the actions of significant adults.

moral behavior—Doing the right thing for the right reason, based on underlying moral values.

moral development—The process whereby individuals reach higher levels of moral reasoning through learning and experience.

moral dilemmas—Life events that create questions about right versus wrong and how they should be decided.

moral reasoning—The process people use in deciding what is the right thing to do.

norms—Accepted and expected standards of behavior.

prosocial behaviors—Actions that benefit others, such as cooperating, sharing, and empathizing.

reinforcement—Using rewards and punishment to modify behavior.

social learning—A psychological theory proposing that children become aware of and learn culturally valued behaviors or social norms as they are socialized into adulthood.

sportsmanship—Acting in ways that promote fairness and mutual respect in competition, even when these actions allow strategic gain by the opponent.

violence—Rough or injurious physical force.

Summary Points

1. Sportsmanship and moral behavior are not automatically developed through youth sport participation.

2. Youth sport has the potential to help athletes develop socially and morally, but only if the program is structured and delivered in appropriate ways.

3. The term *character* is vague and hard to define, so practitioners should focus on enhancing sportsmanship, moral behavior, and life skills in youth sport participants.

4. Sportsmanship and moral behavior are caught by children through effective modeling, taught through clear reinforcement, and bought through the development of mature moral reasoning skills.

5. The idea that aggression is useful in releasing inner tension so that more violent aggression can be avoided is a myth.

6. As children become more cognitively mature, they develop the capacity to move to higher levels of moral reasoning.

7. Athletes have lower moral reasoning skills than nonathletes, with team sport athletes, male athletes, and high-contact sport athletes showing the lowest levels of moral reasoning.

8. Lower moral reasoning levels are related to aggression by athletes.

9. Intervention programs have successfully enhanced the moral reasoning and life skills of youth athletes.

10. Youth sport leaders can use simple, practical strategies to build and enhance sportsmanship, moral behavior, and life skills in young athletes.

Study Questions

1. Explain the difference between the terms *life skills, sportsmanship,* and *moral behavior.*

2. Why is it impossible to answer the question "Does sport build character?"

3. What is aggression, and why is it confused with aggressiveness?

4. Explain how powerful norms in society influence children's sport behavior, and provide research examples of this reinforcement.

5. What does the term *catharsis* mean, and why is the idea of catharsis misunderstood in sports like ice hockey, American football, and lacrosse?

6. Discuss several reasons why athletes are lower in moral reasoning than nonathletes.

7. What do we mean when we say that sportsmanship or moral behaviors are *caught by* and *taught to* youth athletes? Explain what each term means, and provide examples of how a youth sport coach can teach moral skills to athletes in this way.

8. Explain what it means when we say sportsmanship, or moral behaviors, is bought by youth athletes. How is this different from the caught and taught ways of learning?

9. Describe a specific example of how youth sport coaches can use a naturally occurring moral dilemma in sport to enhance the moral reasoning of young athletes, and explain how the coach can help the athletes work through the moral dilemma.

10. Explain how an athlete might think at each of the five levels of the moral reasoning staircase and provide a sport example.

Reflective Learning Activities

1. Search the Internet for quotes by famous athletes about sportsmanship. Discuss how you could use these quotes to help youth athletes learn important life lessons.

2. Read the following three scenarios. Decide how you would handle each, particularly in creating a moral dialogue with the athletes. The aim of the dialogue would be to help your athletes reason through the dilemma to encourage them to internalize mature moral values.

   a. The two best players on your basketball team of 9- and 10-year-olds state in a team meeting that they don't agree with your rule that everyone plays significant minutes in games. They say they know the team could win more games if this rule were relaxed a little so that they and the other more skilled kids could play more.

   b. You are the coach of a middle school tennis team, and your players ask you about how they should call their lines during play. Everyone cheats a little, they say—and since their opponents sometimes call a line in their own favor on a crucial point, shouldn't they be doing the same thing?

   c. A parent of one of your 9-year-old hockey players is constantly yelling at his son directives such as "Take him out" and "Knock his block off" during play. He expresses frustration with you as the coach for not emphasizing toughness in the players. In front of the players, he tells you that he would like to talk to the team at the next practice, because he knows some tricks that can be used on the ice to get away with illegal moves without the referees noticing.

4. Develop five moral dilemmas that could occur in your particular sport. Design these as case studies that athletes could read and discuss in small groups.

5. Using the five levels of moral reasoning from figure 16.1, read the following two scenarios and discuss (a) what level of moral reasoning was used in this situation, and (b) your agreement or disagreement with the situation, including pros and cons.

   a. Kentucky's high school athletic association issued a directive in 2013 advising teams not to organize postgame handshake lines, citing the fact that in the past three years such lines had led to more than two dozen fights.

   b. Kenbriel Hearn from Lubbock, Texas, missed the 2013 season of high school football (his senior season), having spent three weeks close to death in a coma and on life support due to two strokes and bleeding in his brain. He had regained his ability to jog by the time of the team's last home game. His coach asked him to suit up for the game, and with the team trailing 35-0 in the final minute, sent Hearn in. The two teams had agreed to give Hearn an opportunity to carry the ball and score a touchdown if the game outcome had already been decided. He received the handoff and scored, and teammates mobbed and hugged him and opposing players shook his hand. Coaches, parents, teammates, and Hearn himself all shed tears and agreed that they would never forget this memorable touchdown run.

Resource Guide

The First Tee Life Skills Experience (YouTube) (www.youtube.com/watch?v=FUesKzkkMZc). This 5-minute clip shows how First Tee uses golf as a vehicle to teach life skills to kids participating in the program.

Sportsmanship, NFHS free online course (www.nfhslearn.com).

EPILOGUE

What part of your tour of knowledge about youth sport made the biggest impression on you? What ideas stuck with you the most? Most importantly, how will you use the knowledge that you've gained?

Consider how you could respond to these questions by integrating what you've learned:

1. How did youth sport become what it is today? What are the positive outcomes, as well as the negative outcomes, from this evolution?

2. What are the many unique characteristics of child and adolescent athletes that make coaching and teaching them different from coaching and teaching adults?

3. How do we get kids interested in joining youth sport, get them to fall in love with it, and get them to continue to be physically active throughout their lives?

4. What would you recommend to the parents of talented and passionate youth athletes as the best way to facilitate their sport potential and overall well-being?

5. What are the most important things coaches can do to make youth sport work best? How about parents? How about youth sport program directors?

Many of our students tell us that of all the things they've learned, they will definitely remember the mantra "It's all about the kid." That's probably because we repeat it so much in class! But we agree that it's a good thing to keep in the forefront of our minds when teaching, coaching, directing, officiating, or parenting in youth sport.

We hope that you will be a strong proponent of developmentally appropriate practice. Actually, if you're not a DAP disciple after reading this book, we haven't done our job as authors very well! We hope you'll use the DAP principle when planning programs; designing practices; teaching skills; providing feedback; modifying activities; and deciding how early, how much, how long, and how intense when it comes to youth sport participation. Your big challenge is to stick to the DAP principle in the face of strong resistance resulting from entrenched traditional thinking, or "the way it's always been." We understand that this is a difficult challenge, often with lots of blowback. But you can be confident in the evidence presented here when making developmentally appropriate decisions. Remember that best practice for youth sport is always developmentally appropriate practice.

We believe in youth sport. We believe that youth sport can and often does provide quality experiences for young people. But we realize that we can always do things better. The intent of this book has been to educate and inspire you to find ways to do it better. Toward that end, we advocate that you adopt a solution-focused approach. It's very common to focus on the problems in youth sport and to wring our hands over the audacious behavior of some misguided adults. A solution-focused approach means that we identify the problems but that our energy focuses on solutions and the implementation of important changes to make youth sport work better and be more developmentally appropriate. Youth sport will and should always be a work in progress. We want to be a part of that progress, and we hope that you do as well.

APPENDIX A
The 100-Points Exercise

Below is a list of possible objectives for youth sport programs. You have 100 points that you can divide across the objectives to represent how important that objective is to you in relation to youth sport.

You can add your own objectives if those that are important to you are not on this list. When you are finished, your points should add up to 100.

How important is this objective of youth sport to you?

_____   Have fun

_____   Be physically fit

_____   Be with or make friends or both

_____   Win

_____   Develop physical skills

_____   Learn life lessons

_____   Earn a college athletic scholarship

_____   Entertain parents

_____   Provide a feeder system

_____   Encourage lifetime participation

_____   Gain self-confidence and feelings of mastery

_____   Learn how to compete

_____   Other (specify): _____

_____   Other (specify): _____

_____   Other (specify): _____

100   Total

From R.S. Vealey and M.A. Chase, 2016, *Best practice for youth sport* (Champaign, IL: Human Kinetics). Adapted, by permission, from J. Thompson, 2009, *Positive sports parenting* (Portola Valley, CA: Balance Sports Publishing), 56.

APPENDIX B
Sample Issues to Consider
When Developing Your Principles

Following is a list of issues common in youth sport. Consider your position on these issues to help you identify important principles for your program.

Remember that your principles logically follow from your philosophy and objectives. These provide you with predetermined guidelines about how you'll make decisions, interact with your athletes, and model your philosophy.

1. Winning versus athlete participation

2. Winning versus skill development and mastery

3. Talent development for all participants versus enhanced talent development for the better skilled

4. Athlete centered versus adult centered

5. Play versus work

6. Autocratic leadership versus participative (shared decision making) leadership

7. Sport for all versus sport for the gifted or talented

8. Child-only versus parent involvement

9. Pyramid model versus palm community model

10. Use of praise as a motivator versus use of punishment as a motivator

From R.S. Vealey and M.A. Chase, 2016, *Best practice for youth sport* (Champaign, IL: Human Kinetics). Based on Martens 2001; adapted from Martens 2000.

APPENDIX C
Case Studies on Growth and Maturation

CASE STUDY 1

Aaron is 13 years old and in 8th grade. He is currently 5 feet 7 inches and weighs 145 pounds. Within the past six months, he hasn't changed much in height, but his body shape and composition have really changed. His shoulders have broadened; he has considerably more muscle mass than he did last year; and he has lost some of the pudgy fat on his trunk and stomach. His voice has deepened, and the hair on his arms and legs has increased in amount and the color has darkened. He's had an outstanding middle school football season as a running back, as he is faster and stronger than many of his peers.

CASE STUDY 2

Hannah is 11 years old and in 5th grade. She is 5 feet 1 inch tall and weighs 125 pounds. She achieved menarche at 10.5 years. Within the last two years, she has grown about 6 inches and gained about 20 pounds. She is self-conscious about her body because she has become more pear shaped than her friends the same age, with bigger breasts and hips. She is considering dropping out of club swimming, which she has enjoyed since the age of 8.

CASE STUDY 3

Keisha is 13 years old and in 7th grade. She currently stands 5 feet 2 inches and weighs 105 pounds. She has a linear build, with no significant muscle mass or body fat. She shows no obvious signs of secondary sex characteristics development. She hasn't grown much in height over the past four months, but her hands and feet have grown bigger. Keisha is an outstanding soccer player and 400-meter runner, and she enjoys other sports and being physically fit.

CASE STUDY 4

Nate is 14 years old and in 8th grade. He is 5 feet 4 inches and weighs 115 pounds. He is extremely skinny, and he has huge feet. He has not grown significantly for a few months and is shorter than his friends on the community recreational basketball team. He didn't make his 8th-grade school basketball team, mainly because he lacks strength, power, and size. He is showing no signs of puberty (hair on legs and arms, deepening voice) at all, and is discouraged because he desperately wants to play high school basketball. His mother is 6 feet 1 inch and his dad is 6 feet 4 inches, and Nate wonders why he is so short when he has such tall parents.

From R.S. Vealey and M.A. Chase, 2016, *Best practice for youth sport* (Champaign, IL: Human Kinetics).

APPENDIX D

Sample Letter to Parents
Explaining Readiness Evaluation Session

[Date]

Dear youth basketball parents,

Welcome to this year's Oxford Parks and Recreation (OPR) youth basketball season! We are excited to provide your child with an enjoyable learning experience in the great game of basketball. The purpose of this letter is to give you more detailed information about player evaluations for the league.

All players who wish to participate in the basketball league this year **MUST** attend **ONE** of three scheduled evaluation sessions (all at Grant Elementary School) for their age group:

October 22, 23, or 24 (Please plan to attend ONE of these sessions.)

    Girls, 8 and 9 years old—6:00-7:00 p.m.

    Boys, 8 years old—7:00-8:00 p.m.

    Boys, 9 years old—8:00-9:00 p.m.

When you arrive in the lobby of the Grant Elementary School gymnasium, **please check your child in at the registration table.** We will assign your child an evaluation number and measure your child's height and weight. You can then proceed into the gym, and our staff members will direct your child to his or her group.

This is an evaluation, **not a tryout.** Every child who signs up for OPR basketball will be placed on a team. We use evaluations to create teams that are as even as possible in terms of players' skills, height, weight, and experience. All of the coaches in the program will observe and assess the players during the evaluation. Based on this evaluation, coaches will select players for their teams through a draft system. This evaluation and draft system has been successful in eliminating lopsided league standings and "stacked" teams, and has been shown to provide the most equitable experience possible for the players.

We suggest that you explain to your child that this is not a tryout. They should come to play and have fun. There will be some time for scrimmage, or game play, but they will also go through some dribbling, passing, shooting, rebounding, and defensive drills. If they don't have any or much experience with basketball, that's okay. We plan to teach them these skills. Our number-one priority for this program is to teach your child the skills of basketball in an enjoyable introductory competitive format.

Thanks for being a part of OPR basketball!

Zoe Griffith, Sports Coordinator

From R.S. Vealey and M.A. Chase, 2016, *Best practice for youth sport* (Champaign, IL: Human Kinetics).

APPENDIX E
Why I Play Sports Survey

Why do you play sports? Following is a list of reasons that kids have given for why they play sport. Look at each reason and decide how much you agree with it in terms of why YOU play sport. Check ONE box for each reason, depending on if you agree, if you are not sure, or if you disagree.

There are no right or wrong answers. We're interested in YOUR REASONS FOR WHY YOU PLAY.

	Strongly agree	Agree	Not sure	Disagree	Strongly disagree
1. To be active					
2. To learn new skills					
3. To have fun					
4. My parents want me to play					
5. To be on a team					
6. To compete against others					
7. I'm good at it					
8. It's exciting					
9. To win					
10. To meet friends					
11. To become a good athlete					
12. It makes me feel special					
13. To be healthy					
14. So I can play sports in college					
15. To be with friends					
16. It gives me confidence					
17. I love my sport					
18. To improve my skills					
19. To show how good I am					
20. To learn self-control					
21. I like my coach					
22. It helps me look good					
23. My parents like it					

Now, look over this list and your answers, and write down the **three** most important reasons that you play your sport.

1. _____
2. _____
3. _____

From R.S. Vealey and M.A. Chase, 2016, *Best practice for youth sport* (Champaign, IL: Human Kinetics). Adapted, by permission, from S. Murphy, 1999, *The cheers and the tears: A healthy alternative to the dark side of youth sport* (San Francisco, CA: Jossey-Bass), 70-71.

APPENDIX F

Motivational Climate Scale for Youth Sports

Read each statement below and think about **how true you think it is about YOUR COACH.** For each statement, **circle one number.**

There are no right or wrong answers. **You do NOT have to sign your name on this paper,** and **no one will know** that these are your responses. Please be honest. **Your coach wants honest feedback** to help him or her understand how to be the best coach possible.

	Very true		Somewhat true		Not at all true
1. Coach made players feel good when they improved a skill.	5	4	3	2	1
2. Coach said that teammates should help each other improve their skills.	5	4	3	2	1
3. Winning games was the most important thing for Coach.	5	4	3	2	1
4. Coach paid most attention to the best players.	5	4	3	2	1
5. Coach encouraged us to learn new skills.	5	4	3	2	1
6. Coach spent less time with the players who weren't as good.	5	4	3	2	1
7. Coach told us to try to be better than our teammates.	5	4	3	2	1
8. Coach told us that trying our best was the most important thing.	5	4	3	2	1
9. Players were taken out of games if they made a mistake.	5	4	3	2	1
10. Coach said that all of us were important to the team's success.	5	4	3	2	1
11. Coach told us which players on the team were best.	5	4	3	2	1
12. Coach told players to help each other get better.	5	4	3	2	1

Scoring Instructions for the Motivational Climate Scale for Youth Sports (MCSYS)

1. On a blank copy of the MCSYS, label each item with a T or E to designate it as Task or Ego.

   Task-involved climate items: 1, 2, 5, 8, 10, 12

   Ego-involved climate items: 3, 4, 6, 7, 9, 11

2. On each questionnaire, add up the numbers for Task items and divide by 6 to get the mean (average) score. Do the same for the Ego items. Write the Task and Ego mean on each questionnaire.

3. Add up all the Task scores (one for each questionnaire), and then divide this number by the number of questionnaires (your overall mean score for Task-Involved Climate). Do the same to come up with your overall Ego-Involved Climate score.

4. Consider your two scores. Do you think they are accurate? If not, how are the scores different from what you perceive you do as a coach?

5. If you want more information, you could also score each item, and then create means for each item to help you understand how your players view your coaching behavior. You could insert the numbers in an Excel spreadsheet to quickly compute the different means of the items.

6. If you talk to your players about the scores, be sure to be grateful for their feedback and not resentful about any of their responses. You could have a discussion about ways in which both coaches and athletes could enhance the motivational climate for the team.

APPENDIX G
Motivation Case Studies

CASE STUDY 1

Ethan joins the summer swim team at his community pool when he is 11. He can swim freestyle, but has yet to learn backstroke, breaststroke, and butterfly. Lanes 1 and 2 of the pool are reserved for beginners and newcomers to the program, with an emphasis on learning correct stroke technique. But almost all the kids in these beginning lanes are younger than age 9, and Ethan's friends and other swimmers his age are in lanes 3 through 6. The swim program has the philosophy that anyone can join at any time, and beginners all start in lanes 1 and 2. Ethan comes home and tells his parents that he doesn't want to swim anymore because he's in the "baby lanes" and not with his friends. What steps might his parents take to help keep Ethan motivated and in the swim program?

CASE STUDY 2

Caitlyn is a high school freshman volleyball player who plays the middle hitter position. She has had a solid year playing full-time on both the freshman and junior varsity squads. Her skills have improved significantly; her confidence and love of the game have blossomed, and she enjoys the friendships and camaraderie on these teams. Due to a freak number of injuries to middle hitters in the program, Caitlyn is told she will play for the varsity for the rest of the season. Although initially excited, she is so nervous and afraid before the varsity match that she feels sick. When she gets into the game, she performs adequately, but she repeatedly plays it safe by tipping the ball instead of spiking it. At home after the match, Caitlyn sobs and tells her parents that she doesn't feel she fits in with the varsity girls (all juniors and seniors) and that she doesn't feel she's good enough to play on the varsity. Her parents are perplexed because they think she should be overjoyed by the opportunity to play at the varsity level. How would you explain Caitlyn's responses based on her underlying motivational orientations? How could her parents and coach help her in this situation?

CASE STUDY 3

Middle school athletic director Ms. Jefferson has received several complaints about Coach Bates, who coaches the 8th-grade girls' basketball team. Coach Bates knows the game very well, having played and coached at both the high school and college levels. She is intent on building a strong program and has implemented a conditioning regimen that requires players to attend every morning at 6 a.m. during July and August, before school starts. She has implemented a fitness test (distance run for time) that all girls must pass before they are allowed to try out for the team, which has scared many girls away from trying out. She teaches complex offensive sets, and the players struggle to learn and remember what do on the floor. They look robotic, timid, and hesitant when they play. Coach Bates really wants to develop a strong program and is confused about why her players don't like basketball and why parents are complaining. How could Ms. Jefferson help Coach Bates?

From R.S. Vealey and M.A. Chase, 2016, *Best practice for youth sport* (Champaign, IL: Human Kinetics).

APPENDIX H

Talent Development Environment Questionnaire for Sport (Selected Items Only)

Read each statement below and think about **how much you agree** that it describes your sport situation in this program. For each statement, **circle one number** to represent **how much you agree or disagree** with the statement in relation to your sport program.

There are no right or wrong answers. **You do NOT have to sign your name on this paper,** and **no one will know** that these are your responses. Please be honest.

	Strongly agree	Agree	Agree a little bit	Disagree a little bit	Disagree	Strongly disagree
1. My coach emphasizes the need for constant work on fundamental and basic skills.	6	5	4	3	2	1
2. The more experienced I get, the more my coach encourages me to take responsibility for my own development and learning.	6	5	4	3	2	1
3. My development plan incorporates a variety of physical preparation exercises, such as fitness, flexibility, agility, coordination, balance, and strength training.	6	5	4	3	2	1
4. My training sessions are normally beneficial and challenging.	6	5	4	3	2	1
5. My coach plans training to incorporate a wide variety of useful skills and attributes, such as techniques, physical abilities, tactical skills, mental skills, and decision making.	6	5	4	3	2	1
6. My coach is good at helping me understand my strengths and weaknesses.	6	5	4	3	2	1
7. My training is specifically designed to help me develop effectively in the long term.	6	5	4	3	2	1
8. My coach emphasizes that what I do in training and competition is far more important than winning.	6	5	4	3	2	1

	Strongly agree	Agree	Agree a little bit	Disagree a little bit	Disagree	Strongly disagree
9. My coach allows me to learn through making my own mistakes.	6	5	4	3	2	1
10. My coach is good at helping me understand what I am doing and why I am doing it.	6	5	4	3	2	1
11. I would be given good opportunities even if I experienced a dip in performance.	6	5	4	3	2	1
12. I am encouraged to participate in other sports, cross-train, or both.	6	5	4	3	2	1
13. My coach makes time to talk to my parents about me and what I am trying to achieve.	6	5	4	3	2	1
14. The advice my parents give me fits well with the advice I get from my coaches.	6	5	4	3	2	1
15. My progress and personal performance are reviewed regularly on an individual basis.	6	5	4	3	2	1
16. I am regularly told that winning and losing just now does not indicate how successful I will be in the future.	6	5	4	3	2	1
17. I have access to a variety of different types of professionals to help my sports development.	6	5	4	3	2	1
18. My coach shows that she or he is concerned about my well-being.	6	5	4	3	2	1
19. I am taught how to balance training, competing, and recovery.	6	5	4	3	2	1
20. I am involved in most decisions about my sport development.	6	5	4	3	2	1

Instructions for Scoring and Using the Abbreviated Talent Development Environment Questionnaire for Sport (TDEQS)

1. Because this questionnaire contains only selected items from the TDEQS for brief practical use, there are no subscales to compute. We suggest that you look at scores on the individual items to get feedback about specific aspects of your talent development program. If you've administered questionnaires to a group of athletes, you could compute mean scores for each item to assess strengths and weaknesses of your program.

2. All items are worded so that 6 is the highest score and 1 is the lowest score.

3. If you talk to athletes in your program about the scores, be sure to be grateful for their feedback and not resentful about any of their responses. You could have a discussion about ways in which both coaches and athletes could enhance the talent development climate in the program.

4. Items in this questionnaire focus mainly on key aspects of long-term talent development. Other subscales in the complete version of the TDEQS include quality preparation, communication, understanding the athlete, support network, and challenging and supportive environment.

5. If you wish to use the TDEQS for research purposes or as a comprehensive evaluation project, we recommend that you use its complete version. The complete TDEQS may be found in the research article (see reference at the end of this appendix) or is typically available from the first author of the article.

From R.S. Vealey and M.A. Chase, 2016, *Best practice for youth sport* (Champaign, IL: Human Kinetics). Adapted, by permission, from R.J.J. Martindale et al., 2010, "Development of the talent development environment questionnaire for sport," *Journal of Sport Sciences* 28(11): 1209-1221.

APPENDIX I
Reactions to Playing Sports

Many athletes get tense or nervous before or during games, meets, or matches. This happens even to pro athletes.

Please read each question. Then, **circle the number that says how you USUALLY feel before or while you compete in sport.** There are no right or wrong answers. Please be as truthful as you can.

	Not at all	A little bit	Pretty much	Very much
Before or while I compete in sport . . .	1	2	3	4
1. my body feels tense.	1	2	3	4
2. I worry that I will not play well.	1	2	3	4
3. I worry that I will let others down.	1	2	3	4
4. I feel tense in my stomach.	1	2	3	4
5. I worry that I will not play my best.	1	2	3	4
6. my muscles feel shaky.	1	2	3	4
7. I worry that I will mess up during the game.	1	2	3	4
8. my muscles feel tight because I am nervous.	1	2	3	4
9. I worry that I will play badly.	1	2	3	4
10. my stomach feels upset.	1	2	3	4

Scoring Instructions for the Sport Anxiety Scale-2 (SAS-2)

1. Notice that the title on the scale used with athletes is Reactions to Playing Sports. This is because we don't want athletes to read that it is a measure of anxiety, which might affect the way they answer the questions.

2. Two different aspects of trait anxiety are measured in the SAS-2. *Physical anxiety* is the degree to which athletes feel tense, tight, and shaky. *Worry* is the degree to which athletes are concerned about not playing well and letting others down.

3. The items that make up the Physical Anxiety scale are 1, 4, 6, 8, and 10. The items that make up the Worry scale are 2, 3, 5, 7, and 9.

4. Add up the athlete's scores for each scale to compute a total Physical Anxiety score and a separate total Worry score. These two scores should range from 5 to 20. Here is a crude way to interpret the athlete's scores:

    17-20: Extremely high; very anxious

    13-16: Higher anxiety than average

    9-12: Average range of anxiety

    5-8: Low anxiety

5. The different scores tell you the degree to which the athlete experiences anxiety in terms of physical symptoms of nervousness, as well as mental anxiety (or worry).

6. Kids that have been tested using the SAS-2 scored on average about 8 in Physical Anxiety and about 9 or 10 in Worry.

7. If you wish to use the SAS-2 for research purposes, we recommend that you use the complete version of the SAS-2, which also contains a subscale called Concentration Disruption. The complete SAS-2 is available in the reference article cited at the end of this appendix.

From R.S. Vealey and M.A. Chase, 2016, *Best practice for youth sport* (Champaign, IL: Human Kinetics). Adapted, by permission, from R.E. Smith et al., 2006, "Measurement of multidimensional sport performance anxiety in children and adults: The Sport Anxiety Scale-2," *Journal of Sport and Exercise Psychology* 28: 479-501.

APPENDIX J
Focusing on Your Controllables

1. This is an active coping exercise for youth athletes. It helps them identify their "controllables" and their "uncontrollables" in terms of the things that influence their performance.

2. Give athletes the form provided on the next page. Ask them to think about the upcoming competitive event and to identify the things that can affect their performance but are beyond their personal control. They should write these things inside the circle labeled My Uncontrollables. (Don't tell them what to write, but these are typically things like my opponent, weather, officials, teammates, whether I win or not, whether my parents approve or not, and my coach's reactions.)

3. Then ask them to think about the upcoming competition and identify the things that can affect their performance and are within their own personal control. They should write these things inside the circle labeled My Controllables. (Again, don't tell them what to write, but these are typically very sport-specific things—for basketball, for example, they could write being active and hard to guard on offense, following my routine on free throws, aggressively fronting cutters on post defense, boxing out every time a shot is taken, focusing on my job each moment, and focusing on the next play after I make a mistake).

4. Then lead a discussion about the exercise, with athletes providing some examples of their controllables and uncontrollables. Often, with young athletes, you have to help them move some things from one circle to the other. For example, young athletes often assume they control winning or a certain performance outcome (e.g., placing in the top three of the race). Help them understand that they can't control performance outcomes.

5. When the discussion is concluded, have them take their pencils (and they should use pencils!), and put a big X over the My Uncontrollables circle. Remind them that when they start thinking or worrying about these uncontrollables during competition they should mentally X them out in their minds.

6. They should now read over their controllables, and particularly just before competition, to remind themselves to keep their focus on these things. They can remind themselves when they start to worry during competition to think "control the controllables" and X out the rest.

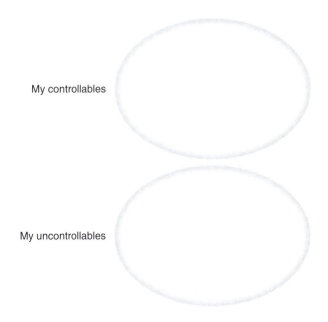

My controllables

My uncontrollables

From R.S. Vealey and M.A. Chase, 2016, *Best practice for youth sport* (Champaign, IL: Human Kinetics).

APPENDIX K
Emergency Action Plan

Team name: _____

Head coach: _____ Phone: _____

Assistant coach: _____ Phone: _____

Park supervisor: _____ Phone: _____

Athletic director: _____ Phone: _____

Emergency Medical Services (EMS) phone number: _____
(or call 911)

EMS Protocol

When you call EMS, provide your name and position, current address, telephone number, explanation-condition of injury and how it occurred, age of injured athlete, and specific directions to the site.

Meet the EMS personnel and ensure their navigation to the exact site of the injured athlete.

Facility Addresses

Name of facility   Address

_____   _____

_____   _____

_____   _____

_____   _____

_____   _____

Hospital Information

Name: _____ Phone: _____

Directions to hospital: _____

_____

_____

Emergency Task Assignments   **Assigned To:**

Care person (immediate care of injured athlete) _____

Communications person (call and direct EMS and inform parents) _____

Charge person (control site)   _____

First-aid kit on-site   _____

Ice on-site   _____

Athlete medical emergency forms on-site and secure _____

Team Roster With Emergency Contact and Athlete Information

For emergency use only; do not publish or distribute this information.

Athlete	Emergency phone #	Emergency contact	Special conditions and medications

From R.S. Vealey and M.A. Chase, 2016, *Best practice for youth sport* (Champaign, IL: Human Kinetics). Adapted, by permission, from National Alliance for Youth Sports.

APPENDIX L
Coaching Appraisal Form

Coach name _____ Sport _____ Date _____

Team _____ Appraiser _____ Minutes observed ____

	Poor	Could improve	Adequate	Good	Excellent
Knowledge of sport (rules, skills, strategies)	1	2	3	4	5
Teaching of skills	1	2	3	4	5
Correcting errors	1	2	3	4	5
Organization and use of time	1	2	3	4	5
Involvement of all athletes	1	2	3	4	5
Provides clear instructions	1	2	3	4	5
Listens to others	1	2	3	4	5
Uses appropriate language	1	2	3	4	5
Provides safe environment	1	2	3	4	5
Sensitive to children's needs	1	2	3	4	5
Physical appearance	1	2	3	4	5
Control of emotions	1	2	3	4	5
Relationships with parents	1	2	3	4	5
Relationships with officials	1	2	3	4	5
Relationships with athletes	1	2	3	4	5
Shows enthusiasm for coaching	1	2	3	4	5
Appropriate perspective on winning	1	2	3	4	5
Appropriate coaching style	1	2	3	4	5

Specific Feedback for Coaches:

_____

_____

_____

_____

_____

From R.S. Vealey and M.A. Chase, 2016, *Best practice for youth sport* (Champaign, IL: Human Kinetics). Adapted, by permission, from R. Martens, 2001, *Directing youth sports programs* (Champaign, IL: Human Kinetics).

APPENDIX M

Athlete Evaluation of Coach

Coach name _____ Team _____ Date _____

A. This season, playing for my coach, I . . .

	Not at all		Somewhat		Very much
Had fun	1	2	3	4	5
Learned how to play the sport better	1	2	3	4	5
Improved my physical fitness	1	2	3	4	5
Learned to cooperate with teammates	1	2	3	4	5
Increased motivation to play this sport	1	2	3	4	5
Learned sportsmanship	1	2	3	4	5
Learned better how to compete	1	2	3	4	5

B. How did your coach do on the following?

	Not so good		Just okay		Very well
Treated you fairly	1	2	3	4	5
Helped you feel good about yourself	1	2	3	4	5
Encouraged and recognized you	1	2	3	4	5
Taught the skills of the sport	1	2	3	4	5
Organized practices	1	2	3	4	5
Coached you and the team in competition	1	2	3	4	5
Kept winning in perspective	1	2	3	4	5
Took appropriate safety precautions	1	2	3	4	5
Talked and listened to you	1	2	3	4	5
Controlled emotions, showed self-control	1	2	3	4	5

C. What did you like best about your coach?

_____

_____

_____

D. What could your coach improve on to be a better coach?

_____

_____

_____

From R.S. Vealey and M.A. Chase, 2016, *Best practice for youth sport* (Champaign, IL: Human Kinetics). Reprinted, by permission, from R. Martens, 2001, *Directing youth sports programs* (Champaign, IL: Human Kinetics).

REFERENCES

Abbott, A., Button, C., Pepping, G., & Collins, D. (2005). Unnatural selection: Talent identification and development in sport. *Nonlinear Dynamics, Psychology and Life Sciences, 9,* 61-88.

Abbott, A., & Collins, D. (2002). A theoretical and empirical analysis of a "state of the art" talent identification model. *High Ability Studies, 13,* 157-178.

Abramson, L.Y., Seligman, M.E.P., & Teasdale, J.D. (1978). Learned helplessness in humans: Critique and reformulation. *Journal of Abnormal Psychology, 87,* 49-74.

Adie, J.W., Duda, J.L., & Ntoumanis, N. (2012). Perceived coach-autonomy support, basic need satisfaction and the well- and ill-being of elite youth soccer players: A longitudinal investigation. *Psychology of Sport and Exercise, 13,* 51-59.

Adirim, T.A., & Cheng, T.L. (2003). Overview of injuries in the young athlete. *Sports Medicine, 33,* 75-81.

Agassi, A. (2009). *Open.* New York: Knopf.

Alexander, B. (2014, May 11). Tommy John surgery doesn't boost performance: Study. Retrieved June 10, 2015 from www.nbcnews.com/tommy-john-surgery-doesn't-boost-performance-study-n48771.

American Academy of Pediatrics. (2000). Intensive training and sports specialization in young athletes. *Pediatrics, 106,* 154-157.

American Academy of Pediatrics. (2011). Policy statement – climatic heat stress and exercising children and adolescents. *Pediatrics, 128,* 1-9.

American College of Sports Medicine. (2007). The female athlete triad. *Medicine and Science in Sports and Exercise, 39,* 1867-1882.

Amorose, A.J., & Horn, T.S. (2000). Intrinsic motivation: Relationships with collegiate athletes' gender, scholarship status, and perceptions of their coaches' behavior. *Journal of Sport & Exercise Psychology, 22,* 63-84.

Anderson, C., & Petrie, T.A. (2012). Prevalence of disordered eating and pathogenic weight control behaviors among NCAA Division I female collegiate gymnasts and swimmers. *Research Quarterly for Exercise and Sport, 83,* 120-124.

Anderson, K. (2013, July 22). Eat, play, dunk. *Sports Illustrated,* pp. 28-32.

Ankersen, R. (2012). *The gold mine effect.* London: Icon Books.

Araujo, D., Fonseca, C., Davids, K., Garganta, J., Volossovitch, A., Brandao, R., & Krebs, R. (2010). The role of ecological constraints on expertise development. *Talent Development and Excellence, 2,* 165-179.

Arias, J.L., Argudo, F.M., & Alonso, J.I. (2012). Effect of ball mass on dribble, pass, and pass reception in 9-11-year-old boys' basketball. *Research Quarterly for Exercise and Sport, 83,* 407-412.

Armstrong, N., & Barker, A.R. (2011). Endurance training and elite young athletes. In N. Armstrong & A.M. McManus (Eds.), *The elite young athlete* (pp. 59-83). New York: Karger.

Arthur, C.A., Woodman, T., Ong, C.W., Hardy, L., & Ntoumanis, N. (2011). The role of narcissism in moderating the relationship between coaches' transformational leader behaviors and athlete motivation. *Journal of Sport & Exercise Psychology, 33,* 3-19.

Arthur-Cameselle, J.N., & Quatromoni, P.A. (2011). Factors related to the onset of eating disorders reported by female collegiate athletes. *Sport Psychologist, 25,* 1-17.

Athletic Footwear Association. (2012, January 26). Youth sports statistics. Retrieved April 20, 2015, from www.statisticbrain.com/youth-sports/statistics.

Australia Bureau of Statistics. (2011). Australian social trends June 2011: Sport and physical recreation. Retrieved April 20, 2015, from www.ausstats.abs.gov.au/ausstats/subscriber.nsf/LookupAttach/4102.0Publication29.06.111/$File/41020_ASTJun2011.pdf.

AZ Quotes. (2015). Retrieved May 15, 2015, from www.azquotes.com/quote/741001.

Bailey, R., Collins, D., Ford, P., MacNamara, A., Toms, M., & Pearce, G. (2010). Participant development in sport: An academic review. Sports Coach UK and Sport Northern Ireland. Retrieved March 29, 2015, from www.academia.edu/3002845/Participant_Developmentin_Sport.

Baker, J. (2012). Do genes predict potential? Genetic factors and athletic success. In J. Baker, S. Cobley, & J. Schorer (Eds.), *Talent identification and development in sport: International perspectives* (pp. 13-24). New York: Routledge.

Baker, J., Cote, J., & Abernathy, B. (2003). Sport-specific practice and the development of expert decision-making in team ball sports. *Journal of Applied Sport Psychology, 15,* 12-25.

Baker, J., Cote, J., & Deakin, J. (2005). Expertise in ultra-endurance triathletes: Early sport involvement, training structure, and the theory of deliberate practice. *Journal of Applied Sport Psychology, 17,* 64-78.

Baker, J., & Schorer, J. (2010). Identification and development of talent in sport – introduction to the special issue. *Talent Development and Excellence, 2,* 119-121.

Baker, J., & Young, B. (2014). 20 years later: Deliberate practice and the development of expertise in sport. *International Review of Sport and Exercise Psychology, 7,* 135-157.

Balyi, I., & Way, R. (2011). The role of monitoring growth in LTAD. Canadian Sport for Life, Canadian Sport Centres, Vancouver. Retrieved March 29, 2015, from www.canadiansportforlife.ca/resources/role-monitoring-growth-ltad.

Balyi, I., Way, R., & Higgs, C. (2013). *Long-term athlete development.* Champaign, IL: Human Kinetics.

Bamman, M.M. (2010). Does your "genetic" alphabet soup spell "runner"? *Journal of Applied Physiology, 108,* 1452-1453.

Bandura, A. (1977). *Social learning theory.* Englewood Cliffs, NJ: Prentice-Hall.

Bandura, A., Ross, D., & Ross, S.A. (1961). Transmission of aggression through imitation of aggressive models. *Journal of Abnormal and Social Psychology, 63,* 575-582.

Barnett, L.M., van Beurden, E., Morgan, P.J., Brooks, L.O., & Beard, J.R. (2010). Gender differences in motor skill proficiency from childhood to adolescence: A longitudinal study. *Research Quarterly for Exercise and Sport, 81,* 162-170.

Barnsley, R.H., Thompson, A.H., & Barnsley, P.E. (1985). Hockey success and birthdate: The relative age effect. *Canadian Association for Health, Physical Education, and Recreation, 51,* 23-28.

Bartholomew, K.J., Ntoumanis, N., & Thogersen-Ntoumani, C. (2010). The controlling interpersonal style in a coaching context: Development and initial validation of a psychometric scale. *Journal of Sport & Exercise Psychology, 32,* 193-216.

Bass, B.M. (1985). *Leadership and performance beyond expectations.* New York: Free Press.

Baumeister, R. (1984). Choking under pressure: Self-consciousness and paradoxical effects of incentives on skillful performance. *Journal of Personality and Social Psychology, 16,* 610-620.

Baumeister, R., & Leary, M.R. (1995). The need to belong: Desire for interpersonal attachments as a fundamental human motive. *Psychological Bulletin, 117,* 497-529.

Baumrind, D. (1989). Rearing competent children. In W. Damon (Ed.), *Child development today and tomorrow* (pp. 349-378). San Francisco: Jossey-Bass.

Baxter-Jones, A.D.G., Mirwald, R.L., Faulkner, R.A., Kowalski, K.C., & Bailey, D.A. (2009). Does the positive effect of physical activity during childhood and adolescence on bone mass accrual persist into early adult life? In T. Jurimae, N. Armstrong, & J. Jurimae (Eds.), *Children and exercise XXIV: The proceedings of the 24th pediatric work physiology meeting* (pp. 47-50). New York: Routledge.

Bell, J.J., Hardy, L., & Beattie, S. (2013). Enhancing mental toughness and performance under pressure in elite young cricketers: A 2-year longitudinal intervention. *Sport, Exercise, and Performance Psychology, 2,* 281-297.

Bengoechea, E.G., Sabiston, C.M., Ahmed, R., & Farnoush, M. (2010). Exploring links to unorganized and organized physical activity during adolescence: The role of gender, socioeconomic status, weight status, and enjoyment of physical education. *Research Quarterly for Exercise and Sport, 81,* 7-16.

Bennett, T. (2011, August 20). Special report: The development of football in China. The Youth Radar. Retrieved March 29, 2015, from http://theyouthradar.com/2011/08/20/special-report-the-development-of-football-in-china.

Berberoglu, M. (2009). Precocious puberty and normal variant puberty: Definition, etiology, diagnosis and current management. *Journal of Clinical Research in Pediatric Endocrinology, 1,* 164-174.

Berry, J., Abernathy, B., & Cote, J. (2008). The contribution of structured activity and deliberate play to the development of expert perceptual and decision-making skill. *Journal of Sport & Exercise Psychology, 30,* 685-708.

Berryman, J.W. (1996). The rise of boys' sports in the United States, 1900 to 1970. In F.L. Smoll & R.E. Smith (Eds.), *Children and youth in sport: A biopsychosocial perspective.* Madison, WI: Brown & Benchmark.

Beunen, G., Malina, R.M., Van't Hoff, M.A., Simons, J., Ostyn, M., Renson, R., & Van Gerven, D. (1988). *Adolescent growth and motor performance: A longitudinal study of Belgian boys.* Champaign, IL: Human Kinetics.

Beverly, J. (2011, June 26). Should kids run long? *Runner's World.* Retrieved March 29, 2015, from www.runnersworld.com/high-school-training/should-kids-run-long.

Bigelow, B., Moroney, T., & Hall, L. (2001). *Just let the kids play: How to stop older adults from ruining your child's fun and success in youth sports.* Deerfield Beach, FL: Health Communications.

Blanchard, K. (1995). *The anthropology of sport: An introduction.* Westport, CT: Bergin & Garvey.

Blazo, J.A., Carson, S., Czech, D.R., & Dees, W. (2014). A qualitative investigation of the sibling sport achievement experience. *Sport Psychologist, 28,* 36-47.

Bloom, B.S. (1985). *Developing talent in young people.* New York: Ballantine.

Bonci, C.M., Bonci, L.J., Granger, L.R., Johnson, C.L., Malina, R.M., Milne, L.W., Ryan, R.R., & Vanderbunt, E.M. (2008). National athletic trainers' association position statement: Preventing, detecting, and managing disordered eating in athletes. *Journal of Athletic Training, 43,* 80-108.

Bouchard, C., Sarzynski, M.A., Rice, T.K., Kraus, W.E., Church, T.S., Sung, Y.J., Rao, D.C., & Rankinen, T. (2010). Genomic predictors of the maximal O$_2$ uptake response to standardized exercise training programs. *Journal of Applied Physiology, 110,* 1160-1170.

Bowker, A., Bocknoven, B., Nolan, A., Bauhaus, S., Glover, P., Powell, T., & Taylor, S. (2009). Naturalistic observations of spectator behavior at youth hockey games. *Sport Psychologist, 23,* 301-316.

Bowlby, J. (1988). *A secure base: Parent-child attachment and healthy human development.* New York: Basic Books.

Boyce, B.A., Gano-Overway, L.A., & Campbell, A.L. (2009). Perceived motivational climate's influence on goal orientations, perceived competence, and practice strategies across the athletic season. *Journal of Applied Sport Psychology, 21,* 381-394.

Brackenridge, C.H., Bishopp, D., Moussalli, S., & Tapp, J. (2008). The characteristics of sexual abuse in sport: A multidimensional scaling analysis of events described in media reports. *International Journal of Sport and Exercise Psychology, 6,* 385-406.

Bredemeier, B.J., & Shields, D.L. (1986). Game reasoning and interactional morality. *Journal of Genetic Psychology, 147,* 257-275.

Bredemeier, B.J., Weiss, M.R., Shields, D.L., & Cooper, B.A.B. (1986). The relationship of sport involvement with children's moral reasoning and aggression tendencies. *Journal of Sport Psychology, 8,* 304-318.

Brenner, J.S. (2007). Overuse injuries, overtraining, and burnout in child and adolescent athletes. *Pediatrics, 119,* 1242-1245.

Bruce, L., Farrow, D., & Raynor, A. (2013). Performance milestones in the development of expertise: Are they critical? *Journal of Applied Sport Psychology, 25,* 281-297.

Bukato, D., & Daehler, M.W. (2012). *Child development: A thematic approach* (6th ed.). Belmont, CA: Wadsworth.

Bullock, N., Gulbin, J.P., Martin, D.T., Ross, A., Holland, T., & Marino, F. (2009). Talent identification and deliberate programming in skeleton: Ice novice to winter Olympian in 14 months. *Journal of Sports Sciences, 27,* 397-404.

Burke, B. (2013, September 2). To Russia, with love. *Sports Illustrated,* p. 166.

Burke, M. (2001). Obeying until it hurts: Coach-athlete relationships. *Journal of the Philosophy of Sport, 28,* 227-240.

Burton, D., & Weiss, C. (2008). The fundamental goal concept: The path to process and performance success. In T.S. Horn (Ed.), *Advances in sport psychology* (3rd ed., pp. 339-376). Champaign, IL: Human Kinetics.

Buszard, T., Farrow, D., Reid, M., & Masters, R.S.W. (2014). Modifying equipment in early skill development: A tennis perspective. *Research Quarterly for Exercise and Sport, 85,* 218-225.

Callahan, T. (2006, June). Earl was right. *Golf Digest,* p. 100.

Camire, M. (2014). Youth development in North American high school sport: Review and recommendations. *Quest, 66,* 495-511.

Camire, M., Trude, P., & Bernard, D. (2013). A case study of a high school sport program designed to teach athletes life skills and values. *Sport Psychologist, 27,* 188-200.

Caron, J.G., Bloom, G.A., Johnston, K.M., & Sabiston, C.M. (2013). Effects of multiple concussions on retired National Hockey League players. *Journal of Sport & Exercise Psychology, 35,* 168-179.

Caspersen, C.J., Powell, K.E., & Christenson, G.M. (1985). Physical activity, exercise, and physical fitness: Definitions and distinctions for health-related research. *Public Health Reports, 100,* 126-131.

Ceci, S.J., Barnett, S.M., & Kanaya, T. (2003). Developing childhood proclivities into adult competencies: The overlooked multiplier effect. In R.J. Sternberg & E.L. Grigorenko (Eds.), *The psychology of abilities, competencies, and expertise* (pp. 70-92). New York: Cambridge University Press.

Centers for Disease Control and Prevention. (2015). Childhood obesity facts. Retrieved January 2015, from www.cdc.gov/healthyyouth/obesity/facts.htm.

Cervello, E.M., Escarti, A., & Guzman, J.F. (2007). Youth sport dropout from the achievement goal theory. *Psicothema, 19,* 65-71.

Chandler, J.B. (2011, March 1). Pitching in youth baseball: Is overuse leading to elbow injuries? Retrieved March 29, 2015, from www.leaguelineup.com/khobaseball/files/pitching.pdf.

Chase, M.A. (2001). Children's self-efficacy, motivational intentions, and attributions in physical education and sport. *Research Quarterly for Sport and Exercise, 72,* 47-54.

Chase, M.A., Ewing, M.E., Lirgg, C.D., & George, T.R. (1994). The effects of equipment modification on children's self-efficacy and basketball shooting performance. *Research Quarterly for Exercise and Sport, 65,* 159-168.

Chase, W.G., & Simon, H.A. (1973). The mind's eye in chess. In W.G. Chase (Ed.), *Visual information processing* (pp. 215-281). San Diego: Academic Press.

Chen, A. (2014, December 15). The Mo'ne effect. *Sports Illustrated,* pp. 151-154.

Cheon, S.H., Reeve, J., & Moon, I.S. (2012). Experimentally based, longitudinally designed, teacher-focused intervention to help physical education teachers be more autonomy-supportive toward their students. *Journal of Sport & Exercise Psychology, 34,* 365-396.

Chiari, M. (2014, March 19). Team wears hijab headscarves in support of Muslim teammate banned from match. Retrieved March 29, 2015, from bleacherreport.com/articles/1998766-team-wears-hijab-headscarves-in-support.

Chugani, H.T. (1998). A critical period of brain development: Studies of cerebral glucose utilization with PET. *Preventive Medicine, 27,* 184-188.

Clark, J.E., & Metcalf, J.M. (2002). The mountain of motor development: A metaphor. In J.E. Clark & J.H. Humphrey (Eds.), *Motor development: Research and reviews* (Vol. 2, pp. 163-190). Reston, VA: National Association for Sport and Physical Education.

Clark, W. (2008). *Kids' sports.* Ottawa: Statistics Canada.

Coakley, J. (1992). Burnout among adolescent athletes: A personal failure or social problem? *Sociology of Sport Journal, 9,* 271-285.

Coakley, J. (2009). *Sports in society: Issues and controversies* (10th ed.). New York: McGraw-Hill.

Coatsworth, J.D., & Conroy, D.E. (2006). Enhancing the self-esteem of youth swimmers through coach training: Gender and age effects. *Psychology of Sport and Exercise, 7,* 173-192.

Coatsworth, J.D., & Conroy, D.E. (2009). The effects of autonomy-supportive coaching, need satisfaction, and self-perceptions on initiative and identity in youth swimmers. *Developmental Psychology, 45,* 320-328.

Cobley, S., Baker, J., Wattie, N., & McKenna, J. (2009). A meta-analytical review of relative age effect in sport: The emerging picture. *Sports Medicine, 39,* 235-256.

Cobley, S., Schorer, J., & Baker, J. (2012). Identification and development of sport talent. In J. Baker, S. Cobley, & J. Schorer (Eds.), *Talent identification and development in sport: International perspectives* (pp. 1-10). New York: Routledge.

Collins, J. (2001, January). Level 5 leadership. *Harvard Business Review,* pp. 115-136.

Colvin, G. (2008). *Talent is overrated.* New York: Portfolio.

Compas, B.E., Connor-Smith, J.K., Saltzman, H., Harding Thomsen, A., & Wadsworth, M.E. (2001). Coping with stress during childhood and adolescence: Problems, progress, and potential in theory and research. *Psychological Bulletin, 127,* 87-127.

Connaughton, D., Wadey, R., Hanton, S., & Jones, G. (2008). The development and maintenance of mental toughness: Perceptions of elite performers. *Journal of Sports Sciences, 26,* 83-95.

Conroy, D.E., Willow, J.P., & Metzler, J.N. (2002). Multidimensional fear of failure measurement: The Performance Failure Appraisal Inventory. *Journal of Applied Sport Psychology, 14,* 76-90.

Cooke, G. (2006). No shortcut to the top for naturally gifted. *Sports Coach, 29* (1). Retrieved February 10, 2014, from www.ausport.gov.au/sportscoachmag/coaching-processes.

Copple, C. (2010). *Developmentally appropriate practice in early childhood programs.* Washington, DC: National Association for Education of Young Children.

Cote, J. (1999). The influence of the family in the development of talent. *Sport Psychologist, 13,* 395-417.

Cote, J., Baker, J., & Abernathy, B. (2003). From play to practice: A developmental framework for the acquisition of expertise in team sports. In J.L. Starkes & K.A. Ericsson (Eds.), *Expert performance in sports: Advances in research on sport expertise* (pp. 89-113). Champaign, IL: Human Kinetics.

Cote, J., Baker, J., & Abernathy, B. (2007). Practice and play in the development of sport expertise. In G. Tenenbaum & R.C. Eklund (Eds.), *Handbook of sport psychology* (3rd ed., pp. 184-202). New York: Wiley.

Cote, J., Erickson, K., & Abernathy, B. (2013). Play and practice during childhood. In J. Cote & R. Lidor (Eds.), *Conditions of children's talent development in sport* (pp. 9-20). Morgantown, WV: Fitness Information Technology.

Cote, J., Strachan, L., & Frasier-Thomas, J. (2008). Participation, personal development, and performance through youth sport. In N.L. Holt (Ed.), *Positive youth development through sport* (pp. 34-45). New York: Routledge.

Covey, S.R. (2013). *The 7 habits of highly effective people: Powerful lessons in personal change.* New York: Simon & Schuster.

Coyle, D. (2007, March 4). How to grow a super-athlete. *New York Times.* Retrieved March 29, 2015, from www.nytimes.com/2007/03/04/sports/playmagazine/04play-talent.html.

Coyle, D. (2009). *The talent code.* New York: Bantam.

Coyle, D. (2012). *The little book of talent.* New York: Bantam.

Cross, T., Bazron, B., Dennis, K., & Isaacs, M. (1999). *Towards a culturally competent system of care.* Washington, DC: National Institute of Mental Health, Child and Adolescent Service System Program Technical Assistance Center, Georgetown University Child Development Center.

Csikszentmihalyi, M. (1990). *Flow: The psychology of optimal experience.* New York: Harper & Row.

Cybergolf. (2014, April 21). The continuing tale of Sean O'Hair. Retrieved March 29, 2015, from www.cybergolf.com/golf_news/the_continuing_tale_of_sean_ohair.

Daniels, E.A. (2009). Sex objects, athletes, and sexy athletes: How media representations of women athletes can impact adolescent girls and college women. *Journal of Adolescent Research, 24,* 399-422.

Danish, S., Nellen, V., & Owens, S. (1996). Community-based life skills programs: Using sports to teach life skills to adolescents. In J. Van Raalte & B. Brewer (Eds.), *Exploring sports and exercise psychology* (pp. 205-225). Washington, DC: APA Books.

Darling, N., & Steinberg, L. (1993). Parenting style in context: An integrative model. *Psychological Bulletin, 113,* 487-496.

d'Arripe-Longueville, F., Pantaleon, N., & Smith, A.L. (2006). Personal and situational predictors of sportspersonship in young athletes. *International Journal of Sport Psychology, 37,* 38-57.

Davids, K., & Baker, J. (2007). Genes, environment and sport performance: Why the nature-nurture dualism is no longer relevant. *Sports Medicine, 37,* 961-980.

Davies, P.L., & Rose, J.D. (2000). Motor skills of typically developing adolescents: Awkwardness or improvement? *Physical & Occupational Therapy in Pediatrics, 20,* 19-42.

Davis, R. (2010). *Teaching disability sport* (2nd ed.). Champaign, IL: Human Kinetics.

Deci, E.L., Koestner, R., & Ryan, R.M. (1999). A meta-analytic review of experiments examining the effects of extrinsic rewards on intrinsic motivation. *Psychological Bulletin, 125,* 627-668.

Deci, E.L., & Ryan, R.M. (1985). *Intrinsic motivation and self-determination in human behavior.* New York: Plenum.

Del Campo, D.G.D., Vicedo, J.C.P., Villora, S.G., & Jordan, O.R.C. (2010). The relative age effect in youth soccer players from Spain. *Journal of Sports Science and Medicine, 9,* 190-198.

Deutsch, M. (2000). Cooperation and competition. In M. Deutsch & P. Coleman (Eds.), *Handbook of conflict resolution: Theory and practice* (pp. 21-40). San Francisco: Jossey-Bass.

Dharamsi, A., & LaBella, C. (2013). Prevention of ACL injuries in adolescent female athletes. *Contemporary Pediatrics, 30,* 12-20.

Diaz, J. (2014, July). Rickie Inc. *Golf Digest,* pp. 102-128.

Dicicco, T., & Hacker, C. (2002). *Catch them being good.* New York: Penguin.

Dohrman, G. (2010). *Play their hearts out.* New York: Ballantine.

Donnelly, P. (1993). Problems associated with youth involvement in high-performance sport. In B.R. Cahill & A.J. Pearl (Eds.), *Intensive participation in children's sport* (pp. 95-126). Champaign, IL: Human Kinetics.

Dunton, G., McConnell, R., Jerrett, M., Wolch, J., Lam, C., Gilliland, F., & Berhane, K. (2012). Organized physical activity in young school children and subsequent 4-year change in body mass index. *Archives of Pediatric and Adolescent Medicine, 166,* 713-718.

Dweck, C.S. (2006). *Mindset: The new psychology of success.* New York: Ballantine.

Dyck, N. (2012). *Fields of play: An ethnography of children's sports.* Toronto: University of Toronto Press.

Eckert, H.M. (1987). *Motor development* (3rd ed.). Berkeley, CA: Benchmark.

Ehrmann, J. (2011). *InSideOut coaching.* New York: Simon & Schuster.

Elling, S. (2005, January 21). Price of success? *Golf Digest.* Retrieved March 29, 2015, from www.golfdigest.com/golf-tours-news/2006-01/gw20050121elling?printable=true.

Elliott, M. (2012, October 17). Legends at home: Se Ri Pak. Retrieved September 9, 2013, from www.lpga.com/news/pak-legends-feature.

Ellis, A., & Dryden, W. (1987). *The practice of rational emotive therapy.* New York: Springer.

Elmore, T. (2014). *12 huge mistakes parents can avoid: Leading your kids to succeed in life.* Eugene, OR: Harvest Home.

Engh, F. (2002). *Why Johnny hates sports.* Garden City Park, NY: Square One.

Entzion, B.J. (1991). A child's view of fair play. *Strategies, 4,* 16-19.

Epstein, D. (2013). *The sports gene: Inside the science of extraordinary athletic performance.* New York: Current.

Eradi, J. (1998, May 30). Want to be Griffey Jr.? Start early. *Cincinnati Enquirer,* pp. D6.

Ericsson, K.A., Krampe, R.T., & Tesch-Romer, C. (1993). The role of deliberate practice in the acquisition of expert performance. *Psychological Review, 100,* 363-406.

ESPN. (2012, March 28). It's been a confounding journey for Michelle Wie. Retrieved March 20, 2015, from Espn.go.com/espnw/news-commentary/article/7749190/elliott-confounding-journey-michelle-wie.

Evert, C. (2010). Evert: The family business. Retrieved March 29, 2015, from espn.go.com/sports/tennis/news/story?id=5276426.

Faigenbaum, A.D., Kraemer, W.J., Blimkie, C.J.R., Jeffreys, I., Micheli, L.J., Nitka, M., & Rowland, T.W. (2009). Youth resistance training: Updated position statement paper from the National Strength and Conditioning Association. *Journal of Strength and Conditioning Research, 23,* S60-S79.

Faigenbaum, A., & Westcott, W. (2009). *Youth strength training.* Champaign, IL: Human Kinetics.

Fairclough, S.J., & Ridgers, N.D. (2010). Relationships between maturity status, physical activity, and physical self-perceptions in primary school children. *Journal of Sports Sciences, 28,* 1-9.

Farber, M. (2008, October 13). Why good teams fight. *Sports Illustrated,* pp. 56-62.

Farrey, T. (2008). *Game on: The All-American race to make champions of our children.* New York: ESPN Books.

Farrow, D. (2010). A multi-factorial examination of the development of skill expertise in high performance netball. *Talent Development and Excellence, 2,* 123-135.

Farrow, D., & Reid, M. (2010). The effect of equipment scaling on the skill acquisition of beginning tennis players. *Journal of Sports Sciences, 28,* 723-732.

Fedewa, A.L., & Ahn, S. (2011). The effects of physical activity and physical fitness on children's achievement and cognitive outcomes: A meta-analysis. *Research Quarterly for Exercise and Sport, 82,* 521-535.

Feltz, D.L., Hepler, T.J., Roman, N., & Paiement, C. (2009). Coaching efficacy and volunteer youth sport coaches. *Sport Psychologist, 23,* 24-41.

Fields, R.D. (2005). Myelination: An overlooked mechanism of synaptic plasticity? *Neuroscientist, 11,* 528-531.

Fine, G. (1987). *With the boys: Little League baseball and preadolescent culture.* Chicago: University of Chicago Press.

Fink, W.J., Costill, D.L., & Pollock, M.L. (1977). Submaximal and maximal working capacity of elite distance runners. Part II: Muscle fiber composition and enzyme activities. *Annals of the New York Academy of Sciences, 301,* 323-327.

Flett, M.R., Gould, D., Griffes, K.R., & Lauer, L. (2013). Tough love for underserved youth: A comparison of more or less effective coaching. *Sport Psychologist, 27,* 325-337.

Floyd, I. (2013). *Opening the gate: Stories & activities about athletes with disabilities.* Lexington, KY: CreateSpace Independent Publishing Platform.

Fraser-Thomas, J., Cote, J., & Deakin, J. (2008a). Examining adolescent sport dropout and prolonged engagement from a developmental perspective. *Journal of Applied Sport Psychology, 20,* 318-333.

Fraser-Thomas, J., Cote, J., & Deakin, J. (2008b). Understanding dropout and prolonged engagement in adolescent competitive sport. *Psychology of Sport and Exercise, 9,* 645-662.

Fredricks, J.A., & Eccles, J.S. (2004). Parental influences on youth involvement in sport. In M.R. Weiss (Ed.), *Developmental sport and exercise psychology: A lifespan perspective* (pp. 145-164). Morgantown, WV: Fitness Information Technology.

Fredricks, J.A., & Eccles, J.S. (2005). Family socialization, gender, and sport motivation and involvement. *Journal of Sport & Exercise Psychology, 27,* 3-31.

French, K.E., Spurgeon, J.J., & Nevett, M.E. (2007). Anthropometric characteristics of Columbia, South Carolina, youth baseball players and Dixie Youth World Series players. *Research Quarterly for Exercise and Sport, 78,* 179-188.

Fry, M.D., & Duda, J.L. (1997). A developmental examination of children's understanding of effort and ability in the physical and academic domains. *Research Quarterly for Exercise and Sport, 68,* 331-344.

Fuhrman, J. (2011, May 6). Girls' early puberty: What causes it, and how to avoid it. *Huffington Post.* Retrieved September 17, 2013, from www.huffingtonpost.com/joel-fuhrman-md/girls-early-puberty.

Gabbard, C.P., & Shea, C.H. (1980). Effects of varied goal height practice on basketball foul shooting performance. *Coach and Athlete, 42,* 10-11.

Gagne, F. (2009). Building gifts into talents: Detailed overview of the DMGT 2.0. In B. MacFarlane & T. Stambaugh (Eds.), *Leading change in gifted education: The festschrift of Dr. Joyce Van Tassel-Baska* (pp. 61-80). Waco, TX: Prufrock.

Gallahue, D.L., Ozmun, J.C., & Goodway, J. (2012). *Understanding motor development: Infants, children, adolescents, adults.* New York: McGraw-Hill.

Garnier-Ombrelle and Canadian Soccer Association team up to protect and educate Canadian youth. (2013, May 27). Retrieved March 29, 2015, from www.newswire.ca/en/story/1172671/garnier-ombrelle-and-canadian-soccer-association-team-up-to-protect-and-educate-canadian-youth.

Gems, G.R., Borish, L.J., & Pfister, G. (2008). *Sports in American history: From colonization to globalization.* Champaign, IL: Human Kinetics.

Gervis, M., & Dunn, N. (2004). The emotional abuse of elite child athletes by their coaches. *Child Abuse Review, 13,* 215-223.

Giedd, J.N., Blumenthal, J., Jeffries, N.O., Castellanos, F.X., Liu, H., Zijdenhos, A., Paus, T., Evans, A.C., & Rapoport, J.L. (1999). Brain development during childhood and adolescence: A longitudinal MRI study. *Nature Neuroscience, 2,* 861-863.

Gilman, R., & Ashby, J.S. (2006). Perfectionism. In G.G. Bear & K.M. Minke (Eds.), *Children's needs III: Development, prevention, and intervention* (pp. 303-312). Bethesda, MD: National Association of School Psychologists.

Ginsburg, K.R. (2007). The importance of play in promoting healthy child development and maintaining strong parent-child bonds. *Pediatrics, 119,* 182-191.

Ginsburg, R.D., Durant, S., & Baltzell, A. (2006). *Whose game is it, anyway?* Boston: Houghton Mifflin.

Ginsburg, R.D., Smith, S.R., Danforth, N., Ceranoglu, T.A., Durant, S.A., Kamin, H., Babcock, R., Robin, L., & Masek, B. (2014). Patterns of specialization in professional baseball players. *Journal of Clinical Sport Psychology, 8,* 261-275.

Glamser, F.D., & Vincent, J. (2004). The relative age effect among elite American youth soccer players. *Journal of Sport Behavior, 27,* 31-38.

Goleman, D. (2005). *Emotional intelligence.* New York: Bantam.

Goodwin, D. (2009). The voices of students with disabilities: Are they informing inclusive physical education practice? In H. Fitzgerald (Ed.), *Disability and youth sport* (pp. 53-75). New York: Routledge.

Gould, D. (2015). Goal setting for peak performance. In J.M. Williams & V. Krane (Eds.), *Applied sport psychology: Personal growth to peak performance* (7th ed., pp. 188-206). New York: McGraw-Hill.

Gould, D., & Carson, S. (2010). The relationship between perceived coaching behaviors and developmental benefits of high school sports participation. *Hellenic Journal of Psychology, 7,* 298-314.

Gould, D., Lauer, L., Rolo, C., Jannes, C., & Pennisi, N. (2008). The role of parents in tennis success: Focus group interviews with junior coaches. *Sport Psychologist, 22,* 18-37.

Gould, D., Tuffey, S., Udry, E., & Loehr, J. (1996). Burnout in competitive junior tennis players: II. Qualitative analysis. *Sport Psychologist, 10,* 322-340.

Gould, D., Tuffey, S., Udry, E., & Loehr, J. (1997). Burnout in competitive junior tennis players: III. Individual differences in the burnout experience. *Sport Psychologist, 11,* 257-276.

Gould, D., & Voelker, D.K. (2010). Youth sport leadership development: Leveraging the sports captaincy experience. *Journal of Sport Psychology in Action, 1,* 1-14.

Green, K. (2010). *Key themes in youth sport.* London: Routledge.

Gregory, S. (2010, February 8). The problem with football. *Time,* pp. 36-43.

Gregory, S. (2014, September 29). 'It didn't cross my mind that I wouldn't see him come off that field:' The tragic risks of an American obsession. *Time,* pp. 32-39.

Griffin, L., Mitchell, S., & Oslin, J. (1997). *Teaching sport concepts and skills: A tactical games approach.* Champaign, IL: Human Kinetics.

Grohmann, K. (2013, March 28). Soccer-German youth work, a success story for club and country. Retrieved June 5, 2013, from articles.chicagotribune.com/2013-3-28/news/sns-rt-soccer-academiesgermany-pix-tvl3n-0ci2fj-20130328_1_youth-work-clubs-academies.

Guivernau, M., & Duda, J.L. (2002). Moral atmosphere and athletic aggression tendencies in young soccer players. *Journal of Moral Education, 31,* 67-85.

Gulbin, J. (2012). Applying talent identification programs at a system-wide level: The evolution of Australia's national program. In J. Baker, S. Cobley, & J. Schorer (Eds.), *Talent identification and development in sport: International perspectives* (pp. 147-165). New York: Routledge.

Gulbin, J.P., Oldenziel, K.E., Weissensteiner, J.R., & Gagne, F. (2010). A look through the rear mirror: Developmental experiences and insights of high performance athletes. *Talent Development and Excellence, 2,* 149-164.

Gustafsson, H., Kentta, G., Hassmen, P., & Lundqvist, C. (2007). Prevalence of burnout in competitive adolescent athletes. *Sport Psychologist, 21,* 21-37.

Hadhazy, A. (2008, August 18). What makes Michael Phelps so good? *Scientific American.* Retrieved August 21, 2013, from www.scientificamerican.com/article/what-makes-michael-phelps-so-good.

Haefner, J. (2015). A basketball coaching guide – how to work with parents the "right way" and avoid unpleasant problems. Retrieved March 29, 2015, from www.breakthroughbasketball.com/coaching/dealing-with-parents.html.

Haibach, P.S., Reid, G., & Collier, D.H. (2011). *Motor learning and development.* Champaign, IL: Human Kinetics.

Hale, C.J. (1956). Physiological maturity of Little League baseball players. *Research Quarterly, 27,* 276-283.

Halstead, M.E., & Walter, K.D. (2010). American Academy of Pediatrics: Clinical report – sport-related concussion in children and adolescents. *Pediatrics, 126,* 597-615.

Hammond, J., & Smith, C. (2006). Low compression tennis balls and skill development. *Journal of Sports Science and Medicine, 5,* 575-581.

Hancock, D.J., Ste-Marie, D.M., & Young, B.W. (2013). Coach selections and the relative age effect in male youth ice hockey. *Research Quarterly for Exercise and Sport, 84,* 126-130.

Hannon, J., Soohoo, S., Reel, J., & Ratliffe, T. (2009). Gender stereotyping and the influence of race in sport among adolescents. *Research Quarterly for Exercise and Sport, 80,* 676-684.

Hanton, S., Cropley, B., Neil, R., Mellalieu, S.D., & Miles, A. (2007). Experience in sport and its relationship with competitive anxiety. *International Journal of Sport and Exercise Psychology, 5,* 28-53.

Harris, B.S., & Watson, J.C. (2014). Developmental considerations in youth athlete burnout: A model for youth sport participants. *Journal of Clinical Sport Psychology, 8,* 1-18.

Harter, S. (1978). Effectance motivation reconsidered. *Human Development, 21,* 34-64.

Harter, S. (1999). *The construction of the self: A developmental perspective.* New York: Guilford.

Harwood, C., & Biddle, S. (2002). The application of achievement goal theory in youth sport. In I.M. Cockerill (Ed.), *Solutions in sport psychology* (pp. 58-74). London: Thomson.

Harwood, C., & Knight, C. (2009). Understanding parental stressors: An investigation of British tennis parents. *Journal of Sports Sciences, 27,* 339-351.

Harwood, C.G., & Knight, C.J. (2015). Parenting in youth sport: A position paper on parenting expertise. *Psychology of Sport and Exercise, 16,* 24-35.

Harwood, C., Spray, C.M., & Keegan, R. (2008). Achievement goal theories in sport. In T.S. Horn (Ed.), *Advances in sport psychology* (3rd ed., pp. 157-186). Champaign, IL: Human Kinetics.

Haywood, K.M., & Getchell, N. (2001). *Learning activities for life span motor development* (3rd ed.). Champaign, IL: Human Kinetics.

Haywood, K.M., & Getchell, N. (2009). *Life span motor development* (5th ed.). Champaign, IL: Human Kinetics.

Hellison, D. (2011). *Teaching personal and social responsibility through physical activity* (3rd ed.). Champaign, IL: Human Kinetics.

Hellstedt, J. (1987). The coach/parent/athlete relationship. *Sport Psychologist, 1,* 151-160.

Helsen, W.F., Hodges, N.J., Van Winckel, J., & Starkes, J.L. (2000). The roles of talent, physical precocity and practice in the development of soccer expertise. *Journal of Sports Sciences, 18,* 727-736.

Helsen, W.F., & Starkes, J.L. (1999). A multidimensional approach to skilled perception and performance in sport. *Applied Cognitive Psychology, 13,* 1-27.

Helsen, W.F., Starkes, J.L., & Hodges, N.J. (1998). Team sports and the theory of deliberate practice. *Journal of Sport & Exercise Psychology, 20,* 13-35.

Henriksen, K., Larsen, C.H., & Christensen, M.K. (2014). Looking at success from its opposite pole: The case of a talent development golf environment in Denmark. *International Journal of Sport and Exercise Psychology, 12,* 134-149.

Henriksen, K., Stambulova, N., & Roessler, K.K. (2011). Riding the wave of an expert: A successful talent development environment in kayaking. *Sport Psychologist, 25,* 341-362.

Herman, K.N., Paukner, A., & Suomi, S.J. (2011). Gene X environment interactions in social play: Contributions from Rhesus Macaques. In A.D. Pellegrini (Ed.), *The Oxford handbook of the development of play* (pp. 58-69). Oxford, UK: Oxford University Press.

Hill, A.P. (2013). Perfectionism and burnout in junior soccer players: A test of the 2 X 2 model of dispositional perfectionism. *Journal of Sport & Exercise Psychology, 35,* 18-29.

Hodges, N.J., & Starkes, J.L. (1996). Wrestling with the nature of expertise: A sport specific test of Ericsson, Krampe and Tesch-Romer's (1993) theory of deliberate practice. *International Journal of Sport Psychology, 27,* 400-424.

Hofferth, S., & Sandberg, J. (2001). How American children spend their time. *Journal of Marriage and Family, 62,* 295-308.

Holt, N.L., Sehn, Z.L., Spence, J.C., Newton, A.S., & Ball, G.D.C. (2012). Physical education and sport programs at an inner city school: Exploring possibilities for positive youth development. *Physical Education and Sport Pedagogy, 17,* 97-113.

Hong, F. (2008). China. In B. Houlihan & M. Green (Eds.), *Comparative elite sport development: Systems, structures and public policy* (pp. 26-52). Boston: Elsevier.

Hong, F., & Zhouxiang, L. (2013). *The politicization of sport in modern China.* New York: Routledge.

Horn, T.S. (2004). Developmental perspectives on self-perceptions in children and adolescents. In M.R. Weiss (Ed.), *Developmental sport and exercise psychology: A lifespan perspective* (pp. 101-144). Morgantown, WV: Fitness Information Technology.

Horn, T.S., & Butt, J. (2014). Developmental perspectives on sport and physical activity participation. In A. Papaioannou & D. Hackfort (Eds.), *Fundamental concepts in sport and exercise psychology* (pp. 4-19). New York: Taylor & Francis.

Horn, T.S., & Horn, J.L. (2007). Family influences on children's sport and physical activity participation, behavior, and psychosocial responses. In G. Tenenbaum & R.C. Eklund (Eds.), *Handbook of sport psychology* (3rd ed., pp. 685-711). New York: Wiley.

Horn, T.S., Lox, C.L., & Labrador, F. (2015). The self-fulfilling prophecy theory: When coaches' expectations become reality. In J.M. Williams (Ed.), *Applied sport psychology: Personal growth to peak performance* (7th ed., pp. 78-100). New York: McGraw-Hill.

Horton, S. (2012). Environmental influences on early development in sports experts. In J. Baker, S. Cobley, & J. Schorer (Eds.), *Talent identification and development in sport: International perspectives* (pp. 39-50). New York: Routledge.

Howe, M.J.A., Davidson, J.W., & Sloboda, J.A. (1998). Innate talents: Reality or myth? *Behavioral and Brain Sciences, 21,* 339-442.

Howie, E.K., & Pate, R.R. (2012). Physical activity and academic achievement in children: A historical perspective. *Journal of Sport and Health Science, 1,* 160-169.

Huggan, J. (2013, September 9). The cat in the hat. *GolfWorld,* pp. 32-38.

Human Rights Watch. (2012). IOC/Saudi Arabia: End ban on women in sport. Retrieved April 20, 2015, from www.hrw.org/news/2012/02/15/locsaudi-arabia-end-ban-women-sport.

Hyde, J.S. (2005). The gender similarities hypothesis. *American Psychologist, 60,* 581-592.

Hyman, M. (2009). *Until it hurts: America's obsession with youth sports and how it harms our kids.* Boston: Beacon Press.

Impact report. Retrieved March 29, 2015, from www.thefirsttee.org/impact.

Imtiaz, F., Hancock, D.J., Vierimaa, M., & Cote, J. (2014). Place of development and dropout in youth ice hockey. *International Journal of Sport and Exercise Psychology, 12,* 234-244.

International Olympic Committee. (2008). Consensus statement: Sexual harassment and abuse in sport. *International Journal of Sport and Exercise Psychology, 6,* 444-446.

Issaacs, L.D., & Karpman, M.B. (1981). Factors affecting children's basketball shooting performance: A log-linear analysis. *Carnegie Research Papers,* pp. 29-32.

Janelle, C.M., & Hillman, C.H. (2003). Expert performance in sport: Current perspectives and critical issues. In J.L. Starkes & K.A. Ericsson (Eds.), *Expert performance in sports: Advances in research on sport expertise* (pp. 19-47). Champaign, IL: Human Kinetics.

Jansen, D. (1999). There's more to life than skating around in a circle. In J. Naber (Ed.), *Awaken the Olympian within* (pp. 3-14). Torrance, CA: Griffin.

Johnson, D.W., & Johnson, R. (2003). *Cooperative, competitive, and individualistic efforts: An update of the research.* Research Report, Cooperative Learning Center, University of Minnesota, Minneapolis.

Jones, G., & Hanton, S. (1996). Interpretations of competitive anxiety symptoms and goal attainment expectations. *Journal of Sport & Exercise Psychology, 18,* 144-157.

Junior player survey. (2010, December 16). *Sports Illustrated,* p. 42.

Juntumma, B., Keskivaara, P., & Punamaki, R. (2005). Parenting, achievement strategies and satisfaction in ice hockey. *Scandinavian Journal of Psychology, 46,* 411-420.

Kachel, K., Buszard, T., & Reid, M. (2015). The effect of ball compression on the match-play characteristics of elite junior tennis players. *Journal of Sports Sciences, 33,* 320-326.

Kalyvas, V., & Reid, G. (2005). Sport adaptation, participation, and enjoyment of students with and without physical disabilities. *Adapted Physical Activity Quarterly, 20,* 1-17.

Kavussanu, M. (2006). Motivational predictors of pro-social and antisocial behavior in football. *Journal of Sports Sciences, 24,* 575-588.

Kaye, M.P., Conroy, D.E., & Fifer, A.M. (2008). Individual differences in incompetence avoidance. *Journal of Sport & Exercise Psychology, 30,* 110-132.

Keegan, R., Spray, C., Harwood, C., & Lavallee, D. (2010). The motivating atmosphere in youth sport: Coach, parent, and peer influences on motivation in specializing sport participants. *Journal of Applied Sport Psychology, 22,* 87-105.

Kentta, G., & Hassmen, P. (1998). Overtraining and recovery: A conceptual model. *Sports Medicine, 26,* 1-16.

Kerr, G.A., & Stirling, A.E. (2012). Parents' reflections on their child's experiences of emotionally abusive coaching practices. *Journal of Applied Sport Psychology, 24,* 191-206.

Kirk, D., Macdonald, D., & O'Sullivan, M. (2006). *Handbook of physical education.* Thousand Oaks, CA: Sage.

Klakk, H., Chinapaw, M., Heidemann, M., Andersen, L.B., & Wedderkopp, N. (2013). Effect of four additional physical education lessons on body composition in children aged 8-13 years. *BMC Pediatrics, 13,* 170-178.

Klawans, H.L. (1996). *Why Michael couldn't hit: And other tales of the neurology of sports.* New York: Freeman.

Knight, C.J., Boden, C.M., & Holt, N.L. (2010). Junior tennis players' preferences for parental behaviors. *Journal of Applied Sport Psychology, 22,* 377-391.

Knight, C.J., & Holt, N.L. (2014). Parenting in youth tennis: Understanding and enhancing children's experiences. *Psychology of Sport and Exercise, 15,* 155-164.

Knight, C.J., Neely, K.C., & Holt, N.L. (2011). Parental behaviors in team sports: How do female athletes want parents to behave? *Journal of Applied Sport Psychology, 23,* 76-92.

Knudsen, E. (2004). Sensitive periods in the development of the brain and behavior. *Journal of Cognitive Neuroscience, 16,* 1412-1425.

Kohlberg, L. (1984). *Essays on moral development: Vol. 2. The psychology of moral behavior.* San Francisco: Harper & Row.

Krane, V., & Williams, J.M. (2010). Psychological characteristics of peak performance. In J.M. Williams (Ed.), *Applied sport psychology: Personal growth to peak performance* (6th ed., pp. 169-188). New York: McGraw-Hill.

Krogman, W.M. (1959). Maturation age of 55 boys in the Little League World Series, 1957. *Research Quarterly, 29,* 54-57.

Kucera, K.L., Klossner, D., Colgate, B., & Cantu, R.C. (2014). *Annual survey of football injury research.* Waco, TX: American Football Coaches Association.

Laby, D.M., Kirschen, D.G., & Pantall, P. (2011, May). The visual function of Olympic-level athletes–an initial report. *Eye and Contact Lens, 37,* 116-122.

Laby, D.M., Rosenbaum, A.L., Kirschen, D.G., Davidson, J.L., Rosenbaum, L.J., Strasser, C., & Mellman, M.F. (1996). The visual function of professional baseball players. *American Journal of Ophthalmology, 122,* 476-485.

LaCaze, J., & Dalrymple, D. (2011). *The athletic body puzzle.* Charlotte, NC: Vivify.

Lally, P., & Kerr, G. (2008). The effects of athlete retirement on parents. *Journal of Applied Sport Psychology, 20,* 42-56.

Lambert, B.G., Rothschild, B.F., Altland, R., & Green, L.B. (1972). *Adolescence: Transition from childhood to maturity* (2nd ed.). Monterey, CA: Brooks/Cole.

Lancaster, S., & Teodorescu, R. (2008). *Athletic fitness for kids.* Champaign, IL: Human Kinetics.

Landers, M.A., & Fine, G.A. (1998). Learning life's lessons in tee ball: The reinforcement of gender and status in kindergarten sport. *Sociology of Sport Journal, 13,* 87-93.

Larsen, C.H., Alfermann, D., Henriksen, K., & Christensen, M.K. (2013). Successful talent development in soccer: The characteristics of the environment. *Sport, Exercise, and Performance Psychology, 2,* 190-206.

Larson, E.J., & Guggenheimer, J.D. (2013). The effects of scaling tennis equipment on the forehand groundstroke performance of children. *Journal of Sport Sciences and Medicine, 12,* 323-331.

Lauer, L., Gould, D., Roman, N., & Pierce, M. (2010a). How parents influence junior tennis players' development: Qualitative narratives. *Journal of Clinical Sport Psychology, 4,* 69-92.

Lauer, L., Gould, D., Roman, N., & Pierce, M. (2010b). Parental behaviors that affect junior tennis player development. *Psychology of Sport and Exercise, 11,* 487-496.

Lauer, L., & Paiement, C. (2004). The playing tough and clean hockey program. *Sport Psychologist, 23,* 543-561.

Law, M.P., Cote, J., & Ericsson, K.A. (2007). Characteristics of expert development in rhythmic gymnastics: A retrospective study. *International Journal of Exercise and Sport Psychology, 5,* 82-103.

Lefevre, J., Beunen, G., Steens, G., Claessens, A., & Renson, R. (1990). Motor performance during adolescence and age thirty as related to age at peak height velocity. *Annals of Human Biology, 17,* 423-435.

Lerner, R.M., Fisher, C.B., & Weinberg, R.A. (2000). Toward a science for and of the people: Promoting civil society through the application of developmental science. *Child Development, 71,* 11-20.

Li, C., Wang, C.K.J., & Pyun, D.Y. (2014). Talent development environmental factors in sport: A review and taxonomic classification. *Quest, 66,* 433-447.

Liang, G., Housner, L., Walls, R., & Yan, Z. (2013). Failure and revival: Physical education and youth sport in China. *Asia Pacific Journal of Sport and Social Science, 1,* 48-59.

Lidor, R., Cote, J., & Hackfort, D. (2009). ISSP position stand: To test or not to test? The use of physical skill tests in talent detection and in early phases of sport development. *International Journal of Sport and Exercise Psychology, 7,* 131-146.

Lidor, R., & Ziv, G. (2013). Physical and skill testing in early phases of talent development. In J. Cote & R. Lidor (Eds.), *Conditions of children's talent development in sport* (pp. 85-98). Morgantown, WV: Fitness Information Technology.

Light, R. (2011). Accessing youth sport in Australia: Schools and clubs. In S. Georgakis & K. Russell (Eds.), *Youth sport in Australia* (pp. 59-70). Sydney: Sydney University Press.

Loh, S. (2011, April 24). Club sports is king in Europe. *Patriot-News,* Pennsylvania. Retrieved June 3, 2013, from blog.pennlive.com/patriotnews-sports/2011/04/club_sports_is_king_in_ europe.html.

Lohmander, L.S., Englund, P.M., Dahl, L.L., & Roos, E.M. (2007). The long-term consequences of anterior cruciate ligament and meniscus injuries: Osteoarthritis. *American Journal of Sports Medicine, 35,* 1756-1769.

Long, T., Pantaleon, N., Bruant, G., & d'Arripe-Longueville, F. (2006). A qualitative study of moral reasoning of young elite athletes. *Sport Psychologist, 20,* 330-347.

Lonsdale, C., Hodge, K., & Rose, E.A. (2008). The Behavioral Regulation in Sport Questionnaire (BRSQ): Instrument development and initial validity evidence. *Journal of Sport & Exercise Psychology, 30,* 323-355.

Loud, K.J., Gordon, C.M., Micheli, L.J., & Field, A.E. (2005). Correlates of stress fractures among preadolescent and adolescent girls. *Pediatrics, 115,* e399-e406.

Loyola University Health System. (2013, April 19). Intense, specialized training in young athletes linked to serious overuse injuries. *ScienceDaily.* Retrieved February 16, 2014, from www.sciencedaily.com/releases/2013/04/130419132508.htm.

Lucia, D. (2009, October). It's time to go back to the future for skill development. *USA Hockey Magazine,* p. 40.

Luvmour, J. (2007). *Everyone wins! Cooperative games and activities.* Gabriola Island, Canada: New Society.

MacDonald, D., Cheung, M., Cote, J., & Abernathy, B. (2009). Place but not date of birth influences the development and emergence of athletic talent in American football. *Journal of Applied Sport Psychology, 21,* 80-90.

MacDonald, D., King, J., Cote, J., & Abernathy, B. (2009). Birthplace effects on the development of female athletic talent. *Journal of Science and Medicine in Sport, 12,* 234-237.

MacNamara, A., Button, A., & Collins, D. (2010a). The role of psychological characteristics in facilitating the pathway to elite performance: Part 1: Identifying mental skills and behaviors. *Sport Psychologist, 24,* 52-73.

MacNamara, A., Button, A., & Collins, D. (2010b). The role of psychological characteristics in facilitating the pathway to elite performance: Part 2: Examining environmental and stage-related differences in skills and behaviors. *Sport Psychologist, 24,* 74-96.

MacNamara, A., & Collins, D. (2012). Building talent development systems on mechanistic principles. In J. Baker, S. Cobley, & J. Schorer (Eds.), *Talent identification and development in sport: International perspectives* (pp. 25-38). New York: Routledge.

Mageau, G., & Vallerand, R.J. (2003). The coach-athlete relationship: A motivational model. *Journal of Sports Sciences, 21,* 883-904.

Magill, R.A., & Anderson, D.I. (1996). Critical periods as optimal readiness for learning sport skills. In F.L. Smoll & R.E. Smith (Eds.), *Children and youth in sport: A biopsychosocial perspective* (pp. 57-72). Indianapolis: Brown & Benchmark.

Magra, M., Caine, D., & Maffulli, N. (2007). A review of epidemiology of paediatric elbow injuries in sports. *Sports Medicine, 37,* 717-735.

Magra, M., & Maffulli, N. (2005). The epidemiology of injuries to the elbow in sport. *International Sports Medicine Journal, 6,* 25-33.

Malcom, N.L. (2006). "Shaking it off" and "toughing it out": Socialization to pain and injury in girls' softball. *Journal of Contemporary Ethnography, 35,* 495-525.

Malina, R.M. (2013). Motor development and performance. In J. Cote & R. Lidor (Eds.), *Conditions of children's talent development in sport* (pp. 61-83). Morgantown, WV: Fitness Information Technology.

Malina, R.M. (2014). Top 10 research questions related to growth and maturation of relevance to physical activity, performance, and fitness. *Research Quarterly for Exercise and Sport, 85,* 157-173.

Malina, R.M., Bouchard, C., & Bar-Or, O. (2004). *Growth, maturation, and physical activity* (2nd ed.). Champaign, IL: Human Kinetics.

Malina, R.M., Eisenmann, J.C., Cumming, S.P., Ribeiro, B., & Aroso, J. (2004). Maturity-associated variation in the growth and functional capacities of youth football (soccer) players 13-15 years. *European Journal of Applied Physiology, 91,* 555-562.

Malina, R., Morano, P.J., Barron, M., Miller, S.J., Cumming, S.P., Kontos, A.P., & Little, B.B. (2007). Overweight and obesity among youth participants in American football. *Journal of Pediatrics, 151,* 378-382.

Mamassis, G., & Doganis, G. (2004). The effects of a mental training program on juniors' precompetitive anxiety, self-confidence, and tennis performance. *Journal of Applied Sport Psychology, 16,* 118-137.

Manoyan, D. (2012, July 7). A 1998 victory in the U.S. that still resonates in South Korea. *New York Times.* Retrieved September 27, 2013, from www.nytimes.com/2012/07/8/sports/golf/south-korean-players-are-dominating-the-lpga-tour.html.

Marano, H.E. (2008). *A nation of wimps: The high cost of invasive parenting.* New York: Broadway Books.

Marshall, S.J., Biddle, S.J.H., Gorely, T., Cameron, N., & Murdey, I. (2004). Relationships between media use, body fatness and physical activity in children and youth: A meta-analysis. *International Review of Obesity, 28,* 1238-1246.

Martens, R. (1975). *Social psychology and physical activity.* New York: Harper-Collins.

Martens, R. (1978). *Joy and sadness in children's sports.* Champaign, IL: Human Kinetics.

Martens, R. (2001). *Directing youth sport programs.* Champaign, IL: Human Kinetics.

Martens, R. (2012). *Successful coaching* (4th ed.). Champaign, IL: Human Kinetics.

Martens, R., Rivkin, F., & Bump, L. (1984). A field study of traditional and nontraditional children's baseball. *Research Quarterly for Exercise and Sport, 55,* 351-355.

Martens, R., & Seefeldt, V. (1979). *Guidelines for children's sports.* Washington, DC: American Alliance for Health, Physical Education, Recreation and Dance.

Martens, R., Vealey, R.S., & Burton, D. (1990). *Competitive anxiety in sport.* Champaign, IL: Human Kinetics.

Martin, E.M., & Horn, T.S. (2013). The role of athletic identity and passion in predicting burnout in adolescent female athletes. *Sport Psychologist, 27,* 338-348.

Martin, S.B., Dale, G.A., & Jackson, A.W. (2001). Youth coaching preferences of adolescent athletes and their parents. *Journal of Sport Behavior, 24,* 197-212.

Martindale, R.J.J., Collins, D., Wang, J.C.K., McNeill, M., Lee, K.S., Sproule, J., & Westbury, T. (2010). Development of the Talent Development Environment Questionnaire for Sport. *Journal of Sports Sciences,* 1-13, *iFirst* article.

Martinek, T., & Hellison, D. (2009). *Youth leadership in sport and physical education.* New York: Palgrave Macmillan.

Matos, N., & Winsley, R.J. (2007). Trainability of young athletes and overtraining. *Journal of Sports Science and Medicine, 6,* 353-367.

Matosic, D., Cox, A.E., & Amorose, A.J. (2014). Scholarship status, controlling coach behavior, and intrinsic motivation in collegiate swimmers: A test of cognitive evaluation theory. *Sport, Exercise, and Performance Psychology, 3,* 1-12.

May, R.A.B. (2001). The sticky situation of sportsmanship: Contexts and contradictions in sportsmanship among high school boys basketball players. *Journal of Sport and Social Issues, 25,* 372-389.

McCollum, J. (2013, February 25). Laker chaos. *Sports Illustrated,* pp. 36-40.

McCormick, J., & Begley, S. (1996, December 9). How to raise a tiger. *Time,* pp. 52-59.

McDowell, M.A., Brody, D.J., & Hughes, J.P. (2007). Has age at menarche changed? *Journal of Adolescent Health, 40,* 227-231.

McGrath, J.E. (1970). Major methodological issues. In J.E. McGrath (Ed.), *Social and psychological factors in stress* (pp. 19-49). New York: Holt, Rinehart & Winston.

McGraw, P.B. (2013, May 17). Sky's Delle Donne relies on strong family ties. *Daily Herald.* Retrieved March 29, 2015, from www.dailyherald.com/article/20130517/sports/705179674/.

McLeod, B.D., Wood, J.J., & Weisz, J.R. (2007). Examining the association between parenting and childhood anxiety: A meta-analysis. *Clinical Psychology Review, 27,* 155-172.

Mikulic, P., & Ruzic, L. (2008). Predicting the 1000m rowing ergometer performance in 12-13-year-old rowers: The basis for selection process? *Journal of Science and Medicine in Sport, 11,* 218-226.

Miller, S.L. (2009). *Why teams win.* Toronto: Jossey-Bass.

Mirtle, J. (2012, October 3). Bauer takes on sagging minor hockey enrolment. The Globe and Mail. Retrieved May 15, 2013 from www.theglobeandmail.com/sports/hockey/bauer-takes-on-sagging-minor-hockey-enrolment/article45878997.

Miserandino, M. (1998). Attributional retraining as a method of improving athletic performance. *Journal of Sport Behavior, 21,* 286-297.

Moceanu, D. (2012). *Off balance.* New York: Touchstone.

Monsaas, J.A. (1985). Learning to be a world-class tennis player. In B.S. Bloom (Ed.), *Developing talent in young people* (p. 211-269). New York: Ballantine.

Monsma, E.V. (2008). Puberty and physical self-perceptions of competitive female figure skaters II: Maturational timing, skating context, and ability status. *Research Quarterly for Exercise and Sport, 79,* 411-416.

Mooney, A. (2012, August 3). The bodies of champion gymnasts. Retrieved February 10, 2014, from www.boston.com/sports/blogs/statsdriven/2012/08/the_bodies_of_champion_gymnast.html.

Morfit, C. (2012, December). That's my boy! *Golf Magazine,* pp. 64-65.

Morris, R.L., & Kavussanu, M. (2009). The role of approach-avoidance versus task and ego goals in enjoyment and cognitive anxiety in youth sport. *International Journal of Sport and Exercise Psychology, 7*, 185-202.

Moser, R.S. (2012). *Ahead of the game: The parents' guide to youth sports concussion*. Hanover, NH: Dartmouth College Press.

Mugno, D.A., & Feltz, D.L. (1985). The social learning of aggression in youth football in the United States. *Canadian Journal of Applied Sport Science, 10*, 26-35.

Murphy, S. (1999). *The cheers and the tears: A healthy alternative to the dark side of youth sport*. San Francisco: Jossey-Bass.

Myer, G.D., Ford, K.R., & Hewett, T.E. (2004). Rationale and clinical techniques for anterior cruciate ligament injury prevention among female athletes. *Journal of Athletic Training, 39*, 352-364.

NASPE Newsletter. (Fall, 1997). *Youth sports: What every parent should know*. Reston, VA: SHAPE America.

Nater, S. (2010). *You haven't taught until they have learned: John Wooden's teaching principles and practices*. Morgantown, WV: Fitness Information Technology.

National Association for Sport and Physical Education. (2010). *Guidelines for participation in youth sport programs: Specialization versus multiple-sport participation*. Reston, VA: American Alliance for Health, Physical Education, Recreation and Dance.

National Federation of State High School Associations. (2014). 2013-14 high school athletics participation survey. Retrieved July 13, 2013, from www.nfhs.org.participationstatistics/pdf/2013-14_Participation_Survey_pdf.pdf.

National Sporting Goods Association. (2012). Sports participation 2011: Series I. Mount Prospect, IL.

Negriff, S., & Susman, E.J. (2011). Pubertal timing, depression, and externalizing problems: A framework, review, and examination of gender differences. *Journal of Research on Adolescence, 21*, 717-746.

Nevett, M.E., & French, K.E. (1997). The development of sport-specific planning, rehearsal, and updating of plans during defensive youth baseball game performance. *Research Quarterly for Exercise and Sport, 68*, 203-214.

Nicholls, A.R., Perry, J.L., Jones, L., Morley, D., & Carson, F. (2013). Dispositional coping, coping effectiveness, and cognitive social maturity among adolescent athletes. *Journal of Sport & Exercise Psychology, 35*, 229-238.

Nicholls, J.G. (1989). *The competitive ethos and democratic education*. Cambridge, MA: Harvard University Press.

Nordstrom, A., Tervo, T., & Hostrom, M. (2011). The effect of physical activity on bone accrual, osteoporosis and fracture prevention. *Open Bone Journal, 3*, 11-21.

Novotney, A. (2012, October). Parenting that works. *Monitor on Psychology*, pp. 44-47.

O'Connor, D. (2011). Factors influencing talent identification and athlete development in youth sport. In S. Georgakis & K. Russell (Eds.), *Youth sport in Australia* (pp. 193-210). Sydney: Sydney University Press.

Okazaki, F.H.A., Keller, B., Fontana, F.E., & Gallagher, J.D. (2011). The relative age effect among female Brazilian youth volleyball players. *Research Quarterly for Exercise and Sport, 82*, 135-139.

Oliver, K.L., & Hamzeh, M. (2010). "The boys won't let us play": Fifth-grade mestizos challenge physical activity discourse at school. *Research Quarterly for Exercise and Sport, 81*, 38-51.

Omli, J., & Wiese-Bjornstal, D.M. (2011). Kids speak: Preferred parental behavior at youth sport events. *Research Quarterly for Exercise and Sport, 82*, 702-711.

Ommundsen, Y., Roberts, G.C., Lemyre, P.N., & Treasure, D. (2003). Perceived motivational climate in male youth soccer: Relations to social-moral functioning, sportspersonship and team norm perceptions. *Psychology of Sport and Exercise, 4*, 397-413.

Opening remarks at a meeting on developing children's physical education and youth sport. (2013, March 13). Retrieved May 6, 2014, from en.kremlin.ru/events/president/transcripts/17667.

Orlick, T. (2006). *Cooperative games and sports*. Champaign, IL: Human Kinetics.

O'Rourke, D.J., Smith, R.E., Smoll, F.L., & Cumming, S.P. (2011). Trait anxiety in young athletes as a function of parental pressure and motivational climate: Is parental pressure always harmful? *Journal of Applied Sport Psychology, 23*, 398-412.

Owens, T. (2006, Fall). 2-4-6-HATE. *Teaching Tolerance*, pp. 23-27.

Patterson, J. (2013, June). Four rules for teaching juniors. *Golf Digest*, p. 56.

Payne, U.G., & Isaacs, L.D. (2008). *Human motor development: A lifespan approach* (7th ed.). Boston: McGraw-Hill.

Pelletier, L.G., Dion, S., Tuson, K., & Green-Demers, I. (1999). Why do people fail to adopt environmentally protective behaviors? Toward a taxonomy of environmental amotivation. *Journal of Applied Social Psychology, 29,* 2481-2504.

Penhune, V.B. (2011). Sensitive periods in human development: Evidence from musical training. *Cortex, 47,* 1126-1137.

Petitpas, A.J., Van Raalte, J.L., Cornelius, A.E., & Presbrey, J. (2004). A life skills development program for high school student-athletes. *Journal of Primary Prevention, 24,* 325-334.

Petranek, L.J., & Barton, G.V. (2011). The over-arm-throwing pattern among U-14 ASA female softball players: A comparative study of gender, culture, and experience. *Research Quarterly for Exercise and Sport, 82,* 220-228.

Pickhardt, C.E. (2009). Parental pride and adolescence. *Psychology Today.* Retrieved May 20, 2014 from www.psychologytoday.com/blog/surviving-your-childs-adolescence/200910/parental-pride-and-adolescence.

Plunkett Research Ltd. (2013). Sports industry overview. Retrieved March 29, 2015, from www.plunkettresearch.com/sports-recreation-leisure-market-research/industry-statistics.

Pomerantz, E.M., Grolnick, W.S., & Price, C.E. (2005). The role of parents in how children approach achievement: A dynamic process perspective. In A.J. Elliot & C.S. Dweck (Eds.), *Handbook of competence and motivation* (pp. 259-278). New York: Guilford Press.

Power, T.G., & Woolger, C. (1994). Parenting practices and age-group swimming: A correlational study. *Research Quarterly for Exercise and Sport, 65,* 59-66.

Price, M.S., & Weiss, M.R. (2013). Relationships among coach leadership, peer leadership, and adolescent athletes' psychosocial and team outcomes: A test of transformational theory. *Journal of Applied Sport Psychology, 25,* 265-279.

Quick, S., Simon, A., & Thornton, A. (2010). PE and sport survey 2009/10. U.K. Department for Education Research Report DFE-RR032. Retrieved May 2, 2014, from www.gov.uk/government/publications/pe-and-sport-survey-2009-to-2010.

Raedeke, T.D. (1997). Is athlete burnout more than just stress? A sport commitment perspective. *Journal of Sport & Exercise Psychology, 19,* 396-417.

Raedeke, T.D., & Smith, A.L. (2004). Coping resources and athlete burnout: An examination of stress mediated and moderation hypotheses. *Journal of Sport & Exercise Psychology, 26,* 525-541.

Raglin, J., Sawamura, S., Alexiou, S., Hassmen, P., & Kentta, G. (2000). Training practices and staleness in 13-18-year-old swimmers: A cross-cultural study. *Pediatric Exercise Science, 12,* 61-70.

Ratey, J.J. (2008). *Spark: The revolutionary new science of exercise and the brain.* New York: Little, Brown, and Company.

Rees, T., Ingedew, D.K., & Hardy, L. (2005). Attribution in sport psychology: Seeking congruence between theory, research, and practice. *Psychology of Sport and Exercise, 6,* 189-204.

Reeves, C.W., Nicholls, A.R., & McKenna, J. (2009). Stressors and coping strategies among early and middle adolescent premier league academy soccer players: Differences according to age. *Journal of Applied Sport Psychology, 21,* 31-48.

Reuters. (2013, March 30). Saudi Arabia to allow women's sports clubs. Retrieved May 10, 2014, from www.reuters.com/article/2013/03/30/us-saudi-women-sports.

Richardson, S., Andersen, M., & Morris, T. (2008). *Overtraining athletes.* Champaign, IL: Human Kinetics.

Rideout, V.J., Foehr, U.G., & Roberts, D.F. (2010). *Generation M2: Media in the lives of 8- to 19-year-olds.* Menlo Park, CA: Kaiser Family Foundation.

Riess, S.A. (1991). *City games: The evolution of American urban society and the rise of sports.* Urbana and Chicago: University of Illinois Press.

Rinehart, R.E. (2008). Exploiting a new generation: Corporate branding and the co-optation of action sport. In M.D. Giardina & M.K. Donnelly (Eds.), *Youth culture and sport: Identity, power, and politics* (pp. 71-90). New York: Routledge.

Rink, J.E., & Hall, T.J. (2008). Research on effective teaching in elementary school physical education. *Elementary School Journal, 108,* 207-218.

Roberts, S. (2010, November 22). Learning by example. *Sports Illustrated,* p. 102.

Rolex Women's World Golf Rankings. Retrieved June 10, 2015 from www.rolexrankings.com.

Rowland, T.W. (2005). *Children's exercise physiology* (2nd ed.). Champaign, IL: Human Kinetics.

Russell, B., & Branch, T. (1979). *Second wind: The memoirs of an opinionated man.* New York: Random House.

Rutherford, M.B. (2009). Children's autonomy and responsibility: An analysis of childrearing advice. *Qualitative Sociology, 32,* 337-353.

Ryan, E.D. (1980). Attribution, intrinsic motivation, and athletes: A replication and extension. In C.H. Nadeau, W.R. Halliwell, K.M. Newell, & G.C. Roberts (Eds.), *Psychology of motor behavior and sport, 1979* (pp. 19-26). Champaign, IL: Human Kinetics.

Ryan, R.M., & Deci, E.L. (2002). Overview of self-determination theory: An organismic dialectical perspective. In E.L. Deci & R. Ryan (Eds.), *Handbook of self-determination research* (pp. 3-33). Rochester, NY: University of Rochester Press.

Sabo, D., & Veliz, P. (2008). *Go out and play: Youth sports in America.* East Meadow, NY: Women's Sports Foundation.

Sagar, M. (2009, May). Todd Marinovich: The man who never was. *Esquire.* Retrieved April 20, 2015, from www.esquire.com/features/the-game/tdd-marinovich-0509.

Sagar, S.S., Busch, B.K., & Jowett, S. (2010). Success and failure, fear of failure, and coping responses of adolescent academy football players. *Journal of Applied Sport Psychology, 22,* 213-230.

Sagar, S.S., Lavallee, D., & Spray, C.M. (2007). Why young elite athletes fear failure: Consequences of failure. *Journal of Sports Sciences, 25,* 1171-1184.

Sallis, J.F., Prochaska, J.J., & Taylor, W.C. (2000). A review of correlates of physical activity of children and adolescents. *Medicine and Science in Sports and Exercise, 32,* 963-975.

Salter, R.B., & Harris, W.R. (1963). Injuries involving the epiphyseal plate. *Journal of Bone and Joint Surgery, 45,* 587-622.

Sampras, P. (2008). *A champion's mind: Lessons from a life in tennis.* New York: Three Rivers Press.

Sampson, C. (2013, April 8). Life in the big pool. *GolfWorld,* pp. 48-56.

Sapakoff, G. (1995, October 30). Little league's civil war. *Sports Illustrated.* Retrieved July 27, 2015, from www.si.com/vault/1995/10/30/207729/little-leagues-civil-war.

Sapieja, K.M., Dunn, J.G.H., & Holt, N.L. (2011). Perfectionism and perceptions of parenting styles in male youth soccer. *Journal of Sport & Exercise Psychology, 33,* 20-39.

Satern, M.N., Messier, S.P., & Keller-McNulty, S. (1989). The effects of ball size and basket height on the mechanics of a basketball free throw. *Journal of Human Movement Studies, 16,* 123-137.

Scammon, R.E. (1930). The measurement of the body in childhood. In J.A. Harris, C.M. Jackson, D.G. Paterson, & R.E. Scammon (Eds.), *The measurement of man* (pp. 173-215). Minneapolis: University of Minnesota Press.

Scanlan, T.K., Carpenter, P.J., Schmidt, G.W., Simons, J.P., & Keeler, B. (1993). An introduction to the sport commitment model. *Journal of Sport & Exercise Psychology, 15,* 1-15.

Schaerlaeckens, L. (2012, January 19). How to improve U.S. soccer. Retrieved March 7, 2014, from espn.go.com/sports/soccer/news/_?id?7468594/prominent-us-coaches-discuss-problems-american-soccer.

Schafer, A. (2010, February 25). Why you shouldn't say "I'm so proud of you." Retrieved March 29, 2015, from www.alysonschafer.com/why-you-shouldnt-say-im-so-proud-of-you.

Scituate "Green Death" soccer coach resigns. (2009, March 31). *Patriot Ledger.* Retrieved March 29, 2015, from www.patriotledger.com/archive/x575725578/-Green-Death-coach-resigns.

Seefeldt, V. (1980). Developmental motor patterns: Implications for elementary school physical education. In C. Nadeau, W. Halliwell, K. Newell, & G. Roberts (Eds.), *Psychology of motor behavior and sport, 1979* (pp. 314-323). Champaign, IL: Human Kinetics.

Selby, C.L.B., & Reel, J.J. (2011). A coach's guide to identifying and helping athletes with eating disorders. *Journal of Sport Psychology in Action, 2,* 100-112.

Sey, J. (2008). *Chalked up.* New York: Morrow.

Shields, D.L.L., & Bredemeier, B.J.L. (1995). *Character development and physical activity.* Champaign, IL: Human Kinetics.

Shields, D.L., & Bredemeier, B.L. (2007). Advances in sport morality research. In G. Tenenbaum & R.C. Eklund (Eds.), *Handbook of sport psychology* (3rd ed., pp. 662-684). Hoboken, NJ: Wiley.

Shields, D.L., & Bredemeier, B.L. (2009). *True competition.* Champaign, IL: Human Kinetics.

Shields, D.L., LaVoi, N.M., Bredemeier, B.L., & Power, F.C. (2007). Predictors of poor sportpersonship in youth sports: Personal attitudes and social influences. *Journal of Sport & Exercise Psychology, 29,* 747-762.

Sifers, S.K., & Shea, D.N. (2013). Evaluations of girls on the run/girls on track to enhance self-esteem and well-being. *Journal of Clinical Sport Psychology, 7,* 77-85.

Silvers, H.J., & Mandelbaum, B.R. (2007). Prevention of anterior cruciate ligament injury in the female athlete. *British Journal of Sports Medicine, 41,* 52-59.

Simon, H.A., & Chase, W.G. (1973). Skill in chess. *American Scientist, 61,* 394-403.

Simon, J.A., & Martens, R. (1979). Children's anxiety in sport and nonsport evaluative activities. *Journal of Sport Psychology, 1,* 160-169.

Simonton, D.K. (1999). Talent and its development: An emergenic and epigenetic model. *Psychological Review, 106,* 435-457.

Singer, R.N., & Janelle, C.M. (1999). Determining sport expertise: From genes to supremes. *International Journal of Sport Psychology, 30,* 117-150.

Singh, A., Uijtdewilligen, L., Twisk, J.W.R., Van Mechelen, W., & Chinapaw, M.J.M. (2012). Physical activity and performance at school. *Archives of Pediatric Adolescent Medicine, 166,* 49-55.

Sinnott, K., & Biddle, S. (1998). Changes in attributions, perceptions of success and intrinsic motivation after attribution retraining in children's sport. *International Journal of Adolescence and Youth, 7,* 137-144.

Sit, C.H.P., & Lindner, K.J. (2006). Situational state balances and participation motivation in youth sport: A reversal theory perspective. *British Journal of Educational Psychology, 76,* 369-384.

Smith, A.L., Ullrich-French, S., Walker, E., & Hurley, K.S. (2006). Peer relationship profiles and motivation in youth sport. *Journal of Sport & Exercise Psychology, 28,* 362-382.

Smith, M.D. (1974). Significant others' influence on the assaultive behavior of young hockey players. *International Review of Sport Sociology, 3-4,* 45-46.

Smith, M.D. (1982). Social determinants of violence in hockey: A review. In R.A. Magill, M.J. Ash, & F.L. Smoll (Eds.), *Children in sport* (pp. 294-309). Champaign, IL: Human Kinetics.

Smith, R.E., & Christensen, D.L. (1995). Psychological skills as predictors of performance and survival in professional baseball. *Journal of Sport & Exercise Psychology, 17,* 399-415.

Smith, R.E., Cumming, S.P., & Smoll, F.L. (2008). Development and validation of the Motivational Climate Scale for Youth Sports. *Journal of Applied Sport Psychology, 20,* 116-136.

Smith, R.E., Schutz, R.W., Smoll, F.L., & Ptacek, J.T. (1995). Development and validation of the multidimensional measure of sport-specific psychological skills: The athletic coping skills inventory-28. *Journal of Sport & Exercise Psychology, 17,* 379-398.

Smith, R.E., Shoda, Y., Cumming, S.P., & Smoll, F.L. (2009). Behavioral signatures at the ballpark: Intra-individual consistency of adults' situation-behavior patterns and their interpersonal consequences. *Journal of Research in Personality, 43,* 187-195.

Smith, R.E., & Smoll, F.L. (2002). *Way to go, coach!* Portola Valley, CA: Warde.

Smith, R.E., & Smoll, F.L. (2007). Social-cognitive approach to coaching behaviors. In S. Jowett & D. Lavallee (Eds.), *Social psychology in sport* (75-90). Champaign, IL: Human Kinetics.

Smith, R.E., Smoll, F.L., & Cumming, S.P. (2007). Effects of a motivational climate intervention for coaches on young athletes' sport performance anxiety. *Journal of Sport & Exercise Psychology, 29,* 39-59.

Smith, R.E., Smoll, F.L., & Hunt, E. (1977). A system for the behavioral assessment of athletic coaches. *Research Quarterly, 48,* 401-407.

Soberlak, P., & Cote, J. (2003). The developmental activities of professional ice hockey players. *Journal of Applied Sport Psychology, 15,* 41-49.

Soccer Still Canada's Most-played Sport. Retrieved March 29, 2015, from www.theepochtimes.com/news/8-2-12/65884.html.

Sokolove, M. (2008). *Warrior girls.* New York: Simon & Schuster.

Sowell, E.R., Thompson, P.M., Tessner, K.D., & Toga, A.W. (2001). Mapping continued brain growth and gray matter density in dorsal frontal cortex: Inverse relationships during post adolescent brain maturation. *Journal of Neuroscience, 15,* 8819-8829.

Sparks, W.L. (2012). *Season of change.* Lexington, KY: In His Hands Press.

Sparvero, E., Chalip, L., & Green, B.C. (2008). United States. In B. Houlihan & M. Green (Eds.), *Comparative elite sport development: Systems, structures and public policy* (pp. 242-271). Amsterdam: Elsevier.

Spitznagel, E. (2011, July 14). Child bodybuilding: How jacked is your kid? *Businessweek.* Retrieved February 2, 2014, from www.bloombergcom/bw/magazine/child-bodybuilding-how-jacked-is-your-kid-07142011.html.

Sport New Zealand. (2012a). New Zealand community sport coaching plan 2012-2020. Retrieved April 10, 2013, from www.sportnz.org.nz/assets/uploads/attachments/managing-sport/coaching/New-Zealand-community-sport-coaching-plan-20122020.pdf.

Sport New Zealand. (2012b). Young people's survey. Retrieved April 10, 2013, from www.sportnz.org.nw/managing-sport/research/young-peoples-survey-2011.

Sports and Fitness Industry Association. (2013). 2013 sports, fitness, and leisure activities topline participation report. Retrieved April 2, 2013, from espn.go.com/pdf/2013/1113/espn_otl_sportsreport.pdf.

Sports: When winning is the only thing, can violence be far away? Canadian Centres for Teaching Peace. Retrieved November 23, 2008, from www.peace.ca/sports.htm.

Starkes, J.L. (1993). Motor experts: Opening thoughts. In J.L. Starkes & F. Allard (Eds.), *Cognitive issues in motor expertise* (pp. 3-16). Amsterdam: Elsevier.

Stein, J. (2013, May 20). The new greatest generation. *Time*, pp. 26-34.

Stephens, D.W. (2001). Predictors of aggressive tendencies in girls' basketball: An examination of beginning and advanced participants in a summer skills camp. *Research Quarterly for Exercise and Sport, 72,* 257-266.

Stirling, A.E., & Kerr, G.A. (2007). Elite female swimmers' experiences of emotional abuse across time. *Journal of Emotional Abuse, 7,* 89-113.

Stodden, D.F., Goodway, J.D., Langendorfer, S.J., Roberton, M.A., Rudisill, M.E., Garcia, C., & Garcia, L.E. (2008). A developmental perspective on the role of motor skill competence in physical activity: An emergent relationship. *Quest, 60,* 290-306.

Stone, J., Lynch, C.I., Sjomeling, M., & Darley, J.M. (1999). Stereotype threat effects on black and white athletic performance. *Journal of Personality and Social Psychology, 77,* 1213-1227.

Strachan, L., Cote, J., & Deakin, J. (2009). "Specializers" versus "samplers" in youth sport: Comparing experiences and outcomes. *Sport Psychologist, 23,* 77-92.

Strauss, R. (2007, April 11). Rutgers women send Imus an angry message. *New York Times.* Retrieved March 29, 2015, from www.nytimes.com/2007/04/11/sports/ncaabasketball/11rutgers.html.

Summitt, P. (2013). *Sum it up.* New York: Random House.

Syed, M. (2010). *Bounce.* New York: Harper.

Takeuchi, T., & Inomata, K. (2009). Visual search strategies and decision making in baseball batting. *Perceptual and Motor Skills, 108,* 971-980.

Tamminen, K.A., & Holt, N.L. (2010). A meta-study of qualitative research examining stressor appraisals and coping among adolescents in sport. *Journal of Sports Sciences, 28,* 1563-1580.

Telama, R., Yang, X., Hirvensalo, M., & Raitakari, O. (2006). Participation in organized youth sport as a predictor of adult physical activity: A 21-year longitudinal study. *Pediatric Exercise Science, 17,* 76-88.

Thomas, L. (2013, February 21). The Teammates. Retrieved April 20, 2015, from www.grantland.com/story/_/id/8959568/missy-franklin-olympic-champion-swims-high-school.

Thompson, J. (2003). *The double-goal coach.* New York: HarperCollins.

Thompson, J. (2009). *Positive sports parenting.* Portola Valley, CA: Balance Sports.

Thompson, J. (2010a). *The high school sports parent.* Portola Valley, CA: Balance Sports.

Thompson, J. (2010b). *The power of double-goal coaching.* Portola Valley, CA: Balance Sports.

Thompson, J. (2011). *Elevating your game: Becoming a triple-impact competitor.* Portola Valley, CA: Balance Sports.

Till, K., Cobley, S., O'Hara, J., Chapman, C., & Cooke, C. (2010). Anthropometric, physiological, and selection characteristics in high performance UK junior rugby league players. *Talent Development and Excellence, 2,* 193-207.

Timiras, P.S. (1972). *Developmental physiology and aging.* New York: Macmillan.

Tischler, A., & McCaughtry, N. (2011). PE is not for me: When boys' masculinities are threatened. *Research Quarterly for Exercise and Sport, 82,* 37-48.

Tofler, I., & DiGeronimo, T.F. (2000). *Keeping your kids out front without kicking them from behind.* San Francisco: Jossey-Bass.

True champions. (2014, December 15). *Sports Illustrated,* p. 102.

Ullrich-French, S., & McDonough, M.H. (2013). Correlates of long-term participation in a physical activity-based positive youth development program for low-income youth: Sustained involvement and psychosocial outcomes. *Journal of Adolescence, 36,* 279-288.

Ulrich, B. (1987). Developmental perspectives of motor skill performance in children. In D. Gould & M.R. Weiss (Eds.), *Advances in pediatric sport sciences: Behavioral issues* (Vol. 2, pp. 167-186). Champaign, IL: Human Kinetics.

Ulrich, D. (1985). *Test of gross motor development.* Austin, TX: Pro-Ed.

U.S. Department of Labor. (1972). Title IX, Education Amendments of 1972. Retrieved March 29, 2015, from www.dol.gov/oasam/regs/statutes/titleix.htm.

Vaeyens, R., Gullich, A., Warr, C.R., & Philippaerts, R. (2009). Talent identification and promotion programmes of Olympic athletes. *Journal of Sports Sciences, 27,* 1367-1380.

Vallerand, R.J., Deshaies, P., Cuerrier, J.P., Briere, N.M., & Pelletier, L.G. (1996). Toward a multidimensional definition of sportsmanship. *Journal of Applied Sport Psychology, 8,* 89-101.

Vallerand, R.J., Mageau, G.A., Elliot, A.J., Dumais, A., Demers, M., & Rousseau, F. (2008). Passion and performance attainment in sport. *Psychology of Sport and Exercise, 9,* 373-392.

Valovich McLeod, T.C., Decoster, L.C., Loud, K.J., Micheli, L.J., Parker, J.T., Sandrey, M.A., & White, C. (2011). National athletic trainers' association position statement: Prevention of pediatric overuse injuries. *Journal of Athletic Training, 46,* 206-220.

Vasagar, J. (2010, September 23). School sport is growing, but not fast enough, say ministers. *Guardian.* Retrieved March 19, 2015, from www.guardian.co.uk/education/2010/sep/23/school-sport-growing-but-slowly.

Vealey, R.S. (2005). *Coaching for the inner edge.* Morgantown, WV: Fitness Information Technology.

Vealey, R.S., & Forlenza, S. (2015). Understanding and using imagery in sport. In J.M. Williams & V. Krane (Eds.), *Applied sport psychology: Personal growth to peak performance* (7th ed., pp. 240-273). Boston: McGraw-Hill.

Verducci, T. (2010, April 19). Legend before his time. *Sports Illustrated,* pp. 62-68.

Verducci, T. (2010, June 14). A different kind of perfect. *Sports Illustrated,* pp. 44-48.

Veroff, J. (1969). Social comparison and the development of achievement motivation. In C.P. Smith (Ed.), *Achievement-related motives in children* (pp. 46-101). New York: Russell Sage Foundation.

Wagner, M., Jones, T., & Riepenhoff, J. (2010, August 29). Children may be vulnerable in $5 billion youth-sports industry. *Columbus Dispatch,* Columbus, Ohio. Retrieved March 29, 2015, from www.dispatch.com/content/stories/local/2010/08/29/children-may-be-vulnerable-in-5-billion-youth-sports-industry.html.

Waldron, J.J. (2007). Influence of involvement in the Girls on Track program on early adolescent girls' self-perceptions. *Research Quarterly for Exercise and Sport, 78,* 520-530.

Wall, M., & Cote, J. (2007). Developmental activities that lead to dropout and investment in sport. *Physical Education and Sport Pedagogy, 12,* 77-87.

Walvoord, E.C. (2010). The timing of puberty: Is it changing? Does it matter? *Journal of Adolescent Health, 46,* 1-7.

Ward, T., & Groppel, J. (1980). Sport implement selection: Can it be based upon anthropometric indicators? *Motor Skills: Theory to Practice, 2,* 103-110.

Weight loss in wrestlers [ACSM Current Comment]. (2013). Retrieved February 11, 2014, from www.acsm.org/docs/current-comments/weightlossin-wrestlers.pdf.

Weiner, B. (1986). *An attributional theory of motivation and emotion.* New York: Springer-Verlag.

Weir, P.L., Smith, K.L., Paterson, C., & Horton, S. (2010). Canadian women's ice hockey – evidence of a relative age effect. *Talent Development and Excellence, 2,* 209-217.

Weiss, M.R., & Amorose, A.J. (2008). Motivational orientations and sport behavior. In T.S. Horn (Ed.), *Advances in sport psychology* (3rd ed., pp. 115-156). Champaign, IL Human Kinetics.

Weiss, M.R., & Fretwell, S.D. (2005). The parent-coach/child-athlete relationship in youth sport. *Research Quarterly for Exercise and Sport, 76,* 286-305.

Weiss, M.R., Smith, A.L., & Stuntz, C.P. (2008). Moral development in sport and physical activity. In T.S. Horn (Ed.), *Advances in sport psychology* (3rd ed., pp. 187-210). Champaign, IL: Human Kinetics.

Weiss, M.R., Stuntz, C.P., Bhalla, N.D., Bolter, N.D., & Price, M.S. (2013). "More than a game": Impact of The First Tee life skills program on positive youth development: Project introduction and year 1 findings. *Qualitative Research in Sport, Exercise, and Health, 5,* 214-244.

Weiss, M.R., & Williams, L. (2004). The why of youth sport involvement: A developmental perspective on motivational processes. In M.R. Weiss (Ed.), *Developmental sport and exercise psychology: A lifespan perspective* (pp. 223-268). Morgantown, WV: Fitness Information Technology.

Wertheim, L.J. (2012, January 23). Driving for home. *Sports Illustrated Vault.* Retrieved March 29, 2015, from www.si.com/vault/search?term=driving+for+home.

White, R.W. (1959). Motivation reconsidered: The concept of competence. *Psychological Review, 66,* 297-330.

White, S.H., & O'Brien, J.E. (1999). What is a hero? An exploratory study of students' conceptions of heroes. *Journal of Moral Education, 28,* 81-95.

Whitehead, J., Andree, K.V., & Lee, M.L. (2004). Achievement perspectives and perceived ability: How far do interactions generalize in youth sport? *Psychology of Sport and Exercise, 5,* 291-317.

Whitehead, M., & Murdoch, E. (2006). Physical literacy and physical education: Conceptual mapping. Retrieved August 12, 2014, from www.physical-literacy.org.uk/conceptualmapping2006.php.

Wiersma, L.D. (2000). Risks and benefits of youth sport specialization: Perspectives and recommendations. *Pediatric Exercise Science, 12,* 13-22.

Wiersma, L.D. (2005). Reformation or reclassification? A proposal of a rating system for youth sport programs. *Quest, 57,* 376-391.

Wiersma, L.D., & Fifer, A.M. (2008). "The schedule has been tough but we think it's worth it": The joys, challenges, and recommendations of youth sport parents. *Journal of Leisure Research, 40,* 505-530.

Wiersma, L.D., & Sherman, C.P. (2005). Volunteer youth sport coaches' perspectives of coaching education/certification and parental codes of conduct. *Research Quarterly for Exercise and Sport, 76,* 324-338.

Wiggins, D.K. (2013). A worthwhile effort? History of organized youth sport in the United States. *Kinesiology Review, 2,* 65-75.

Williams, A.M., & Ward, P. (2003). Perceptual expertise: Development in sport. In J.L. Starkes & K.A. Ericsson (Eds.), *Expert performance in sports* (pp. 219-249). Champaign, IL: Human Kinetics.

Williams, N., Whipp, P.R., Jackson, B., & Dimmock, J.A. (2013). Relatedness support and the retention of young female golfers. *Journal of Applied Sport Psychology, 25,* 412-430.

Winner, E. (1996). The rage to master: The decisive case for talent in the visual arts. In K.A. Ericsson (Ed.), *The road to excellence: The acquisition of expert performance in the arts and sciences, sports, and games* (pp. 271-301). Hillsdale, NJ: Erlbaum.

Winnick, J.P. (2011). *Adapted physical education and sport* (5th ed.). Champaign, IL: Human Kinetics.

Woitalla, M. (2014). Coach Egidio's New York success story. Retrieved April 20, 2015, from www.usyouthsoccer.org/coach-egidio's-new-york-success-story.

Wolverton, B. (2006, August 4). Morality play. *Chronicle of Higher Education,* pp. A33-A35.

Women's Sports Foundation. (2011, November). *Progress without equity: The provision of high school athletic opportunity in the United States by gender 1993-94 through 2005-06.* East Meadow, NY: Women's Sports Foundation.

Women's Sports Foundation. (2013, March 18). *Title IX myths and facts.* East Meadow, NY: Women's Sports Foundation.

Wood, E. (2002). The impact of parenting experience on gender-typed toy play of children. *Sex Roles, 47,* 39-50.

Woods, C.B., Moyna, N., Quinlan, A., Tannehill, D., & Walsh, J. (2010). *The children's sport participation and physical activity study.* Research Report No. 1. Dublin City University and the Irish Sports Council, Dublin, Ireland.

Woods, E. (1997). *Training a tiger.* New York: HarperCollins.

Woods, R.B. (2011). *Social issues in sport* (2nd ed.). Champaign, IL: Human Kinetics.

Wrisberg, C.A. (2007). *Sport skill instruction for coaches.* Champaign, IL: Human Kinetics.

Wuerth, S., Lee, M.J., & Alfermann, D. (2004). Parental involvement and athletes' career in youth sport. *Psychology of Sport and Exercise, 5,* 21-33.

Young, B.W., & Salmela, J.H. (2010). Examination of practice activities related to the acquisition of elite performance in Canadian middle distance running. *International Journal of Sport Psychology, 41,* 73-90.

Zarrett, N., Fay, K., Li, Y., Carrano, J., Phelps, E., & Lerner, R.M. (2009). More than child's play: Variable- and pattern-centered approaches for examining effects of sports participation on youth development. *Developmental Psychology, 45,* 368-382.

Zazulak, B.T., Paterno, M., Myer, G.D., Romani, W.A., & Hewett, T.E. (2006). The effects of the menstrual cycle on anterior knee laxity. *Sports Medicine, 36,* 847-862.

INDEX

Note: The fully italicized *See references* refer to a type of heading rather than to specific headings.
Note: The italicized *f* and *t* following page numbers refer to figures and tables, respectively.

A

ABC training 188-189
Abrams, Doug 146
abuse
    emotional abuse 217, 333
    physical abuse 217, 333
    sexual abuse 292-294, 295, 296, 297
academies of sport 9, 10-11, 10*f*, 14, 16, 17-18, 23, 213-214, 225
achievement by proxy (ABP) 332-333, 338
achievement by proxy distortion (ABPD) 333-334, 338, 339
active learning time 159, 169. *See also* practice
adolescence 74, 75, 86, 87. *See also* maturation
Adu, Freddie 212
aerobic fitness
    gender and racial differences 283, 287
    training and trainability 176, 177, 189, 191, 193, 207
African American discrimination and stereotypes in sport 35, 286-287, 288, 313. *See also specific individuals*
Agassi, Andre 217
age. *See also* maturation; specialization
    chronological versus biological age 75, 84, 86, 87
    minimal age restrictions for competition 221-222
    relative age effect 83-86, 84*f*, 85*f*, 87, 88
    starting age considerations 103, 105-109, 108*t*, 112
aggression
    versus aggressiveness 346, 354, 360
    modeling 346-347
    moral reasoning 353
    myth of useful aggression 351, 361
    norms 349-350
    violence 342, 345, 346
agility 188, 189, 191
air push-up record 174
alpha-actinin-3 (ACTN3) gene 207
Amateur Athletic Union (AAU) 36, 52, 93, 222, 324
Amateur Sports Act 36, 37, 39*t*, 41
amenorrhea 177, 178*f*, 191
American Academy of Pediatrics 113, 183
American College of Sports Medicine (ACSM) 181, 194
American Sport Education Program (ASEP) 61-62
Americans with Disabilities Act 291
American Youth Soccer Organization 39*t*, 304
amotivation 129*f*, 130, 137
anabolic steroids 181-182, 191, 193
anaerobic fitness 176, 189, 191, 193
ankle sprains 260-261
anorexia nervosa 178, 192
anterior cruciate ligament (ACL) injuries 252, 261-265, 262*f*, 264*f*, 272
anthropometric measures 71, 201, 201*t*
anticipatory cues 197*t*, 205, 206-207, 222-223, 224, 227
anxiety 233-234, 238, 241, 246, 248, 284-285. *See also* pressure; stress
apophysitis 255-258, 257*t*, 271
Armstrong, Lance 182
arousal 240, 240*f*, 241, 248
athletic position 264-265, 264*f*
athletic proficiency barrier 97-98, 110, 111
Atlas Sport Genetics 207
at-risk youth 28, 40, 47
attachment 320-321, 332-334, 338
attentional focus 240-241
attributions 124-126, 137, 138, 242
Australia
    coaching education programs 302, 303
    participation patterns 16, 20, 23
    talent identification and development 198, 202, 208

authoritarian versus authoritative parenting 323, 323*f*, 338
autonomy
    autonomy-supportive behaviors and strategies 131-132, 136, 310-311, 315, 316
    motivation considerations 128-131, 129*f*, 132-134
    optimal push 331-332, 338, 339
    role in youth sport 128, 137
avulsion fractures 255, 258
awkwardness in adolescence 74

B

balance
    ABC skills and training 188, 189, 192
    growth stages 71, 72*f*, 74, 87
ballistic stretching 188, 192
Barbie 285
Barkley, Charles 347
barriers
    athletic proficiency barrier 97-98, 110, 111
    participation barriers 18-21, 23, 24, 58
baseball. *See also individual players*
    Cannon Street All-Stars 35
    Dixie Youth Baseball 35, 39*t*
    history of the sport 28, 39*t*
    injuries and prevention 144, 254, 255, 256-257, 257*t*, 258, 259, 269, 271
    instructional cues and development strategies 158*t*, 162, 170, 186, 241
    Little League 30, 34, 35, 36, 39*t*, 41, 82, 256-257, 257*t*, 258, 259, 271, 286, 350
    Major League Baseball 221
    Michael Jordan's professional baseball experiment 101
    modifying for youth 144, 146, 147, 148-149
    overarm throw development and proficiency 96, 96*f*, 97, 97*t*, 99, 283
    Pony Baseball 39*t*
    racial segregation and stereotypes 35, 39*t*, 287
    study of cognitive readiness in youth shortstops 104
    talent identification and development 200, 205, 206-207, 208, 219, 221
    tee ball 53-54, 146, 148-149, 235
basketball. *See also individual players and coaches*
    AAU 36, 52, 93, 222, 324
    aggression and sportsmanship 349, 350
    arousal levels 240
    history of the sport 28, 32, 39*t*
    injuries and prevention 253, 255, 262, 263, 264, 265, 272
    instructional cues and development strategies 158, 158*t*, 163, 164, 241
    modifying for youth 106, 142, 143, 147
    NBA 18, 221, 350
    sample physical training session 191*f*
    talent development 208, 221-222
Baumeister, Roy 126
Beckham, David 8, 204, 247
behavior. *See* discipline; moral development
behavioral signature 310, 315
Bench, Johnny 83
Biddy Basketball 39*t*
Bill of Rights For Young Athletes 39*t*, 48, 48*f*
biological age 75, 84, 86
biological clock 73, 74, 75
biomechanics. *See* technique
Bird, Sue 158
birthplace effect 20, 22
bisexual athletes 289-290
bisphenol A (BPA) 77
blocked skill practice 162, 169
Bloom, Benjamin 209-210, 210*t*, 211, 228
Bobo doll experiment 346-347

ABOUT THE AUTHORS

Robin S. Vealey, PhD, is a professor in the department of kinesiology and health at Miami University in Ohio, where she has worked for more than 30 years. She has dedicated nearly her entire adult life to youth sports, whether as a coach, administrator, educator, researcher, or consultant. She is internationally known for her research on the psychological aspects of youth sport and coaching effectiveness. Vealey, who has authored three books, has won several professional awards throughout her academic career, including being named a fellow by the Association for Applied Sport Psychology (AASP) and the National Academy of Kinesiology. She previously was president of AASP, is a certified consultant in sport psychology as recognized by AASP, and is on the U.S. Olympic Committee Sport Psychology Registry. In addition to serving on numerous journal editorial review boards, Vealey is a past editor of *The Sport Psychologist*.

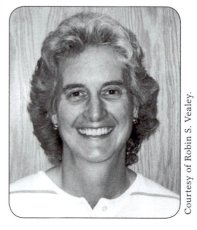

Courtesy of Robin S. Vealey.

In 2011, Vealey was named to the Marshall University Athletic Hall of Fame after a stellar playing career in women's basketball. Vealey went on to serve as a collegiate volleyball and women's basketball coach and an athletics administrator. She currently enjoys playing golf and continues to remain active in various sports as a sport psychology consultant for youth athletes and teams.

Melissa A. Chase, PhD, is a professor in the department of kinesiology and health at Miami University in Ohio, where she has worked for two decades. She specializes in research about coaching efficacy and self-efficacy in children interested in increasing motivation and effectiveness, and she has presented her research across the United States and internationally. She was named a fellow by the Association for Applied Sport Psychology (AASP) and SHAPE America and is a certified consultant in sport psychology as recognized by AASP. Chase was the founding editor of the *Journal of Sport Psychology in Action*, which is an official AASP publication.

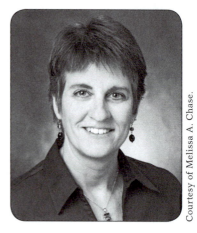

Courtesy of Melissa A. Chase.

Before becoming a professor, Chase gained experience as a physical education teacher at both the elementary and secondary school levels while coaching various levels of basketball, cross-country, track and field, and volleyball for several years. She enjoys running and watching her teenage children participate in youth sports.